Textbook of Real-Time Three Dimensional Echocardiography

Luigi P. Badano · Roberto M. Lang
José Luis Zamorano

(Editors)

Textbook of Real-Time Three Dimensional Echocardiography

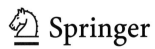 Springer

Editors
Luigi P. Badano
Department of Cardiac, Vascular,
and Thoracic Sciences
University of Padua
Via Giustiniani 2
35128 Padova
Italy

José Luis Zamorano
Hospital Clinico San Carlos
Instituto Cardiovascular
C/Professor Martin Lagos s/n
28040 Madrid
Spain

Roberto M. Lang
Department of Medicine
University of Chicago
Noninvasive Cardiac Imaging Laboratory
Section of Cardiology
MC 5084, S. Maryland Ave. 5841
Chicago IL 60637
USA

ISBN 978-1-84996-494-4   e-ISBN 978-1-84996-495-1
DOI 10.1007/978-1-84996-495-1
Springer London Dordrecht Heidelberg New York

British Library Cataloguing in Publication Data
A catalogue record for this book is available from the British Library

Additional material to this book can be downloaded from http://extra.springer.com.

Library of Congress Control Number: 2010938794

Cover design: eStudioCalamar, Figueres/Berlin

Printed on acid-free paper

Springer is part of Springer Science+Business Media (www.springer.com)

Foreword

No other imaging modality has so much contributed to the development of our knowledge in cardiology such as echocardiography. More than half a century has passed since the first exploration of human cardiac structures was obtained in vivo. In early 1950s two pioneers, I. Edler and CH Hertz, certainly were full of enthusiasm and willingness in pursuing research once they realized that the heart could be explored thanks to a single ultrasound beam oriented in the chest by the hand of a physician, but very unlikely, at that time, they were able to minimally predict both the future extraordinary technological evolution of cardiac ultrasound and its unbelievable impact on the progress of our understanding and recognition of almost every cardiac disease. In half a century of its history and technological evolution echocardiography has been the object of extremely important methodological achievements: the initial simple single beam exploration of the heart has evolved to progressively more and more sophisticated diagnostic potentials such as two dimensional echocardiography, pulsed and continuous Doppler, stress echocardiography, digital storage and treatment of images, transesophageal echocardiography, tissue analysis, contrast echocardiography, etc. Although rich of success and clinical achievements the technological evolution of cardiac ultrasound is still in progress. Three dimensional echocardiography, initially considered a dream of the echo lovers, is nowadays no longer a technological experiment; three dimensional echocardiography is becoming more and more a feasible diagnostic approach and for a progressive percentage of cardiac disease the diagnostic standard. I've had the privilege to live the entire evolution of cardiac ultrasound in the last 35 years and to personally appreciate the enormous impact of each technological achievement since the time of single beam, or also called M-Mode, echocardiography, both in research and patients management. Three dimensional echocardiography is the last achievement and those that are willing to be involved in this last frontier need to be interfaced with the experience of the recognized experts. In this respect the *Textbook of Real-Time Three Dimensional Echocardiography* written by Luigi Badano, Pepe Zamorano and Roberto Lang represents an important contribution since it covers not only the technological peculiarities of this fascinating new diagnostic technique, but also presents its potential in the relevant cardiac conditions that can take advantage from such a new and sophisticated exploration. I'm convinced that L. Badano, P. Zamorano and R. Lang thanks to their expertise and enthusiasm will contribute with their book to the diffusion of this last new fascinating result of the technological evolution of cardiac ultrasound.

Sabino Iliceto, MD
Professor and Chief of Cardiology
University of Padua

Preface

Tremendous improvements in ultrasound electronics and computer technology have led to development of one of the most impressive advancements of the use of ultrasounds to assess cardiac morphology and function: three-dimensional echocardiography (3DE). During the last decade, 3DE has made a dramatic transition from predominantly a research tool used in few large academic medical centers to a technology available in most echo labs, cardiac surgery operating rooms and catheterization and/or electrophysiology labs to address everyday clinical practice and guide interventional procedures.

Nowadays, 3DE is an established technique able to provide intuitive recognition of cardiac structures from any spatial point of view and complete information about absolute heart chamber volumes and function. In particular, 3DE has demonstrated its superiority over current echocardiographic modalities in several clinical applications: (1) assessment of left ventricular size and function whose accuracy compete with cardiac magnetic resonance; (2) Reliable and accurate assessment of right ventricular size and function; (3) Comprehensive visualization and quantitation of heart valve morphology and function leading to improved understanding of their function; (4) Improved display of complex spatial relationships between structures in patients with congenital heart lesions; (5) Guiding and monitoring surgical interventions and interventional procedures in the catheterization and electrophysiology lab. However, there have been few comprehensive books to introduce this new echocardiographic technique. Therefore we planned this book to summarize the experiences collected by several scientists who have contributed to the development of 3DE to provide you with the most recent developments in this emerging field, focusing on the clinical value of transthoracic 3DE and on the expanding role of transesophageal 3DE in guiding and monitoring surgical and interventional procedures. We hope that this book can serve multiple purposes. For echocardiographers who already use 3DE, we have tried to present the more advanced applications of 3DE and also some future developments which are expected to enter soon in the clinical arena. For those who have not yet experience the "third dimension," we have provided hundreds of images and videos in an accompanying DVD to show the beauty and the added clinical value of 3D imaging of cardiac structures. For clinicians, who may want to understand the added clinical value of this new echo modality, we tried to demonstrate the potential values of 3DE in the everyday clinical setting of cardiology practice. We are sure that 3D echo will help them to better understand and diagnose their patients.

The contributors to this book have all been selected for their special expertise in their own fields, their access to outstanding material and their ability to describe the significance of it in an effective and concise way. The Editors are grateful to the outstanding group of Authors for their extraordinary and timely contributions, and pleased to present such a truly international authorship.

Luigi P. Badano
Roberto M. Lang
José L. Zamorano

Contents

Contributors

David H. Adams, MD Department of Medicine, Section of Cardiology,
The University of Chicago Medical Center, Chicago, Illinois, USA

Luigi P. Badano, MD, FESC Head of Noninvasive Imaging Lab,
Department of Cardiology, Vascular and Thoracic Sciences,
University of Padua, Padua, Italy

G. Hamilton Baker, MD Department of Pediatrics, Pediatric Cardiology,
Medical University of South Carolina, Charleston, South Carolina, USA

Jose Alberto de Agustín, MD Unidad de Imagen Cardiovascular,
Hospital Clínico San Carlos, Madrid, Spain

Leopoldo Pérez de Isla. MD, PhD, FESC Unidad de Imagen Cardiovascular,
Instituto Cardiovascular – Hospital Clínico San Carlos,
Universidad Complutense de Madrid, Madrid, Spain

Miguel Angel Garcìa Fernàndez, MD, FESC Director Echocardiographic Laboratory,
Hospital Gregorio Maraňòn, Madrid, Sapin

Benjamin H. Freed, MD Department of Medicine, Section of Cardiology,
University of Chicago Medical Center, Chicago, Illinois, USA

Maurizio Galderisi, MD, FESC Director of Echo-Lab, Cardioangiology with CCU,
Department of Clinical and Experimental Medicine, "Federico II" University, Naples, Italy

Andreas Hagendorff, MD Professor of Medicine, Department of Cardiology-Angiology,
University of Leipzig, Germany

Anthony M. Hlavacek, MD MSCR and G. Hamilton Baker, MD
Department of Pediatrics, Pediatric Cardiology, Medical University of South Carolina,
Charleston, South Carolina, USA

Jarosław D. Kasprzak MD PhD FESC, FACC II Chair and Department of Cardiology,
Medical University of Łódź, Bieganski Hospital Łódź, Poland

James N. Kirkpatrick, MD Assistant Professor of Medicine,
"Cardiovascular Division, Associate Fellow, Center for Bioethics,
University of Pennsylvania, Philadelphia, Pennsylvania, USA

Itzhak Kronzon, MD, FACC, FASE, FAHA, FACP, FCCP, FESC Professor of Medicine,
Director Non invasive Cardiology, NYU School of Medicine, New York, USA

Roberto M. Lang, MD, FACC, FASE, FAHA, FESC, FRCP Professor of Medicine,
Director, Noninvasive Cardiac Imaging Laboratories, Department of Medicine,
Section of Cardiology, University of Chicago Medical Center, Chicago, Illinois, USA

Pedro Marcos-Alberca, MD, PhD Cardiovascular Imaging Unit,
Cardiology Department, Hospital Clínico San Carlos, Universidad Complutense,
Madrid, Spain

Mark Monaghan FRCP(Hon) FESC FACC Honorary Senior Lecturer in Cardiology,
Director of Non-Invasive Cardiology, King's College Hospital, London, United Kingdom

Victor Mor-Avi, PhD Professor, Director of Cardiac Imaging Research,
Department of Medicine, Section of Cardiology, University of Chicago Medical Center,
Chicago, Illinois, USA

Denisa Muraru, MD "Prof. Dr. C.C. Iliescu" Institute of Cardiovascular Diseases,
Bucharest, Romania

Mauro Pepi, MD, FESC Centro Cardiologico Monzino, IRCCS, Institute of Cardiology,
University of Milan, Milan, Italy

Gila Perk, MD Non-Invasive Cardiology, NYU School of Medicine,
New York, New York, USA

Juan Carlos Plana, MD Assistant Professor of Medicine, Director,
Echocardiography Laboratory, Director, Cardiac Imaging, Department of Cardiology,
The University of Texas M.D. Anderson Cancer Center, Houston, Texas, USA

Stein Inge Rabben, MSc, PhD Senior Engineer R&D,
GE Healthcare Cardiovascular Ultrasound, Forskningsparken,
Gaustadalleen 21 N-0349, Oslo, Norway

Fausto Rigo, MD, FESC Non Invasive Cardiology Department,
Dell'Angelo Hospital, Venice, Italy

Vasileios Sachpekidis, MD Non-Invasive Cardiology Department,
King's College Hospital, London, United Kingdom

Ivan S. Salgo, MD, MS Chief, Cardiovascular Investigations, Research & Development,
Ultrasound, Philips Healthcare, Andover, Massachusetts, USA

Muhamed Saric, MD Non-Invasive Cardiology, NYU School of Medicine,
New York, New York, USA

Girish S. Shirali, MBBS Department of Pediatrics, Pediatric Cardiology,
Medical University of South Carolina, Charleston, South Carolina, USA

Lissa Sugeng, MD Associate Professor, Department of Medicine,
Section of Cardiology, University of Chicago Medical Center,
Chicago, Illinois, USA

Gloria Tamborini, MD Centro Cardiologico Monzino, IRCCS, Institute of Cardiology,
University of Milan, Milan, Italy

José Luis Zamorano, MD, FESC Professor of Medicine,
Director Unidad de Imagen Cardiovascular, Hospital Clínico San Carlos, Madrid, Spain

The Evolution of Three-Dimensional Echocardiography: How Did It Happen

Victor Mor-Avi and Roberto M. Lang

From the early days of medical imaging, the concept of three-dimensional (3D) was indisputably perceived as desirable based on the wide recognition that depicting complex 3D systems of the human body in less than three dimensions severely limited the diagnostic value of the information gleaned from these images. Over the last half of the twentieth century, we have witnessed continuous technological developments driven by strong demand from the medical community that allowed the transition from fuzzy single-projection x-ray films to multi-slice tomographic images of exquisite quality depicting anatomical details previously seen only in anatomy atlases. The ability to visualize these details in a living patient had spurred revolutionary changes in how physicians understand disease processes and resulted in new standards in the diagnosis of disease. Today, the diagnosis of multiple disease states heavily relies on information obtained by noninvasive imaging. The ability to virtually slice and dice the human body in any desired plane has boosted the diagnostic accuracy and confidence by orders of magnitude.

Despite the broad appeal of computed tomography (CT) and magnetic resonance imaging (MRI), for several decades, heart disease has remained outside the scope of these sophisticated technologies because of the constant motion of the beating heart. While imaging of stationary organs was conceptually easy to solve by collecting information from different parts or from different angles consecutively, imaging of the beating heart required data collection to occur virtually in real time. While for decades ultrasound imaging had this edge over CT and MRI, it remained limited to a single cut plane. In fact, one may find in textbooks from the early 1970s explanations why real-time 2D imaging of a beating heart is an enormous technological advancement that is unsurpassable because of the limitations imposed by the speed at which sound waves travel inside the human body. Nevertheless, despite the fact that the speed of sound has not changed since then, the combination of the meteoric rise of computing technology with ingenious engineering solutions that increased the efficiency of the process of image formation from ultrasound reflections dispelled this tenet. In the 1990s, we witnessed the increase in imaging frame rates from a crawling few to a blazing hundreds per second, paving the way to 3D echocardiography (3DE).[1] The concept behind this new imaging modality was that it should be possible to image multiple planes in real time, albeit at lower frame rates, similar to those of earlier versions of 2D imaging.

Recently, this vision turned into reality, and today real-time 3DE is booming and gradually capturing an important place in the noninvasive clinical assessment of cardiac anatomy and function.[2-5] The purpose of this chapter is to review the evolution of 3DE and describe the milestones this technology has gone through on its way to today's reality, and to highlight the promises and setbacks that propelled the technological development into the race for the next "base" in the understanding of its full potential.

1.1 Linear Multiplane Scanning

Before technology necessary for real-time scanning of multiple planes was in place, attempts for 3D reconstruction of the heart from echocardiographic images were based on the use of linear step-by-step motion, wherein the transducer was mechanically advanced between acquisitions using a motorized driving device[6] (Fig. 1.1a). However, this simple solution was not applicable for transthoracic echocardiography, because of the need to find inter-costal acoustic windows for each acquisition step. This approach was also implemented in a pull-back transesophageal echocardiography (TEE) transducer, known as "lobster tail" probe (Fig. 1.1b).

1.2 Gated Sequential Acquisition

One developmental aspect crucial for the success of 3D reconstruction from multiplane acquisition was the registration of the different planes, so that they could be combined

V. Mor-Avi (✉)
University of Chicago Medical Center, Section of Cardiology, Chicago, Illinois 60637
e-mail: vmoravi@bsd.uchicago.edu

L.P. Badano et al. (eds.), *Textbook of Real-Time Three Dimensional Echocardiography*,
DOI: 10.1007/978-1-84996-495-1_1, © Springer-Verlag London Limited 2011

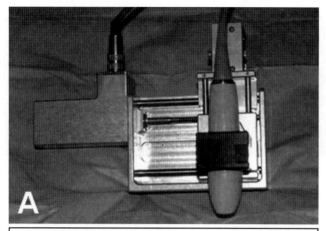

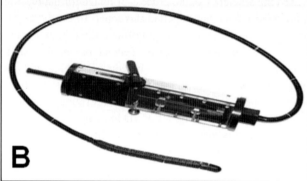

Fig. 1.1 Motorized linear-motion device used to allow acquisition of parallel cut planes for 3D reconstruction using linear step-by-step transducer motion (**a**); pull-back transesophageal probe that utilized the same approach of linear motion (**b**)

together to create a 3D image of the heart. This was achieved by sequential gated acquisition, wherein different cut planes were acquired one-by-one with gating designed to minimize artifacts. To minimize spatial misalignment of slices because of respiration, respiratory gating was used, such that only cardiac cycles coinciding with a certain phase of the respiratory cycle were captured. Similarly, to minimize temporal misalignment because of heart rate variability, ECG gating was used, such that only cardiac cycles within preset limits of R-R interval were included. This methodology became standard in both transthoracic and transesophageal multiplane imaging aimed at 3D reconstruction and was widely used until real-time 3D imaging became possible.

1.3 Transesophageal Rotational Imaging

An alternative approach to linear scanning was to keep the transducer in a fixed position corresponding to an optimal acoustic window, and rotate the imaging plane by internally steering the imaging element in different direction (Fig. 1.2a). This concept of rotational scanning in combination with gated

sequential scanning was implemented into TEE technology and resulted in a probe (Fig. 1.2b, left) that has subsequently become the main source of multiplane images used for 3D reconstruction, both for research and clinical practice.[7,8] This approach provided 3D reconstructions of reasonably good quality due to the high quality of the original 2D images and the fact that the TEE probe is relatively well "anchored" in its position throughout image acquisition, especially in sedated patients. Nevertheless, cardiac structures, such as valve leaflets appeared jagged as a result of stitch artifacts (Fig. 1.2c), reflecting the contributions of individual imaging planes that could not be perfectly aligned during reconstruction, despite the ECG and respiratory gating. Multiple studies demonstrated the clinical usefulness of this approach mostly in the context of the evaluation of valvular heart disease.

1.4 Transthoracic Rotational Imaging

An early transthoracic implementation of rotational approach consisted of a motorized device that contained a conventional transducer, which was mechanically rotated several degrees at a time (Fig. 1.2d), resulting in first transthoracic gated sequential multiplane acquisitions suitable for 3D reconstruction of the heart.[9-11] A later, more sophisticated implementation used a multiplane TEE transducer that was repackaged into a casing suitable for transthoracic imaging (Fig. 1.2c, right). Despite the previously unseen transthoracic 3DE images that excited so many, it quickly became clear that this methodology was destined to remain limited to the research arena because image acquisition was too time-consuming and tedious for clinical use. In addition, the quality of the reconstructed images was limited.

1.5 Transthoracic Free-Hand Imaging

An alternative approach for transthoracic 3DE is known as free-hand scanning.[11-13] This methodology is based on the use of spatial locators (Fig. 1.3), conceptually similar to the global positioning system, widely known today as GPS, except these devices were communicating with a receiver unit located in the exam room, rather than on a satellite revolving around the Earth. Initially, these locators used acoustic technology known as "spark gaps" (Fig. 1.3a,b), which was based on precise measurements of the differences in travel time of sounds emitted by three different sources mounted on the transducer. Subsequently, an electromagnetic version of this technology was used based on phase differences of signals originating from different sources (Fig. 1.3c). Regardless of the underlying technology, these devices could

Fig. 1.2 Rotational approach (**a**) implemented into a transesophageal multiplane transducer (**b**, *left*). Example of a 3D image of the mitral valve reconstructed from multiplane images acquired using this transducer (**c**). A version of the same technology repackaged for transthoracic imaging (**b**, *right*), and an earlier motorized device that mechanically rotated a built-in transthoracic transducer (**d**)

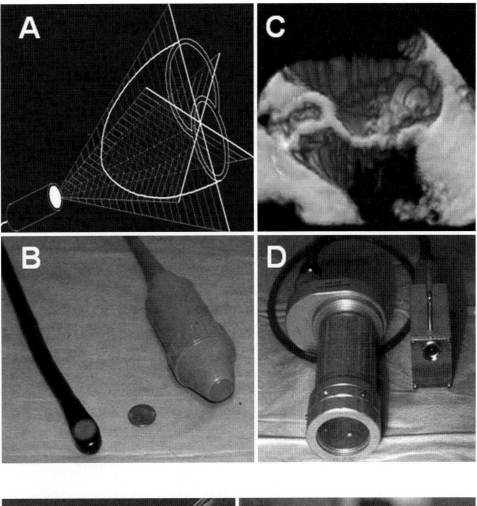

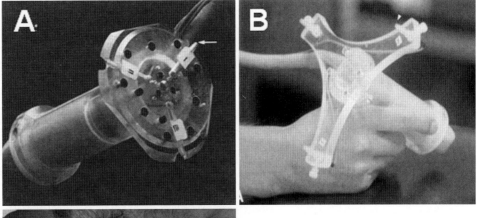

Fig. 1.3 Examples of spatial locators designed for free-hand transthoracic scanning. Imaging transducer was mounted into a holder that communicated with a receiver to provide information on transducer's location and orientation at any given moment: acoustic spark-gaps (**a** and **b**) and a later electromagnetic locator system (**c**)

accurately determine the location and orientation of the transducer at any moment. This information was translated into precise location of the imaging plane, allowing the sonographer to image from any identifiable good acoustic window. These images could be added to the data set eventually used for 3D reconstruction, thus eliminating the problem of using suboptimal images obtained from poor acoustic windows.

Since the number of planes typically acquired using this approach was relatively small (3–8), but nevertheless sufficient for 3D reconstruction of heart chambers and volume quantification, the acquisition was relatively quick. However, the downside of this high speed of acquisition was that there was not enough information to create detailed 3D views of the valves. Another drawback of this methodology was that while the acquired cut-planes could be perfectly aligned in the fixed room coordinates, they were not necessarily aligned anatomically, whenever any patient's body movement occurred between the consecutive acquisitions of individual cut planes. The result again was motion artifacts that frequently necessitated repeated acquisition. Another factor that has limited the use of this methodology in the clinical practice was the relative lack of portability of the locator devices, although conceivably they could be incorporated into the imaging system.

1.6 Transthoracic Real-Time 3D Imaging

The collective experience and the limitations of the gated sequential acquisition and offline 3D reconstruction gradually led developers to the understanding that scanning volumes rather than isolated cut planes would intrinsically resolve many of these limitations.[14,15] This revolutionary idea led to the development of the first real-time 3DE system equipped with a phased-array transducer (Fig. 1.4), in which piezoelectric elements were arranged in multiple rows, rather than one row, allowing fast sequential scanning of multiple planes. The phased array technology, that has been an integral part of the 2D transducers for decades, was modified to electronically change the direction of the beam not only within a single plane to create a fan-shaped scan, but also in the lateral direction to generate a series of such scans. Importantly this was achieved without any mechanical motion, allowing the speeds necessary for volumetric real-time imaging.

The first generation of real-time 3D transducers was bulky due to unprecedented number of electrical connections to the individual crystals, despite the relatively small number of elements in each row. This sparse array matrix transducer consisted of 256 non-simultaneously firing elements and had large footprint, which did not allow good coupling with the chest

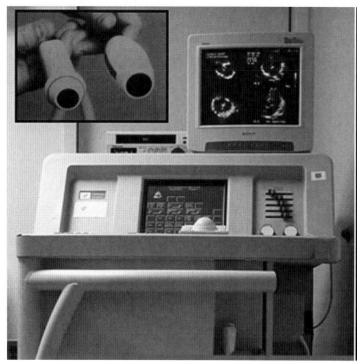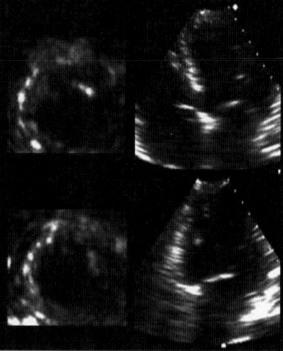

Fig. 1.4 An early real-time 3D echocardiographic imaging system equipped with a sparse matrix array transducer, shown in an insert panel (*top left*) side-by-side with a standard at the time 2D transducer, allowed simultaneous display of multiple planes extracted from the real-time data (*right*)

wall for optimal acoustic windows, and produced 3D images that were suboptimal in any selected plane, when compared to the quality of standard at the time 2D echocardiographic images. Nevertheless, the mere fact of successful real-time 3D imaging was a huge technological breakthrough.

The subsequent generations of fully-sampled matrix array transducers differed from this prototype fist and foremost in the considerably larger number of elements per row, with a total of approximately 3000 elements. This dramatic increase in the number of elements was accompanied by progressive miniaturization of electronic connections, resulting today in 3D transducers with footprints comparable to those of conventional 2D transducers, capable of providing high 3D

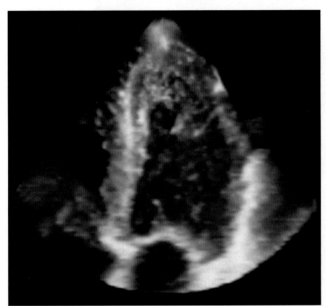

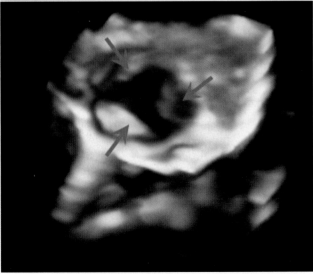

Fig. 1.5 Transthoracic real-time 3DE images of the heart extracted from the pyramidal datasets: apical four-chamber cross-sectional view obtained from a full-volume acquisition (*top*), and zoomed acquisition of the aortic valve in early systole shown from the left ventricular perspective depicting the three aortic valve leaflets (*bottom, arrows*)

resolution images (Fig. 1.5). Cut-planes extracted from these 3D datasets are similar in their quality to 2D images obtained using state of the art 2D transducers.

1.7 From Gated to Single-Beat Acquisition

Until recently, because of the limited size of the 3D scan volume, ECG-gated "full-volume" acquisition mode was used to capture the entire left ventricle section-by-section over several cardiac cycles. The major drawback of this approach was misregistration of the subvolumes manifesting itself as "stitch artifacts" as a result of irregular heart rhythm, respiration, or any movement of the patient or transducer during image acquisition, which frequently needed to be repeated to obtain a high quality dataset. Recent technological developments resulted in the capability to capture the entire heart in a single cardiac cycle (Fig. 1.6). This approach promises to further improve the ease of real-time 3DE evaluation of the left ventricle by improving the speed of acquisition and reducing artifacts.

1.8 Transesophageal Real-Time Imaging

Recently transesophageal imaging has also undergone the transition from gated sequential multiplane acquisition and off-line reconstruction to real-time volumetric scanning. Technological advances have allowed the miniaturization of matrix-array transducers by using integrated circuits that perform most of the beam forming within the transducer, rather than in the imaging system (Fig. 1.7). This modification allowed fitting thousands of piezoelectric elements into the tip of the TEE transducer, resulting in unprecedented views of the heart valves and unparalleled level of anatomic detail virtually in every patient.[16,17] It is becoming increasingly clear that this methodology is poised to assume a leading role in perioperative assessment of patients with valve disease.

1.9 Display of 3D Image Information

Another important part of 3DE, which has gone through its own developmental phases is the display of the 3D information. Regardless of the mode of acquisition, multi-plane reconstruction or real-time imaging, the information needs to be displayed in a way understandable to the user, which should be suited to a specific clinical goal in each case. Thus, evaluation of valvular pathology requires detailed dynamic 3D rendering of the annulus and leaflet surface and an ability to easily manipulate the rendered image in terms view angle.[8] The assessment of the spatial relationships in complex

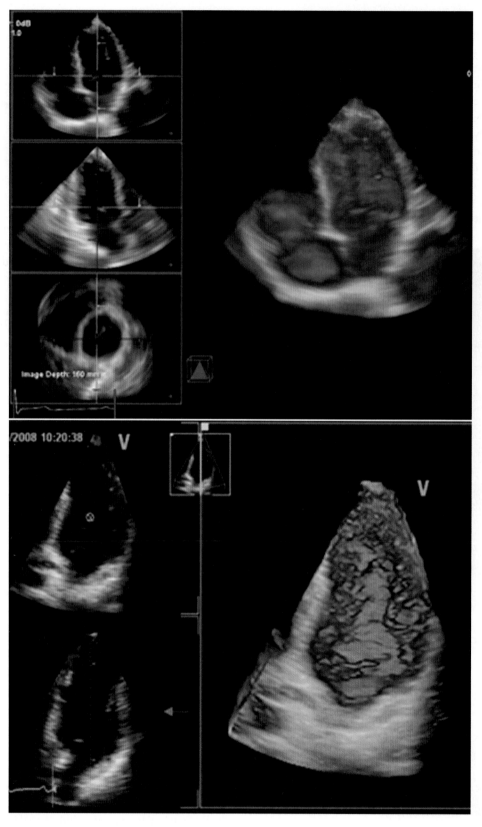

Fig. 1.6 Single-beat acquisition mode, currently available from several vendors (*upper* and *lower panels*), is time saving not only because the entire beating left ventricle can be captured in a single cardiac cycle, but because it reduces motion artifacts, thus eliminating the need for repeated acquisition

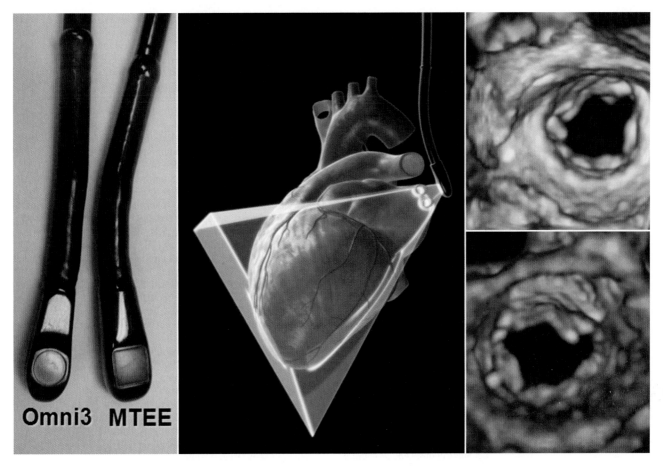

Fig. 1.7 Multiplane Omni-3 and matrix array transesophageal (MTEE) transducers shown side-by-side (*left*). While the dimensions of both transducers are similar, the MTEE probe that utilizes miniaturized beam-forming technology that allows fitting of near 3,000 piezoelectric elements into the head of the probe and thus provides real-time 3D images of the heart (*middle*). Example of 3D TEE views of the mitral valve from the left atrial (*right, top*) and LV (*right, bottom*) perspectives obtained during diastole

congenital heart disease relies on accurate visualization of anatomic detail as well,[18] but also required extensive capabilities of changing the dynamic range of colors and opacity. In contrast, the evaluation of chamber size and function requires a dynamic display of the detected endocardial surface,[19,20] from which chamber volume can be calculated over time and regional abnormalities can be visualized, but understandably does not require the same level of anatomic detail as valve imaging. These specific applications branched off of the original display of simple planes selected from the 3D dataset, and each of them has gone over the last decade through multiple improvements, finally resulting in vivid images tailored to answer a variety of diagnostic questions.

1.10 Volumetric Quantification

It is widely accepted today that quantitative measurements replacing subjective visual interpretation are of significant clinical value, because they allow serial evaluation of the effects of therapy in individual patients as well as inter-subject comparisons essential for objective detection of abnormalities. Nevertheless, the development of quantitative analysis tools for analysis of 3DE images has been and likely will always be lagging behind the continuous progress in the imaging technology. There are several reasons for this, including: (1) analysis tools emerge only after imaging capabilities are tested and proven, (2) developing and testing new analysis tools requires time and resources, (3) proving the clinical usefulness of such tools through publications takes time as initial reports are confirmed by multiple investigators and collective experience is gathered. Also, historically, the manufacturers of ultrasound imaging equipments did not have the resources necessary to develop and market software tools. However, this picture has changed dramatically over the last decade, as most manufacturers, having realized the need for such tools, provide today more and more comprehensive software tools for analysis of 3DE images with their imaging equipment. These tools allow anatomic measurements that aid clinicians in the diagnosis of disease processes, and researchers in collecting information that eventually constitutes the scientific basis for official guidelines and standards.

1.11 Summary

In summary, over the last two decades, echocardiographic community has witnessed technological developments and breakthroughs that have propelled 3DE imaging from an initial concept requiring more technology than was available at the time, to a widespread clinically useful imaging modality. Today, 3DE is gradually establishing itself as the preferred diagnostic method in many clinical scenarios, in which continuing technological refinements steadily improve the user's confidence and lead to better patient outcomes.[4,5] This process is an example of technological development driven by clinical demand that evolves in turn with each increment in technology and pushes the envelope of addressing new, more complex clinical questions.

References

1. Levine RA, Weyman AE, Handschumacher MD. Three-dimensional echocardiography: techniques and applications. *Am J Cardiol.* 1992;69:121H–130H.
2. Roelandt JR. Three-dimensional echocardiography: new views from old windows. *Br Heart J.* 1995;74:4–6.
3. de Castro S, Yao J, Pandian NG. Three-dimensional echocardiography: clinical relevance and application. *Am J Cardiol.* 1998; 81:96G–102G.
4. Lang RM, Mor-Avi V, Sugeng L, Nieman PS, Sahn DJ. Three-dimensional echocardiography: the benefits of the additional dimension. *J Am Coll Cardiol.* 2006;48:2053–2069.
5. Mor-Avi V, Sugeng L, Lang RM. Real-time 3D echocardiography: an integral component of the routine echocardiographic examination in adult patients? *Circulation.* 2009;119:314–329.
6. Matsumoto M, Inoue M, Tamura S, Tanaka K, Abe H. Three-dimensional echocardiography for spatial visualization and volume calculation of cardiac structures. *J Clin Ultrasound.* 1981;9:157–165.
7. Pandian NG, Nanda NC, Schwartz SL, Fan P, Cao QL, Sanyal R, Hsu TL, Mumm B, Wollschlager H, Weintraub A. Three-dimensional and four-dimensional transesophageal echocardiographic imaging of the heart and aorta in humans using a computed tomographic imaging probe. *Echocardiography.* 1992;9: 677–687.
8. Flachskampf FA, Franke A, Job FP, Krebs W, Terstegge A, Klues HG, Hanrath P. Three-dimensional reconstruction of cardiac structures from transesophageal echocardiography. *Am J Cardiol Imaging.* 1995;9:141–147.
9. Vogel M, Losch S. Dynamic three-dimensional echocardiography with a computed tomography imaging probe: initial clinical experience with transthoracic application in infants and children with congenital heart defects. *Br Heart J.* 1994;71:462–467.
10. Ludomirsky A, Vermilion R, Nesser J, Marx G, Vogel M, Derman R, Pandian N. Transthoracic real-time three-dimensional echocardiography using the rotational scanning approach for data acquisition. *Echocardiography.* 1994;11:599–606.
11. Kupferwasser I, Mohr-Kahaly S, Stahr P, Rupprecht HJ, Nixdorff U, Fenster M, Voigtlander T, Erbel R, Meyer J. Transthoracic three-dimensional echocardiographic volumetry of distorted left ventricles using rotational scanning. *J Am Soc Echocardiogr.* 1997;10:840–852.
12. Levine RA, Handschumacher MD, Sanfilippo AJ, Hagege AA, Harrigan P, Marshall JE, Weyman AE. Three-dimensional echocardiographic reconstruction of the mitral valve, with implications for the diagnosis of mitral valve prolapse. *Circulation.* 1989;80:589–598.
13. Gopal AS, Schnellbaecher MJ, Shen Z, Boxt LM, Katz J, King DL. Freehand three-dimensional echocardiography for determination of left ventricular volume and mass in patients with abnormal ventricles: comparison with magnetic resonance imaging. *J Am Soc Echocardiogr.* 1997;10:853–861.
14. von Ramm OT, Smith SW. Real time volumetric ultrasound imaging system. *J Digit Imaging.* 1990;3:261–266.
15. Sheikh K, Smith SW, von Ramm OT, Kisslo J. Real-time, three-dimensional echocardiography: feasibility and initial use. *Echocardiography.* 1991;8:119–125.
16. Sugeng L, Shernan SK, Salgo IS, Weinert L, Shook D, Raman J, Jeevanandam V, DuPont F, Settlemier S, Savord B, Fox J, Mor-Avi V, Lang RM. Live three-dimensional transesophageal echocardiography: initial experience using the fully-sampled matrix array probe. *J Am Coll Cardiol.* 2008;52:446–449.
17. Sugeng L, Shernan SK, Salgo IS, Weinert L, Shook D, Raman J, Jeevanandam V, DuPont F, Settlemier S, Savord B, Fox J, Mor-Avi V, Lang RM. Real-time 3D transesophageal echocardiography in valve disease: comparison with surgical findings and evaluation of prosthetic valves. *J Am Soc Echocardiogr.* 2008;21:1347–1354.
18. Magni G, Cao QL, Sugeng L, Delabays A, Marx G, Ludomirski A, Vogel M, Pandian NG. Volume-rendered, three-dimensional echocardiographic determination of the size, shape, and position of atrial septal defects: validation in an in vitro model. *Am Heart J.* 1996;132:376–381.
19. Gopal AS, Keller AM, Rigling R, King DL, Jr., King DL. Left ventricular volume and endocardial surface area by three-dimensional echocardiography: comparison with two-dimensional echocardiography and nuclear magnetic resonance imaging in normal subjects. *J Am Coll Cardiol.* 1993;22:258–270.
20. Mele D, Maehle J, Pedini I, Alboni P, Levine RA. Three-dimensional echocardiographic reconstruction: description and applications of a simplified technique for quantitative assessment of left ventricular size and function. *Am J Cardiol.* 1998;81:107G–110G.

Technical Principles of Transthoracic Three-Dimensional Echocardiography

Stein Inge Rabben

2.1 Introduction

The last years we have experienced a rapid development in three-dimensional echocardiography (3DE). Along this journey of development, technology battles have been won at many frontiers. Modern 3D scanners are now armed with cutting-edge technology. Breakthroughs in transducer design, beamforming, display technologies, and quantification have been released almost on a yearly basis. These developments have been enabled by the passion of numerous engineers for solving challenging technical problems.

The aim of this chapter is to provide the reader with some basic understanding of the technical principles of current 3D echocardiography.

All current 3D scanners are based on fully sampled 2D phase array transducers. The 3D transducer technology and beamforming will therefore be the topics of Sects. 2.2 and 2.3. Electronic beamforming in 3D is not in itself enough to make 3DE clinically useful. The finite speed of sound in tissue of approximately 1540 m/s limits the number of ultrasound pulses that can be fired per second giving a tough compromise between frame rate, volume size and spatial resolution. Section 2.4 describes different techniques (parallel receive beam forming, ECG gated stitching and real-time zoom) to get clinical acceptable frame rates and volume sizes. After acquiring the 3D data other challenges arise. How can 3D data be displayed in a meaningful manner? The computer screen is 2D in nature, but the examiner needs to get proper depth perception of the structure of interest. Section 2.5 covers the different image displays (slice, volume and surface renderings) made available with 3D ultrasound. The imaging modalities in 3DE ranging from multi-plane imaging (bi and tri-plane) to various types of volumetric 3D imaging and will be discussed in Sect. 2.6. Even though visualization of cardiac anatomy in 3D is important in itself, clinicians need to quantify the cardiac anatomy and function. Different quantification methods available in 3DE are covered in Sect. 2.8.

2.2 3D Transducer Design and Technology

Ultrasound imaging is based on transmitting pulses of mechanical (acoustic) vibrations into the body and then recording the reflected/backscattered mechanical vibrations (echoes) generated by the pulse propagating through the body. By directing the pulse in different steering (beam) directions within the acquisition volume, a volume can be acquired.

The transducer is designed to generate mechanical vibrations on the transducer surface in such a way that the pulses are transmitted in a specified beam direction. To obtain this, the transducer surface consists of an array of piezoelectric elements. Each piezoelectric element either increases or decreases its thickness depending on the polarity of the electrical transmit signal. By applying time delays between the transmit signals of each element the transmitted pulse will sum up in a specified steering direction (Fig. 2.1a). In traditional 2D ultrasound imaging, the transducer consists of 64–128 piezoelectric elements arranged along a single row (1D phase array transducer). Since all elements are arranged along a single row, the steering angles only vary within a single 2D image plane called the azimuth plane.

The piezoelectric elements can also transfer energy from mechanical vibrations into electric signals. Hence, after pulse transmission, the system changes to receive mode and the transducer converts the received echoes into electrical signals for further processing by the receive beamformer.

To steer the beam electronically in 3D (Fig. 2.1b), a 2D array of piezoelectric elements needs to be used in the transducer. Today a typical 2D array transducer consists of 2,000–3,000 elements arranged in rows and columns. Advanced fabrication methods are used to dice the block of piezoelectric material into the 2D array of independent elements and then connect all these elements to the transducer electronics. An example of a diced piezoelectric transducer material is shown in Fig. 2.2a.

S.I. Rabben
Senior Engineer R&D, GE Healthcare Cardiovascular Ultrasound, GE Vingmed Ultrasound AS, Forskningsparken, Gaustadalleen 21, N-0349 OSLO, Norway
e-mail: stein.rabben@med.ge.com

L.P. Badano et al. (eds.), *Textbook of Real-Time Three Dimensional Echocardiography*,
DOI: 10.1007/978-1-84996-495-1_2, © Springer-Verlag London Limited 2011

Fig. 2.1 (**a**) Electronic beam-forming: by applying time delays between the electrical signals applied to the piezoelectric elements (*small grey squares*), the sound waves (*half-circles*) from the elements sum up in a specified steering direction. (**b**) In 3D beamforming, the beams are steered in both azimuthal (Az) and elevation (El) directions by utilizing all elements of the 2D matrix array. In addition to electronic steering in 3D, current 3D systems are able to perform parallel receive beamforming where the system transmits one wide transmit beam and receives on multiple receive beams (in this case 16 receive beams)

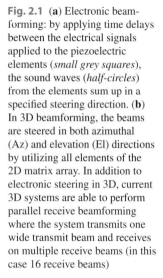
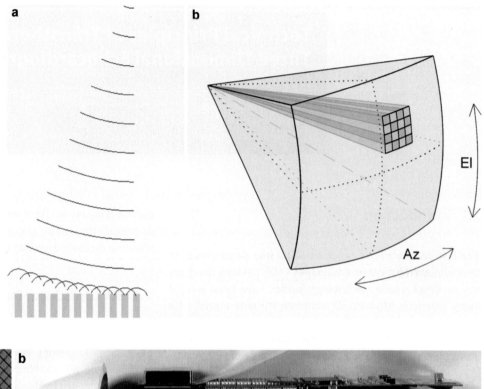

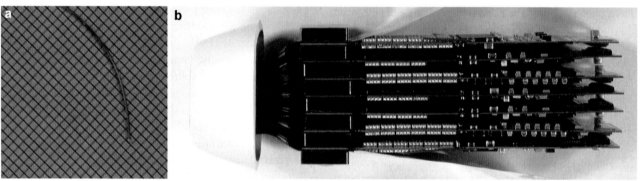

Fig. 2.2 (**a**) Microscopy of a 2D matrix array transducer material. The human hair is shown for size comparisons. (**b**) 3D transducer with fully sampled 2D matrix array, interconnection technology and custom made transmit and receive electronics

The latest generation of 3D ultrasound transducers are all fully sampled[1], as opposed to the sparsely sampled 2D matrix array transducers mentioned in the previous chapter. This means that all elements are active during beamforming. To obtain this, the transducers contain miniaturized interconnection technology between the elements and transmit/receive electronics. Figure 2.2b shows a picture of an opened 3D transducer with fully sampled 2D matrix array, interconnection technology and custom made transmit and receive electronics. The miniaturization of the electronics and the interconnection technology has now come so far that even 3D TEE probes have been developed[2].

In traditional 2D systems, beamforming is done entirely on the ultrasound system. However, using this approach for a fully sampled 2D array transducer, would lead to an unacceptable large diameter of the transducer cable. Furthermore, the ultrasound system would need to contain much more beamformer electronics than today. The cost and power consumption of the system would therefore be extensive. To solve this problem, the current 3D transducers contain beamformer circuitry. By performing pre-beamforming within the transducer, the number of channels between the transducer and the system can be reduced significantly. The 3D beamformer scheme is described in more detail in the next section.

One problem with electronics in the transducer handle is the heat generation during imaging. The temperature at the transducer surface has to be kept below a certain limit and the heat generated by the electronics therefore has to be transported away. Traditionally, this is achieved by carefully designed passive cooling. In some situations passive cooling is not enough and the 3D system has to reduce the transmit power to avoid too high skin temperatures. Lately, 3D transducers with active cooling have been introduced to avoid reducing the transmit power. In these transducers, the heat is transported actively through the transducer cable to the ultrasound system.

To conclude, in the past, the transducers were mainly responsible for converting electrical transmit signals to mechanical vibrations (ultrasound waves) on transmit and vice versa on receive. The control of the electrical signals for steering and focusing the beams was performed by the ultrasound system. With the development of real-time 3DE, the transducer has grown in complexity, both electro-mechanically and electronically. The 3D transducer now contains thousands of active elements and pre-beamforming takes place within the transducer. This increased complexity is the reason for 3D transducers being larger, heavier, and higher priced than traditional 2D transducers. However, these transducers can steer the beam in 3D.

2.3 Beamforming in Three Spatial Dimensions

The 3D beamformer steers in both azimuthal (Az) and elevation (El) directions as illustrated in Fig. 2.1b. By sequentially firing pulses in different directions, a pyramidal shaped volume is build up.

In traditional 2D systems, each transducer element is connected via the cable to a system channel and the beamforming is done on the ultrasound system. On transmit, the electrical pulses with correct time-delays are generated by the system and the transducer converts the electrical signals to mechanical vibrations. On receive, the element signals are amplified, filtered and digitized by analog-to-digital (A/D) convertors. The resulting digital signals are focused using digital delay circuitry and summed together to form the received signal from a desired point within the imaging plane (Fig. 2.1a). All this is done by the ultrasound system.

With 3D transducers containing thousands of elements, this approach becomes unpractical and the beamforming is split into two stages[1]: (1) pre-beamforming by custom made integrated circuits within the transducer handle, and (2)

traditional 128–256 channels digital beamforming within the ultrasound system.

There are alternatives for the pre-beamforming. One alternative is to divide the aperture into sub-apertures. For each sub-aperture, the elements are time-delayed and summed together to form one signal. Since the focusing delays between neighbouring matrix array elements are small, the amount of electronics can be kept to a minimum. The longer delays needed to time align the sub-aperture signals are implemented by digital beamforming on the ultrasound system. Another alternative for pre-beamforming is to use multiplexers that form desired patches of elements according to the desired steering direction.

2.4 Frame Rate, Volume Size and Spatial Resolution

Let us start with a small example. Assume that we want to image down to 16 cm depth, with a volume width of 60 by 60 degrees. As the speed of sound in tissue and blood is close to 1540 m/s and each pulse in this case has to propagate 32 cm, at most 1540/0.32 = 4812 pulses may be fired per second without getting interference between the pulses. If we assume that one degree beam spacing in each dimension is sufficient, we need 3600 beams to spatially resolve the 60 by 60 degrees volume (60 × 60 = 3600). We will then get a frame rate of 4812/3600 = 1.3 Hz.

A frame rate of 1.3 Hz is practically useless in echocardiography and the example above illustrates that the finite speed of sound in tissue and blood is a major challenge to the development of 3DE. So how do we cope with this problem? There are several techniques that have to be utilized. First, parallel beamforming (Fig. 2.1b) has to be implemented. Second, to further improve frame rate, we need to utilize ECG gated stitching of sub-volumes from several cardiac cycles (Fig. 2.3b). Third, a flexible and efficient real-time zoom feature where the operator can keep the frame rate up by reducing the volume size to a minimum needs to be available (Fig. 2.3c).

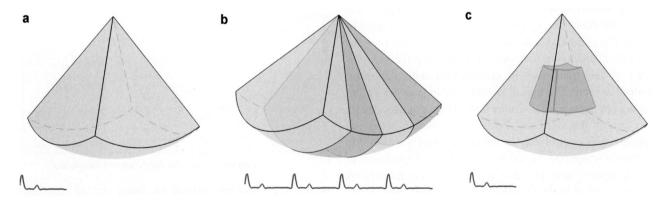

Fig. 2.3 (a) Real-time 3D imaging: a 60 by 60 degrees volume is acquired in real-time. (b) ECG gated stitched 3D imaging: sub-volumes from four consecutive heartbeats are stitched together to a 80 by 80 degrees volume. The stitched volume is displayed in real-time. (c) Real-time 3D zoom: only data within the small region of interest (30 by 30 degrees) is acquired. By reducing the volume size the frame rate can be kept high

Parallel beamforming, or multi-line acquisition as it is also called, is a technique where the system transmits one wide beam and receives on multiple narrow beams in parallel (Fig. 2.1b). This way the frame rate can be increased with a factor equal to the number of receive beams. Current 3D systems are able to process tens of receive beams in parallel. The number of parallel beams increases the amount of beamforming electronics and thereby the size, cost and power consumption of the system.

It may sound like a good idea to increase the number of parallel beams more than what is available in current 3D systems. However, there are challenges to this. When increasing the number of receive beams, the width of the transmit beams must be increased accordingly and the signal-to-noise ratio and contrast resolution may be affected. Since the receive beams are steered farther and farther away from the center of the transmit beam this may give striping or line artifacts in the image. Finally, the transmit beams become so wide that the sound wave pressures generated when the pulse propagates the tissue may become lower than what is needed for generating second harmonic signals. Second harmonic imaging is absolutely needed to make 3DE clinically useful. The future will show how far parallel receive beamforming can be taken.

In 2D imaging there is a well known inverse relation between frame rate and sector width, depth and line density. There is a similar relation in 3D and the following simplified equation describes this:

$$Frame\ Rate = \frac{1540 * Number\ of\ Parallel\ Receive\ Beams}{2 * Volume\ Width^2 * Volume\ Depth * Lateral\ Resolution^2} \quad (2.1)$$

Where 1540 is given by the speed of sound in human tissue, *Volume Width* is the azimuth and elevation widths of the pyramid (assuming equal width in both directions), *Volume Depth* is the maximum depth of the volume and *Lateral Resolution* is the spatial resolution lateral to the beam direction. The spatial resolution determines the detectability of closely spaced tissue inhomogeneities. An examiner can change the frame rate by either controlling volume widths or depth. The optimal (i.e. the highest achievable lateral resolution) is related to the footprint (or more correctly the aperture) of the transducer in combination with the pulse frequency used. The typical lateral resolution at 10–16 cm depth is in the range 1.5–2 mm. The 3D system may offer a user control that decreases the lateral resolution below the optimal. This control may be called line density, resolution or simply frame rate. However, to trade lateral resolution to obtain higher frame rates may not work well in all patients since a decrease in spatial resolution also affects the contrast resolution of the image. It should be pointed out that the spatial resolution in the beam direction (the axial resolution) is not relevant for the above discussion as it is only related to

the pulse length. Increasing the pulse length does not give any frame rate increase. The axial resolution is typically in the range 0.8–1 mm.

The inverse relation between frame rate, volume size and spatial resolution is illustrated in Fig. 2.4. Be aware that the cases shown are based on theoretical considerations and may be difficult to achieve in practice. The solid line represents a case where we have changed the volume width from 20 to 90 degrees, while keeping the depth to 16 cm, the lateral resolution to its theoretical optimal (assuming a frequency of 3 MHz and an aperture of 2 cm) and the number of parallel beams to 16. One striking observation is how favourable it is to decrease the volume width to a minimum to increase frame rate. This illustrates that there are good reasons for using the real-time 3D zoom feature on the systems. We have also calculated a case (dotted line) where the lateral resolution has been reduced from its theoretical optimal down to half of its optimal. In this case, the width is 60 degrees, depth 16 cm and the number of parallel beams 8. In terms of frame rate increase, this clearly shows how favourable it can be to compromise on the lateral resolution, but be aware that the image quality may degrade significantly when reducing the resolution. Figure 2.4 also shows the frame rate effect when changing the depth from 10–20 cm (dashed-dot line). This case (with 60 degrees width, optimal lateral resolution and 32 receive beams) indicates that the volume depth should be kept to a minimum when performing 3DE. However, there is a practical limit to reducing the volume depth, since a too high pulse repetition frequency (PRF) gives reverberations (multiple interfering echoes) destroying the image. The ultrasound system therefore automatically limits the PRF when the user decreases the volume depth below a certain limit. Finally, we have added one case illustrating a system

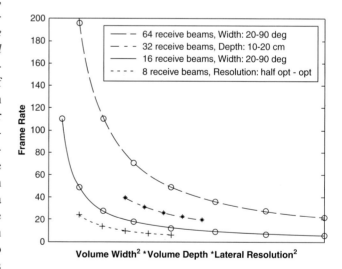

Fig. 2.4 The relation between frame rate, volume size and spatial resolution in different cases. Be aware that the relations shown are based on theoretical considerations and may be difficult to achieve in practice. However, the figure illustrates the trade-offs between frame rate, volume size and lateral resolution

with 64 parallel beams. In this calculation, the volume width is ranging from 20 to 90 degrees, while the depth is 16 and lateral resolution is optimal. With these settings the frame rate is acceptable in all situations, but remember that there are limits to how far parallel beamforming can be taken.

ECG gated stitching of sub-volumes acquired from different cardiac cycles is another technique to increase the volume size, while maintaining the frame rate. The technique is illustrated in Fig. 2.3b where gating over four cardiac cycles gives a full volume acquisition (meaning a large acquisition volume able to cover the complete chamber of interest) with the same frame rate as the smaller sub-volumes. ECG gated stitching is of course prone to motion artifacts caused by transducer movement, respiration and varying heart rate. It is important that the 3D system is able to display the stitched data in real-time so that the examiner, while imaging, can verify that the data is without artifacts[3].

The current 3D systems offer a real-time 3D zoom mode so that the examiner can spend the acquisition resources on only what is needed to answer the clinical question. With a real-time zoom mode, the volume widths and depth can be reduced to a minimum giving the highest achievable frame rate. Figure 2.3c shows a case where the examiner has defined a 30 by 30 degrees region of interest. A beneficial by-product of real-time zooming is that the need for further cropping of the data is reduced. Hence, the examiner may save analysis time after using real-time 3D zoom.

To conclude, in 3DE, the finite speed of sound constitutes a major challenge to obtaining large volumes with adequate frame rate. Vendors have developed several techniques, such as parallel receive beams, sub-volume stitching and real-time 3D zoom, to cope with this challenge. It is important that the examiner utilizes these techniques and optimizes the acquisition to the clinical application at hand. If, for example, the examiner wants to assess a mitral valve prolapse, high frame rate is important because the prolapse may only be visible in a few frames in late systole. In this case, volume size should be reduced to only cover the mitral valve apparatus. On the other hand, if the examiner needs to evaluate if an atrial septal defect is suitable for catheter closure, high frame rates may not be important and the examiner may be happy with a large real-time volume with low frame rate. Finally, if the clinical application at hand is myocardial 3D strain analysis, high frame rate, large volume and high spatial resolution are probably needed. These different examples illustrate how important it is that the 3D system has flexible acquisition setup capabilities.

2.5 3D Displays

The main benefit of 3DE is that the technique gives the examiner access to dense volumetric data, covering the entire structure of interest. In live, but also retrospectively, the examiner can generate various views of the cardiac structures contained in the data.

There are fundamentally three methods of displaying information from volumetric data: (1) the system can cut one or multiple slices through the volume and display these as standard 2D images (Fig. 2.5a), (2) the system can simulate the 3D appearance of the object by showing a volume rendering (Fig. 2.5b), or (3) the cardiac structures can be displayed as a surface rendered model in a 3D scene (Fig. 2.5c).

2.5.1 Slice Rendering

In the slice display, a 2D image is generated from the volume samples intersected by a cross-sectional plane through the

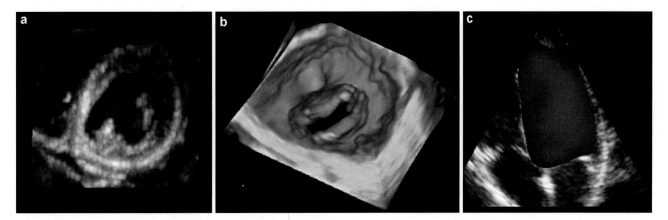

Fig. 2.5 (**a**) A slice rendering of a short axis cross-section of the left ventricle. (**b**) A volume rendering of the mitral valve during diastole. The pixels of the volume rendering are colorized according to the depth from the view plane to the tissue structure. (**c**) A surface rendering of the left ventricle shown together with the apical four-chamber view in a 3D scene

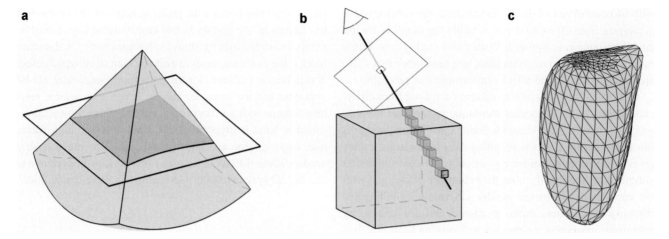

Fig. 2.6 (**a**) Slice principle: a 2D image is generated from the volume samples intersected by a freely adjustable slice plane (illustrated by the horizontal plane that intersects the acquisition volume). (**b**) Volume rendering principle: the volume rendering is generated by casting rays from the view plane through the volume and recording the sample values along each ray. The final ray values recorded at the view plane are a combination of the values of all the samples met along the rays. (**c**) Surface rendering principle: a geometrical description (e.g. a triangulated mesh) of a cardiac structure is generated by manual or automatic boundary outlining. Texture and shading are typically added to the mesh to generate the final surface rendering as seen in Fig. 2.5c

heart (Fig. 2.6a). The real advantage of the slice display is that the examiner can generate the 2D image from any desired cross-section, cross-sections that can be physically unavailable in transthoracic 2D echocardiography (2DE). This way the examiner can obtain the correct standard views of the object and avoid foreshortening. The current 3D systems offer freely adjustable slice planes, also called any-planes. In addition, several slices may be linked together. Either as equidistant parallel slices (paraplane), or as slices rotated around a common rotation axis (rotoplane). As an example, Fig. 2.7 shows a screen layout with three apical slices rotated around a common long axis for the left ventricle together with nine equidistant parallel short axis slices from the base to the apex of the chamber. Another display with linked slices is the mainplane layout that shows three orthogonal planes together. The paraplane, rotoplane and mainplane displays are also called multi-plane reconstruction (MPR). To improve the efficiency of the data analysis, the linked slices typically move together when the examiner navigates in the data.

Be aware that in some applications, to increase the wall visibility, it makes sense to generate slices that are "thicker" than the spatial resolution of the image data would require. Typically, an average or maximum projection will then be used.

2.5.2 Volume Rendering

The computer screen is in nature 2D, but the examiner wants to see the cardiac structures with 3D depth perception. Volume rendering is a well-known technique to produce images with depth perception (Fig. 2.5b). With this technique, the system casts rays from the view plane through the volume and records the sample values along the rays (Fig. 2.6b). The final ray value recorded behind the object is a combination of the values of all the samples met along the ray from the viewpoint to the back plane, thus the name volume rendering. Typically, the combination is the sum of the sample values; each multiplied by a weight called opacity. The opacity is modulated by the grey-level of the sample. Either the ray hits high grey-level samples and renders the pixel opaque (i.e. tissue), or the ray keeps shining through low grey-level samples and renders the pixel transparent (i.e. blood pool). The relation between the grey-level of the sample and the opacity is given by an opacity function. In practice, finding a good opacity function is difficult. To make a high-quality rendering, the opacity function must satisfy the following two requirements: First, it has to be correct with respect to the image data. That is, if the tissue boundary is associated with some grey-level value, the opacity function should give that sample maximum opacity. Second, the opacity for the remaining samples should be assigned in such a way that it minimizes the creation of misleading artifacts in the rendering. Usually the examiner has some control over the opacity function. It is for example common to provide a method to adjust the grey-level threshold for which samples that the algorithm will let contribute to the rendering. The systems also offer some way of controlling the steepness of the opacity function (i.e. the transparency of the data). In addition to the standard grey-level rendering described above, it is possible to add a light source into the ray-casting procedure, and generate a rendered structure with shading. This is done by combining information about the direction of the tissue-blood boundaries (i.e. the spatial grey-level gradients of the data) with the direction of the light source.

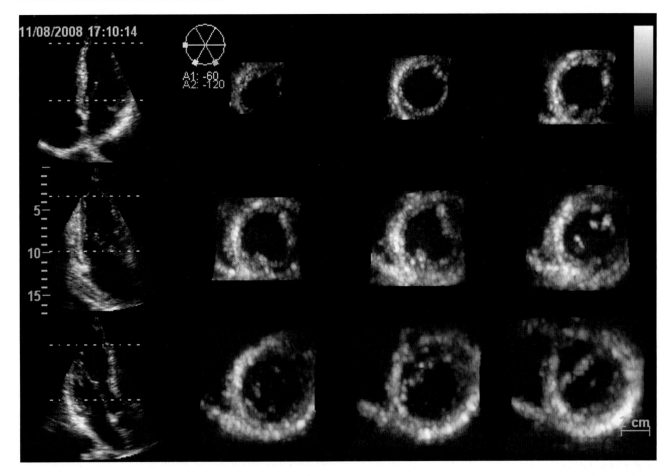

Fig. 2.7 Example of a specialized layout for wall motion assessment with three apical slices rotated about the LV long axis (*rotoplanes*) and nine equidistant parallel short axis slices from apex to base (*paraplanes*)

To improve the depth perception of the traditional volume rendering technique further, depth-encoded renderings have been introduced[4]. The distances from the viewpoint to the different tissue structures are estimated by detecting where along the rays the samples become opaque. By colorizing the data differently according to its depth, the depth perception of the rendering is improved (Fig. 2.5b).

Stereo rendering is also a technique that has been introduced to 3DE. An anaglyph stereo rendering is achieved by rendering the volume from two slightly different viewing angles. Both renderings are combined to a final image by encoding the first rendering using the red color component and the other rendering using green and blue color components. The user has to wear red/cyan glasses to watch the stereo image.

One typical problem with volume renderings is that a structure of interest to the examiner may be hidden behind other structures. For example, the examiner may want to cut away the left atrium to display the surgeon's view of the mitral valve. This is known as cropping, and is typically done by defining a plane within the volume where the part of the volume on one side of that plane is removed from the volume rendering. To simplify the definition of the view and the crop planes, the 3D scanners provide different navigation tools. One way of making the navigation simpler is first to let the system or the examiner align a set of slices to the standard views of the apical or parasternal imaging window. Then the system knows where the different structures are in the data and the user can simply push buttons to choose the structure to render. This is also called auto cropping.

Several alternative algorithms exist for generating the volume rendered images (ray casting, texture mapping or shear warp), and it is now common to exploit the processing power of the graphics card (GPU) on board the system to accelerate the volume-rendering algorithm. A volume rendering is also called a 3D render image, or just a 3D image.

It is worth mentioning that in both the slice and volume rendering displays, the pyramidal 3D ultrasound data acquired in a 3D polar coordinate system, needs to be scan converted to rectangular (Cartesian) space by a 3D scan converter. The scan conversion may be done as an intermediate step before applying the slice or volume rendering algorithms or directly as a part of the rendering algorithms. The box-shaped samples of Cartesian data are usually called voxels (short for volume pixels). In some papers, the authors also use the term voxels to denote the non-box-shaped raw data samples.

2.5.3 Surface Rendering

An alternative way of displaying cardiac structures and still keep the depth perception is to generate surface rendered models in a 3D scene (Fig. 2.5c). The prerequisite for applying this technique is that the system already knows the blood-to-tissue boundaries of the cardiac structures to display. Hence, either manual or automatic outlining of the structure has to be done prior to generating the surface rendering. Once having a geometrical description (e.g. a triangulated mesh) of the structure (Fig. 2.6c), surface rendered images of the anatomy can be generated. To improve the depth perception it is common to add shading before generating the final surface rendering. Typically shading is based on calculating the directions of the object surface (mesh normals) and combining these with the direction of a light source. In this case, the final brightness and color of the surface depends on how perpendicular the light direction is to the rendered surface. For example, if the light direction is perpendicular to the surface, the surface is rendered bright, while if the light direction is parallel to the surface, the surface is rendered dark. Surface renderings may also be called geometrical models.

2.6 3D Imaging Modes

2.6.1 Multi-plane Imaging

In addition to volumetric imaging, the current 3D systems provide multi-plane imaging (Fig. 2.8, left). In this mode[5,6], two (bi-plane) or three (tri-plane) 2D images are acquired simultaneously. With multi-plane imaging, the examiner gets the standard imaging views that he or she is familiar with from 2DE. The learning curve is therefore not as steep as for volumetric 3D imaging. Multi-plane imaging is particularly helpful for acquiring the anatomically correct imaging views, avoiding foreshortening and acquiring images of all relevant views from the very same cardiac cycle. Since the multi-plane modes acquires only two to three times as much data as standard 2D imaging, the frame rate can still be kept at a reasonable level. The 3D systems are now so powerful that the frame rate of the multi-plane recordings is at the level of 2D imaging some years ago. Multi-plane tissue imaging has shown potential in stress echocardiography[7]. The fact that the examiner can image five views from two recordings (parasternal long and short axis images plus three apical images) is time saving. During exercise stress this means that the examiner may be able to acquire the images at higher heart rates, which again may increase the sensitivity of the test. Furthermore, all color Doppler modes, such as color Doppler, tissue Doppler and tissue synchronization imaging, are available in multi-plane imaging.

2.6.2 3D Tissue Imaging

There are fundamentally three different modes for volumetric 3D imaging: real-time 3D imaging (Fig. 2.3a), stitched 3D imaging (Fig. 2.3b) and real-time 3D zoom (Fig. 2.3c). All these modes have been described above in the discussion about frame rate, volume rate and spatial resolution. Earlier, the stitched 3D mode was called full volume imaging. However, with recent breakthroughs, the processing power of the 3D

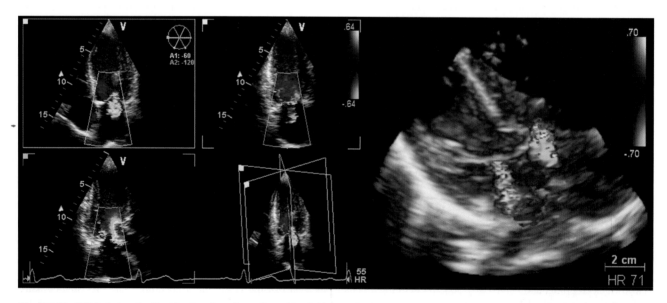

Fig. 2.8 (*Left*) Tri-plane color Doppler imaging of a patient with mitral regurgitation. (*Right*) 3D color Doppler volume rendering of a patient with tricuspid and mitral regurgitations

systems has become so high that they are able to acquire volumes large enough to cover the left ventricle at about 16–18 volumes per second. Full volume imaging is therefore no longer equivalent to stitched 3D imaging. To get higher volume rates or to improve resolution, stitched acquisitions are possible, leading to for instance 75 by 75 degrees at above 50 volumes per seconds. Alternatively, if the examiner would like to focus on a specific structure, volumes rates of more than 100 Hz can be reached by the 3D zoom mode, where the examiner limits the width of the region to acquire to a minimum.

2.6.3 3D Color Doppler Imaging

The current 3D systems also offer 3D color Doppler imaging [8,9]. 3D color Doppler has a role to play since the shape of the jet flows is in nature 3D. Figure 2.8 (right) shows an example of a 3D color Doppler image in a patient with tricuspid and mitral regurgitations. In color Doppler imaging, each velocity estimate is based on firing multiple pulses in the same beam direction. The finite speed of sound therefore becomes a limiting factor for the volume size and resolution. To obtain large enough region of interest, it is necessary to gate over several cardiac cycles. There are still issues that hamper the clinical use of 3D color Doppler imaging. Acquisition over four to seven cardiac cycles makes the technique prone to respiration artifacts. The limited volume size may not allow complete visualization of the jet. Further, to achieve large enough volumes with high enough frame rate, it is common to compromise the 3D tissue image quality.

2.6.4 Contrast Enhanced 3D Imaging

Contrast enhanced imaging is available also in 3DE. As for 2D, the contrast agent increases the visibility of the tissue-blood boundaries for patient with poor image quality and it has been shown that using contrast agents for LV opacification (LVO) during tri-plane [10] or during 3D [12] imaging improve the precision of the LV volume measurement. Contrast enhanced imaging is normally based on firing multiple pulses in each beam direction. Since 3DE is limited by the finite speed of sound, this increases the need for ECG gated stitching. Contrast enhanced 3D imaging therefore may require more cardiac cycles than conventional 3D imaging. One challenge not seen in 2DE is present in 3DE. In contrast-enhanced 2D imaging, the 3D nature of the blood flow ensures fresh supply of non-destructed contrast agent into the imaging sector from frame to frame. In 3DE, this is not necessarily the case as the contrast agent in large parts of the chamber cavity is destructed from frame to frame.

2.7 Image Artifacts

Since 3DE is based on the same physical principles as 2DE, the examiner will experience all the image artifacts usually seen in 2D: (1) reverberations (i.e. multiple reflections between structures) giving false echoes within the acquisition volume, (2) aberrations (i.e. distortions of the ultrasound wave front) generating clutter noise, and (3) shadowing caused by highly echo-reflective structures giving areas of drop-out in the rendered image.

In addition to the common ultrasound artifacts also arising in 2D, there are some image artifacts that relate to 3DE only. First, when using ECG gated stitching of sub-volumes from multiple cardiac cycles, there is a danger of getting motion artifacts caused by respiration and heart rate variability (Fig. 2.9a). It is therefore important to have a real-time display where the examiner can detect stitching artifacts immediately during acquisition [3]. Second, within a (sub) volume, the time difference between first and the last fired beam will be inversely proportional to the frame rate. If the imaged object deforms quickly, geometrical distortions may appear. For example, if using an acquisition setup with a frame rate of 5 Hz, the difference between the first and last fired beam of the volume is 200 ms, and the walls look dyssynchronous (see simulated image shown in Fig. 2.9b) even though they are not. This means that low frame rate setups should not be used for motion assessment. The low frame rate setups should instead be used as a prepare mode to guide the examiner prior to higher frame rate setups or in clinical applications where frame rate is not important. Third, ultrasound data is quite frequently hampered by low-level clutter noise within the object cavities. Since volume-rendering techniques are based on accumulating intensity values along the casted rays, this low level noise might give volume renderings where the true walls are obscured by fog (Fig. 2.9c). Usually the examiner is able to get rid of the noise obscuring the walls by increasing the grey-level threshold for which samples that the algorithm will let contribute to the rendering or by making the whole volume rendering more transparent. Since the grey-levels of the tissue data usually vary a lot within the volume, both these approaches are susceptible to giving volume renderings with artificial holes.

2.8 Measuring in Three Dimensions

2.8.1 Distances and Areas

Current 3D systems offer the possibility of measuring distances and areas directly in the slice images. The distance and area tools are similar to what one is used to from 2D

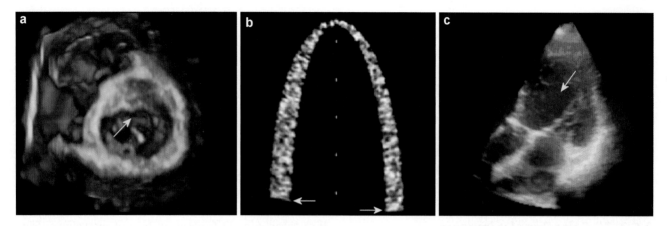

Fig. 2.9 (**a**) Stitching artifact (*arrow*) due to heart rate variability. (**b**) Simulation of 3D imaging using an acquisition setup with 36 by 36 transmit beams, four parallel receive beams and depth of 12.5 cm, giving a frame rate of 4.8 Hz. The deformation of the kinematic model used in the simulation was perfectly symmetric, i.e. the basal walls moved synchronously. Nevertheless, the two imaged walls look asym-metric (*horizontal arrows*) since, due to low frame rate of ~5 Hz, there is ~200 ms difference in acquisition time between the two walls. In phases of the cardiac cycle with high wall motion, this may give apparent depth differences of up to 8 mm. (**c**) Volume rendering where clutter noise in the chamber cavity (*arrow*) obscures the true cardiac wall

imaging. The advantage of using 3D is that the examiner can navigate the slice to the anatomically correct view before performing the distance or area measurement. This in contrast to 2DE where the ribs limit the number of available views of the heart. In some clinical applications, such as mitral valve stenosis evaluation, the free navigation capabilities of 3DE have shown to give more accurate results[11].

It is also possible to perform distance and area measurements directly on the volume rendered image. Ideally, the measurement tools should then take the depth information of the volume rendering into account when providing the measurement results. However, the depth estimation from the volume rendering may be prone to inaccuracies. One common simplification is therefore to provide measurement tools that work directly on the 2D image representing the volume rendering, not taking depth information into account. To avoid projection errors with this approach, it is important that the view direction is perpendicular to the structure that the examiner measures on. Before the examiner can start measuring, the system therefore may move the view plane of the volume rendering parallel to the crop plane intersecting the structure of interest (*En Face* view).

Another potential advantage of 3DE is the possibility to make anatomically correct distance and area measurements also when measuring in different phases of the cardiac cycle. In 2DE, only a part of the true 3D motion of the heart is captured. For example, in a 2D short axis view through the basal part of the left ventricle, there will be severe out-of-plane motion due to the longitudinal shortening and lengthening of the heart during the cardiac cycle. This out-of-plane motion causes new tissue to enter the 2D imaging plane and measurements in later frames will be from different anatomical locations. In 3DE, it is possible to correct for this error by moving the slice during the cardiac cycle.

2.8.2 Left Ventricular (LV) Volumes and Ejection Fraction (EF)

3DE has shown to be superior to 2DE for measuring LV volumes[12,13]. Why is this so? There are several factors: In 2D, volume measurements are based on geometric assumptions, and calculation formulas (e.g. Simpsons method) are used to extrapolate from 2D to 3D. When measuring in 3D, the whole cardiac structure is taken into account and no geometric assumption is needed. Furthermore, the problem of foreshortened views that affect 2D based volume estimate does not occur in 3D.

However, since manual volume measurements in 3D depend on manual tracing in a set of slices intersecting the structure of interest, they are time consuming, and consequently not so much used. The current volume measurement tools are therefore based on automated 3D surface detection algorithms. The automated tools should fulfill the following requirements: high accuracy, efficiency, repeatability and robustness. Given the nature of ultrasound imaging, these requirements are difficult to fulfill and many different surface detection algorithms have been tried out. One possibility is to fit a deformable model, that counteracts stretching and bending, to the tissue boundaries seen in the data. This approach is used because it is robust to boundary dropouts, accommodates large shape variability, supports user interaction and is relatively computational efficient.

Even though the surface detection can be made completely automatic it is important that the measurement tool provides some manual editing capabilities[14]. The reason for this is twofold: (1) the examiner may want to exclude parts of the structure (e.g. papillary muscles) from the volume measurement to comply with clinical conventions at the institution, and (2) ultrasound data often contains acoustic noise, such as multiple reflections, clutter noise, drop-outs and shadows, that may confuse the algorithm. Most surface detection algorithms today are able to incorporate user input.

To make the LV volume measurement tools clinically useful, they must be well integrated in the standard measurement package of the 3D system[15]. Today these tools (Fig. 2.10) provide semi-automatic 3D based end-diastolic volume, end-systolic volume and ejection fraction measurements within a few minutes.

One issue to be aware of is that 3DE has been reported to underestimate LV volumes compared to cardiac magnetic resonance (MRI). There are several sources for this difference[16]. First, the spatial and contrast resolution of current 3D systems are, in most patients, not sufficient for proper visualization of endocardial trabeculae. The trabeculae are therefore lumped together with the myocardium giving a smaller cavity volume than in MRI where the clinical convention is to include the trabeculae in the volume. Simple calculations, for clinically relevant volume sizes (~70 mL), show that a small outward change in endocardial position (~1 mm) can result in a significant change in volume estimate (~10%). To compensate for the poor visualization of trabeculae experienced investigators tend to trace the endocardial boundaries as far outward as possible to include as much endocardial trabeculae as possible in the left ventricular cavity. Second, in MRI, the criteria for inclusion of the basal short-axis slices significantly affect the volume estimate. A common convention is to include all slices in which at least 50% circumference of the left ventricular cavity is surrounded by myocardium. Compared to 3DE, the MRI based volume measurements will therefore be larger.

2.8.3 Other LV Measurements

Besides left ventricular volume measurements, recent studies have shown that 3DE can measure left ventricular mass as accurately and reproducibly as MRI[17]. In left ventricular mass measurements, the epicardium has to be outlined in addition to the endocardial surface. Detecting the epicardial boundary automatically is difficult due to weak boundary signals. The measurement tool therefore needs to offer

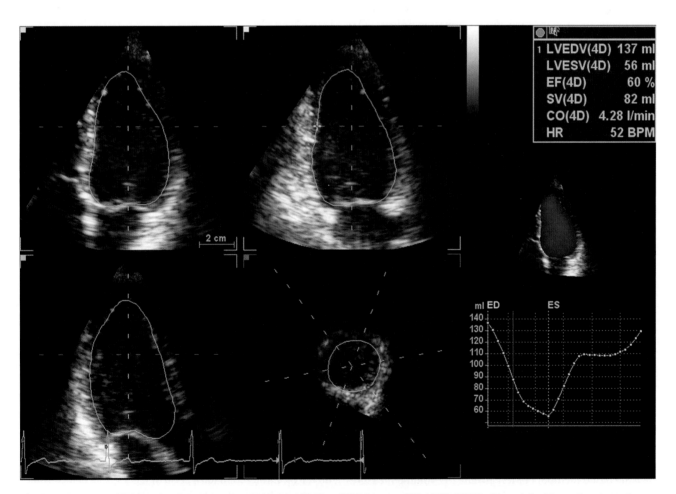

Fig. 2.10 Example of 3D based volume measurements by the 4D Auto LVQ feature of Vivid E9 (GE Healthcare). In this semi-automated measurement tool, the endocardial boundaries are searched for in 4D, i.e. in 3D space plus time

manual editing capabilities. The segmentation algorithm also needs to treat the two surfaces in combination to assure that the endocardium and the epicardium do not intersect.

3DE has also demonstrated potential in the field of cardiac resynchronization therapy[18]. In 3D, the left ventricular cavity and its mesh representation can be divided into 16, 17 or 18 segments/regional volumes. By measuring the deviation between the regional volume curves, the examiner can assess dyssynchronicity in patients considered for bi-ventricular pacing. The underlying assumption of this approach is that the regional volume curve is a surrogate for regional wall motion. This assumption can be disputed since endocardial radial excursion is only one component of the complex motion and deformation of the myocardium.

The true motion of the heart occurs in 3D, and 2D based methods cannot capture the true deformation of the myocardium without combining measurements from a large set of 2D images. Vendors have therefore developed methods for 3D strain estimation in 3D data[19]. Strain estimation can be divided into two steps. First, a tracking algorithm estimates the motion (displacement) field of the myocardium. Then, a 3D strain algorithm estimates regional strain (deformation) from the motion field. The first step (3D tracking) is the most challenging part of the strain estimation process. One possible implementation is to track a huge set of image feature points from frame to frame by using speckle tracking. When going from 2D to 3D the processing requirements of this approach increases dramatically due to the increase in (1) number of points to track, (2) number of search candidates per tracking point, and (3) number of samples in the search kernel. Inventive strategies are therefore applied to obtain an acceptable processing time while keeping the tracking quality. The reader familiar with 2D strain imaging may expect that the low frame rate of 3DE will make 3D strain estimation fail. The main reason for the frame rate recommendation of at least 40 frames per second in 2D strain is to avoid too much out-of-plane motion from frame to frame. In 2D, a high out-of-plane motion will give a large frame-to-frame difference in speckle pattern (high de-correlation), which again will compromise the tracking results. In 3D, however, out-of-plane motion is not an issue since the feature points are searched for in 3D.

2.8.4 Left Atrium and Right Ventricle

3DE has also been reported to measure left atrial[20] and right ventricular volumes[21] accurately. Right ventricle has a complex anatomical shape that can only be correctly assessed by a 3D based method. For left atrium, 3D volume measurements are faster to obtain and more accurate, increasing the clinical value as compared to 2D based volume estimations.

It should be pointed out that both left atrium and right ventricle have their own technical hurdles, as the walls of right ventricle and left atrium are thinner than the left ventricular wall. Also, when imaged from apex, the left atrium is far away from the probe and therefore located in the region of the acquisition geometry with the lowest spatial resolution. For the right ventricle, finding an imaging window that covers all walls may be challenging.

2.8.5 3D Color Doppler Quantification

From 3D color Doppler data it is possible to calculate instantaneous flow rate $Q(t)$ by integrating the velocities of the color Doppler samples over a surface intersecting the orifice. Stroke volume (SV) can then be estimated by integrating the instantaneous flow rate $Q(t)$ over the cardiac cycle[8,9].

2.8.6 Quantification of Mitral Valve Apparatus

3DE has the unique capability of showing the complete morphology of the mitral valve apparatus. This in contrast to 2DE, where the examiner must acquire several imaging planes and mentally reconstruct the shape of the valvular apparatus. With 3DE, the examiner can even quantify the valve apparatus and vendors have therefore developed mitral valve analysis tools for quantifying parameters such as annular diameter, annular nonplanarity, commissural length and leaflet area[2].

2.9 Future Developments

2.9.1 Transducer Technology

The clinical usefulness of modern 3DE was made possible by the development of the fully sampled 2D matrix array transducers. 3D transducer technology is still one of the most active research areas for the large ultrasound companies and further breakthroughs will be made in the years to come. The ultimate goal is to get the same image quality with the 3D transducers, as we currently have with 2D transducers. To obtain this, the 3D transducers must provide higher resolution, sensitivity and frequency bandwidth. In addition, there is a need to improve the ergonomics of the 3D transducers by decreasing size and weight. All these improvements will be driven by further miniaturization of the transducer electronics and the interconnection technology. For example, the custom made integrated circuitry may be placed directly below the transducer material (acoustic stack), making the connection to the elements simpler. Improvements of the high-voltage transmit electronics will probably also be made and 3D transducers with a higher number of piezoelectric elements and new piezoelectric materials will likely be introduced.

It should be pointed out that electronically steered 3D transducers were first introduced in echocardiography and that this type of technology will benefit the ultrasound community at large. In the future, we may see electronically steered 3D transducers also in other fields such as vascular imaging, obstetrics and radiology.

2.9.2 3D Beamforming

Regarding the beamformers, we will likely see two trends in the coming years. First, to increase the frame rate while keeping the volume size, the number of parallel receive-beams will increase. However, as described above, the number of parallel receive beams may have a practical limit. Today it is therefore difficult to say how many parallel receive beams that eventually will become standard in the future 3D systems. Second, the receive beamforming will be moved from dedicated custom made hardware circuitry to more general purpose off-the-shelf electronics such as multi-core CPUs. This will make the beamformer more flexible and in addition to classical beamforming the system may then be able to support alternative beamforming schemes. With general purpose processing units, it will also be easier (and cheaper) to increase the number of parallel receive beams.

2.9.3 Portable 3DE

Further miniaturization of the custom made electronics and shift from dedicated beamformer hardware to general purpose processing units, will make 3DE available on smaller systems. This evolution will eventually enable 3DE even on compact portable systems, making it easier to utilize 3D ultrasound bedside and in interventional settings.

2.9.4 Data Processing

The rapid developments and improvements in computer graphics technology, mainly driven by the gaming industry, opens up for use of more computational intensive data filtering techniques in 3DE. For instance, to reduce noise, while still keeping the details of the tissue, anisotropic diffusion filtering type of processing may be introduced even in

real-time. The technology will also allow computation and display of improved volume rendered images, making it easier to understand the anatomy at a glance.

2.9.5 3D Monitors

Currently only 2D monitors are available on the 3D ultrasound systems. The 2D monitors provides a flat 2D representation of the data and volume and surface rendering techniques have to be applied in order to give the examiner depth perception of the 3D structure. Encouraged by the movie and gaming industry, the monitor vendors now work with developing affordable stereoscopic monitor solutions. Up to now, the main problem with 3D monitors has been their inferior 2D image quality. When this problem is solved, the 3D ultrasound systems will start providing 3D monitors.

2.9.6 Navigation

One challenge with today's 3DE is that the examiner needs to navigate in the 3D data to obtain clinically useful views of the structures of interest. The navigation is time-consuming and new users even get lost in the data. Lately, some of the 3D systems have introduced special navigation tools so that the user more efficiently can select the view of interest. This development will continue and in the future, the clinically interesting views will be detected automatically by the system[22]. In addition, the 3D systems will provide more specialized screen layouts, such as the 9 Slice layout shown in Fig. 2.7, that are tailored for specific clinical applications.

2.9.7 3D Stress Echocardiography

In stress echocardiography, it is important with rapid acquisition of the images. This because ischemia may quickly induce wall motion or thickening abnormalities during the stress level affecting the sensitivity of the test. Furthermore, ischemia induced wall motion abnormalities may quickly resolve after exercise tests have ended. It is also important that the standard views are reproducible, so that the same myocardial segments are compared from stress level to stress level. These requirements favor use of 3D and multi-plane imaging in stress tests. Multi-plane and 3D imaging has therefore been tried out and found useful in stress testing[5,7,23]. The current image quality and frame rates of 3DE are sub-optimal compared to 2DE. Today the examiner therefore uses a 2D transducer in addition to the 3D transducers if acquiring 3D data during the stress test. Future 3D systems will provide 3D imaging with better image quality and higher frame rates than today, reducing the need for using two different transducers during the stress test. Recently 3D imaging has been fully integrated into the stress package of some of the 3D scanners. The stress package now helps the examiner to obtain the same 3D based standard views from stress level to stress level improving the quality and efficiency of the wall motion scoring. These improvements will increase the use of 3DE in stress tests.

2.9.8 Perfusion Imaging

Researchers have started to investigate the potential of 3D perfusion imaging[24]. In 3DE, new perfusion techniques have to be developed, as the flash technique used in 2DE, where a high-energy sound wave is used to destruct the contrast agent in the 2D plane cannot be used directly.

2.9.9 Quantification

Quantification in 3DE is still a very active research field and large projects on complete measurements of the heart's volume, shape, motion, deformation and perfusion are underway. This will make the 3DE examination more comprehensive and grow echocardiography in its role as the primary cardiac imaging modality. New techniques developed within the field of image analysis will eventually benefit 3DE. To make quantification in 3DE work in a clinical setting, the researchers now try to develop fully automatic quantification methods. For example, real-time LV volume measurements have been demonstrated[25]. There is also ongoing work to improve on the limitations of the current quantification methods and we will see a year-by-year improvement of the quantification tools. The automated quantification tools will also benefit from the improved image quality and frame rate of future 3D systems. Furthermore, future 3DE will also provide measurements that are not commonly used today. For instance, the LV shape, characterized by the sphericity parameter[26] (LV volume divided by the volume of a sphere defined by the LV long axis) may be used as a measure of remodelling after myocardium infarctions. Besides global shape, regional wall curvature may be used to measure the extent of the lesion. Combining regional wall curvature with wall thickness and blood pressure may eventually give wall stress estimates.

2.9.10 Image Registration and Fusion

Methods for registration and fusion of 3D ultrasound images with other imaging modalities such as MR and CT are currently under development. Image registration is the process of transforming different image data sets into the same coordinate system so that the examiner is able to compare data from different imaging modalities. Image registration algorithms can be classified into intensity-based and feature-based. Intensity-based methods compare intensity textures such as the speckle pattern, while feature-based methods uses image features such as blood vessels or cardiac chambers. A reliable image registration technique is a prerequisite for successful image fusion. In image fusion, the system combines information from at least two imaging modalities into one single image with the aim of generating an image that are more informative than the two original images. For instance, perfusion from SPECT combined with anatomical information from 3DE [27]. Furthermore, 3DE can be registered with pre-operative model segmentation from CMR and CT and used during interventions to track changes in cardiac function. Since 3DE is the only modality capable of acquiring cardiac 3D data in real-time during interventions, it is a natural complement to cardiac MR and CT. In the future, we will see product features that combine 3DE with other imaging modalities so that the clinical decision-making can be based on more comprehensive information.

2.9.11 Connectivity

The digital image exchange standard DICOM has recently been extended to support digital 3D echocardiographic data. The supplement currently includes: storage of volumetric tissue and Doppler data, definition of multi-plane, rendering and slice views, definition of rotation, translation, pan of view planes, 3D segmentation and crop, handling of stacked ECG waveforms, and blending of the different data types. This will eventually make it possible to review 3D ultrasound data on third-party DICOM viewers. However, be aware that the 3D DICOM supplement currently does not standardize the slice and volume rendering algorithms. Something that will cause the 3D images to look different from viewer to viewer.

In 3D DICOM, each volume is stored as a set of spatially related parallel slices of same size. Prior to storage, the acquired 3DE data therefore has to be scan-converted to rectangular (Cartesian) space. The file sizes and the file transfer times from scanner to server are already a challenge in current us of 3DE. Since scan converted data usually requires more storage space than raw data, the 3D DICOM files will need to be compressed.

In the long run, a well functioning 3D DICOM standard will spread the availability and use of 3DE.

2.10 Concluding Remarks

The last years we have experienced a rapid development in three-dimensional echocardiography. Modern 3D scanners are full of cutting-edge technology. Breakthroughs in transducer design, beamforming, display technologies and quantification have been released almost on a yearly basis. The ultrasound companies currently invest much in research and development in further improvements of 3DE and new inventive break-throughs will be introduced in the years to come. Further miniaturization will improve the image quality and make the 3D systems smaller. New automated image analysis techniques will make the systems simpler, faster to use and extend 3DE into new clinical areas. 3D DICOM will make it easier to integrate 3DE into the daily clinical workflow of the digital echo laboratory. From the current rate of technology breakthroughs, we anticipate a bright future for 3DE. 3DE will become an integral part of the routine echo examinations, making the examinations quicker and more precise.

Acknowledgements The author gratefully acknowledges the reviews by colleagues Kjell Kristoffersen, Olivier Gerard, Geir Haugen, Gunnar Hansen, Jøger Hansegård, Andreas Ziegler, Fredrik Orderud, Lars Linmarker, Luzvilla Anacta and Lea Anne Dantin. Special thanks to Jøger Hansegård and Jan Yee for help with making the figures and to Svein Brekke who let me adapt three of his figures (beamforming, sub-volume stitching and geometrical distortion).

References

1. Savord B, Solomon R. Fully sampled matrix transducer for real time 3D ultrasonic imaging. *Ultrasonics, 2003 IEEE Symposium on*, 2003;Vol 1:945–953.
2. Salgo IS. Three-dimensional echocardiographic technology. *Cardiol Clin*. 2007;25(2):231–239.
3. Brekke S, Rabben SI, Støylen A, Haugen A, Haugen GU, Steen EN, Torp H. Volume stitching in three-dimensional echocardiography: distortion analysis and extension to real time. *Ultrasound Med Biol*. 2007;33(5):782–796.
4. Steen E, Olstad B. Volume rendering of 3D medical ultrasound data using direct feature mapping. *IEEE Trans Med Imaging*. 1994;13(3):517–525.
5. Yang HS, Pellikka PA, McCully RB, Oh JK, Kukuzke JA, Khandheria BK, Chandrasekaran K. Role of biplane and biplane echocardiographically guided 3-dimensional echocardiography during dobutamine stress echocardiography. *J Am Soc Echocardiogr*. 2006;19(9):1136–1143.
6. Nucifora G, Badano LP, Dall'Armellina E, Gianfagna P, Allocca G, Fioretti PM. Fast data acquisition and analysis with real time triplane echocardiography for the assessment of left ventricular size and function: a validation study. *Echocardiography*. 2009;26(1):66–75.
7. Monaghan, M. Multi-plane and four-dimensional stress echocardiography—new solutions to old problems? *European Cardiovascular Disease*. 2006.
8. Berg S, Torp H, Haugen BO, Samstad S. Volumetric blood flow measurement with the use of dynamic 3-dimensional ultrasound color flow imaging. *J Am Soc Echocardiogr*. 2000;13(5):393–402.
9. Pemberton J, Ge S, Thiele K, Jerosch-Herold M, Sahn DJ. Real-time three-dimensional color Doppler echocardiography overcomes the inaccuracies of spectral Doppler for stroke volume calculation. *J Am Soc Echocardiogr*. 2006;19(11):1403–1410.
10. Malm S, Frigstad S, Sagberg E, Steen PA, Skjarpe T. Real-time simultaneous triplane contrast echocardiography gives rapid, accurate, and reproducible assessment of left ventricular volumes and ejection fraction: a comparison with magnetic resonance imaging. *J Am Soc Echocardiogr*. 2006;19(12):1494–1501.
11. Zamorano J, Cordeiro P, Sugeng L, Perez de Isla L, Weinert L, Macaya C, Rodríguez E, Lang RM. Real-time three-dimensional echocardiography for rheumatic mitral valve stenosis evaluation: an accurate and novel approach. *J Am Coll Cardiol* 2004;43: 2091–2096.
12. Jenkins C, Moir S, Chan J, Rakhit D, Haluska B, Marwick TH. Left ventricular volume measurement with echocardiography: a comparison of left ventricular opacification, three-dimensional echocardiography, or both with magnetic resonance imaging. *Eur Heart J*. 2009;30(1):98–106.
13. Jacobs LD, Salgo IS, Goonewardena S, Weinert L, Coon P, Bardo D, Gerard O, Allain P, Zamorano JL, de Isla LP, Mor-Avi V, Lang RM. Rapid online quantification of left ventricular volume from real-time three-dimensional echocardiographic data. *Eur Heart J*. 2006; 27(4):460–468.
14. Muraru D, Badano LP, Piccoli G, Gianfagna P, Del Mestre L, Ermacora D, Proclemer A. Validation of a novel automated border detection algorithm for rapid and accurate quantitation of left ventricular volumes based on three-dimensional echocardiography. *Eur J Echocardiogr*. 2010;11:359–68.
15. Hansegard J, Urheim S, Lunde K, Malm S, Rabben SI. Semi-automated quantification of left ventricular volumes and ejection fraction by real-time three-dimensional echocardiography. *Cardiovasc Ultrasound*. 2009;7:18.
16. Mor-Avi V, Jenkins C, Kühl HP, Nesser HJ, Marwick T, Franke A, Ebner C, Freed BH, Steringer-Mascherbauer R, Pollard H, Weinert L, Niel J, Sugeng L, Lang RM. Real-time 3-dimensional echocardiographic quantification of left ventricular volumes: multicenter study for validation with magnetic resonance imaging and investigation of sources of error. *JACC Cardiovasc Imaging*. 2008; 1(4): 413–423.
17. Pouleur AC, le Polain de Waroux JB, Pasquet A, Gerber BL, Gérard O, Allain P, Vanoverschelde JL. Assessment of left ventricular mass and volumes by three-dimensional echocardiography in patients with or without wall motion abnormalities: comparison against cine magnetic resonance imaging. *Heart*. 2008; 94(8):1050–1057.
18. Kapetanakis S, Kearney MT, Siva A, Gall N, Cooklin M, Monaghan MJ. Real-time three-dimensional echocardiography: a novel technique to quantify global left ventricular mechanical dyssynchrony. *Circulation*. 2005;112(7):992–1000.
19. de Isla LP, Balcones DV, Ferna´ndez-Golfi´n C, Marcos-Alberca P, Almeri´a C, Rodrigo JL, Macaya C, Zamorano J. Three-dimensional-wall motion tracking: a new and faster tool for myocardial strain assessment: comparison with two-dimensional-wall motion tracking. *J Am Soc Echocardiogr*. 2009;22:325–330.
20. Suh IW, Song JM, Lee EY, Kang SH, Kim MJ, Kim JJ, Kang DH, Song JK. Left atrial volume measured by real-time 3-dimensional echocardiography predicts clinical outcomes in patients with severe left ventricular dysfunction and in sinus rhythm. *J Am Soc Echocardiogr*. 2008 May;21(5):439–445.
21. Niemann PS, Pinho L, Balbach T, Galuschky C, Blankenhagen M, Silberbach M, Broberg C, Jerosch-Herold M, Sahn DJ. Anatomically oriented right ventricular volume measurements with dynamic three-dimensional echocardiography validated by 3-Tesla magnetic resonance imaging. *J Am Coll Cardiol*. 2007; 50(17):1668–1676.
22. Orderud F, Torp H, Rabben SI. Automatic alignment of standard views in 3D echocardiograms using real-time tracking. *SPIE Medical Imaging 2009: Ultrasonic Imaging and Signal Processing, Proc. of SPIE*. Vol. 7265, 72650D-1-7.
23. Takeuchi M, Otani S, Weinert L, Spencer KT, Lang RM. Comparison of contrast-enhanced real-time live 3-dimensional dobutamine stress echocardiography with contrast 2-dimensional echocardiography for detecting stress-induced wall-motion abnormalities. *J Am Soc Echocardiogr*. 2006;294–299.

24. Toledo E, Lang RM, Collins KA, Lammertin G, Williams U, Weinert L, Bolotin G, Coon PD, Raman J, Jacobs LD, Mor-Avi V. Imaging and quantification of myocardial perfusion using real-time three-dimensional echocardiography. *J Am Coll Cardiol.* 2006; 47(1):146–154.

25. Orderud F, Hansegård J, Rabben SI. Real-time volume measurements real-time tracking of the left ventricle in 3D echocardiography using a state estimation approach. *MICCAI 2007*, Part I, LNCS 4791, pp. 858–865.

26. Mannaerts HF, van der Heide JA, Kamp O, Stoel MG, Twisk J, Visser CA. Early identification of left ventricular remodelling after myocardial infarction, assessed by transthoracic 3D echocardiography. *Eur Heart J.* 2004;25(8):680–687.

27. Walimbe V., Jaber WA, Garcia MA, Shekhar R. Multimodality cardiac stress testing: combining real-time 3-dimensional echocardiography and myocardial perfusion SPECT. *J Nucl Med.* 2009 February;50(2):226–230.

3D Transesophageal Echocardiographic Technologies

3

Ivan S. Salgo

3.1 Introduction

Seeing is believing. A dramatic evolution in medical imaging has occurred within the past half century. Echocardiography is no exception. The basic, physical nature of ultrasound as a wave propagation phenomenon was well understood for most of the twentieth century. However the ability to control the transmission and reception of sound waves with extraordinary precision has advanced significantly. This coupled with the ability to process, display and quantify enormous amounts of data has progressed echocardiography into modality that will change cardiac intervention. For decades, interpreting ultrasound images was the domain of highly specialized experts. Today, 3D transesophageal echocardiography (3D TEE) has generated near optical cardiac images. The realm of understanding cardiac mechanical motion in all of its spatial and temporal dimensions is elucidating hidden pearls of general physiologic insight for echocardiography as well as precise diagnoses for patients.

This chapter will review the technology used for 3D TEE. First, it is helpful to clarify terminology. We will use the term "dimension" to refer to spatial dimension in 1D for M-mode, 2D for conventional "slices" and 3D for cubic sets of data. The addition of the temporal dimension accommodates movement but we don't call a conventional, moving, 2D spatial echo a "3D echo." We assume any mode that provides one, two or three spatial dimensions of information as having the ability to image dynamically beating hearts. We therefore relegate the usage of "4D echocardiography" as superfluous. Real-time typically refers to the instantaneous generation of an image "as it happens." Alternatively, some users refer to real time in reference to playback speed. Unfortunately, the use of real time in context to playback ignores whether the acquisition was "instantaneous" or gated.

The ability to generate instantaneous 3D echocardiographic images is the most significant advance in the field in the past decade. In order to emphasize this advance, these 3D images are referred to as real-time or live. Gated reconstruction uses images from past acquisitions. Notably, the emerging field of cardiac intervention will depend significantly on this instantaneous 3D imaging capability. Moreover, the miniaturization of application specific integrated circuitry to allow access to the esophagus gives significant acoustic advantages to 3D imaging.

It is expedient to address the technologic advances in terms of the operating sequence in an ultrasound system for TEE. This allows a framework consisting of transduction, beamforming, display, and quantification to be used. Echocardiographic instrumentation is unparalleled with respect to its portability, cost, lack of ionizing radiation and ubiquitous presence.

3.2 Transducer Technology

Amongst imaging modalities, the defining aspect of echocardiography is the transducer. Transduction refers to the ability to convert one form of energy to another. An ultrasound transducer converts electrical into mechanical energy on "transmit" and acts as a microphone on "receive." All ultrasound transducers perform this operation but what sets ultrasound apart is the ability to steer in two or three dimensions. The earliest M-mode transducers created an image consisting of one spatial and one temporal dimension. It is the "element" which is comprised of specialized material that traditionally uses PZT (lead–zirconate–tungsten). Newer single crystal materials that contain homogenous solid state domains are more efficient in the transduction process and have higher bandwidth (more upper and lower frequency content.) This creates a balanced increase of echo penetration and resolution. While M-mode was clearly an advance over the stethoscope, it was limited by its lack of field of view. M-mode used a transmit–listen–wait duty cycle to ascertain the distance of targets along an un-steered scan line and the operator needed to point the transducer to examine different cardiac structures.

I.S. Salgo
Cardiovascular Investigations, Research & Development, Ultrasound, Philips Healthcare, Andover MA 01810
e-mail: ivan.salgo@philips.com

The advent of the phased array methodology allowed scan lines to be steered electronically.

The conventional, "flat" 2D image common in use in echocardiography utilizes transducers with multiple elements. Specifically the elements are oriented in a singular row. These may contain 48–128 elements and each element is electrically isolated from the other. Individual wavefronts are generated by firing elements in a certain sequence. Each element constructively and destructively adds and subtracts pulses to generate an overall wave that has direction. This is the radially propagated scanline. As an example, if the farthest element on the right fires first and a timed sequence propagates along the element to the left, the beam will be steered to the left. Each element fires with a delay in phase with respect to a transmit initiation time. A point of clarification is in order: this 1D array of elements can beamform in two dimensions: radially and azimuthally (laterally). It is this spatiotemporal orientation of elements and their phase timed firing sequence that form the underpinning of any modern phased array system.

Equipped with this knowledge, one can assess the key aspects pertinent to 3D TEE imaging. If one wanted to visualize a static structure not moving in space, one could theoretically sweep a 2D imaging transducer if the third spatial dimension could somehow be registered. Using electromagnetic trackers, early *gated* 3D methodologies used this paradigm. Of course, the 2D images were gated to ECG. This was quite prone to error due to movement or arrhythmias and these lengthy scans could take tens of minutes. Ultimately, high fidelity cardiac imaging requires instantaneous imaging to overcome these limitations. The key difference between a 2D and instantaneous 3D imaging transducer is the arrangement of elements. While a 1D row is used for 2D imaging, a 2D matrix or checkerboard is used to steer an ultrasound scanline in both the azimuthal and elevational directions. A conventional 2D imaging transducer of one row steers energy in the azimuthal plane but unintentionally propagates elevational energy above and below the scanning plane. Early matrix array probes consisted of 5 or 7 electrically dependent rows (e.g. 7×64) whose purpose was to focus elevationally the ultrasound beam better above and below the azimuthal scan-plane. They were not capable of 3D imaging. Modern matrix arrays consist of many rows and columns (e.g. 52×52). This checkerboard pattern allows phasic firing of elements to generate a radially propagated scanline that can be steered in both azimuth and elevation. Hence, the true 3D imaging transducer is born.

In order to realize this paradigm academic research began in the 1980s. A block of PZT material is cut or "diced" by a diamond tipped saw to create the checkerboard pattern. Next, elements are electrically connected to a system. Early systems comprised sparsely sampled arrays, i.e. arrays whose elements were not all electrically active. These sparse arrays created the first instantaneous 3D images and early clinical research was conducted using this type of transducer. It is advantageous to have every element independently active to control the ultrasound beam with more precision. The

spacing or pitch of these elements depends on the desired wavelength of operation (typically lambda/4). Otherwise undesirable diffraction effects such grating lobes appear. This means that higher frequency transducers have finer pitch and increased technologic challenges emerge to create these element connections. The major advance that allowed a fully sampled matrix array to be fabricated was the ability to develop electrical interconnects to every element (Fig. 3.1).

Micro-beamforming splits the steering process into two pieces: coarse and fine steering. This is implemented by putting fine delay circuitry into special application specific integrated circuits (ASICs). The first commercial, fully sampled matrix array transducer utilized this methodology by placing 24–26 ASICs into the transducer handle. Approximately three thousand elements were electrically connected to these ASICs. Fine steering was performed using subsections of the element matrix known as patches. Coarse steering is performed within the system and through a conventional cable. Thus these ASICs allow every element to be electrically active but keep the size of the transducer cable small since a significant portion of beamforming has already taken place in the handle. Early transducers were specialized "3D only probes" but it is now possible to perform all of the transducer functions such as imaging, color flow and Spectral Doppler within the same transducer. Moreover the transducer aperture

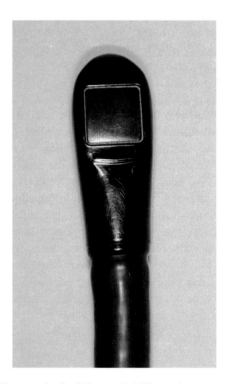

Fig. 3.1 Photograph of a fully sampled 2D matrix array used for 3D beam steering. The 3D TEE probe tip has no moving parts and a square aperture for azimuthal and elevational scan line steering. A conventional 2D multiplane TEE contains a 1-D acoustic array that is mechanically rotated by a mechanical motor. This supports 2D and 3D imaging, and spectral and color Doppler modes

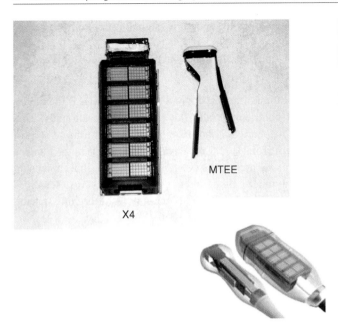

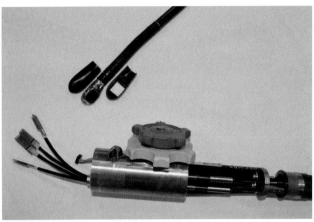

Fig. 3.4 3D TEE probe tip and handle disassembled. The electrical connections to the system are evident. Steering cables are also evident

Fig. 3.2 Example of a fully sampled transthoracic matrix array transducer (*left*) with 24 applications specific integrated circuits. Adjacent (*right*) is a miniaturized sensor with one ASIC. This is used for 3D transthoracic imaging

3.3 Beamforming

3D TEE beamforming comprises the steering and focusing of ultrasound energy both as transmitted and received scan lines so as to create useful signals that can be displayed or quantified. It is both an advanced science and art. Significant advancements continue to occur that maximize frame rate, scanning-volume-size and resolution. Resolution is defined as the ability to distinguish two point targets as distinct. The limiting item in current 3D echocardiographic systems is the speed of sound, not computing power. Ultrasound image quality improves by firing more transmit lines with more closely associated line spacing. Unfortunately, this slows frame rate since there are many more duty cycles for the system to deal with. Parallelism is defined as analyzing more receive lines per transmit line in an effort to extract more signal information. In a sense, a broader volume is interrogated or "listened to" around a transmit scanline. There are limits to parallelism however as insonifying a larger volume means transmitting "blobbier" lines. There are limits as well in signal to noise if you listen too far away from a transmit scanline. Focusing is the ability to concentrate and steer ultrasound energy in a specific direction so as to reduce off axis energy and side-lobe amplitude. All modern ultrasound systems employ "digital beamformers" that convert RF signals to binary information which can be stored. This allows much more sophisticated techniques to manipulate and create multiple receive lines for a given transmit event. Ultimately, the constraint of a system can be described by a triangle whose boundaries are defined by the number of transmit lines that can be fired. Lines widely spaced can increase volume size at the cost of lowering resolution for a constant frame rate. Tight line spacing can be used in zoom modes to increase resolution but at the price of a smaller volume. The number of transmit lines is a key determinant of frame rate: more lines increase resolution but lower frame rate (Fig. 3.5).

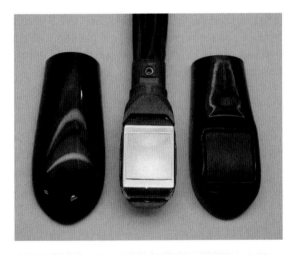

Fig. 3.3 3D Transesophageal transducer distal tip. The active aperture is 10 mm. The external housing has been removed

should be large enough to allow sufficient lateral and elevational resolution but small enough to "fit" into the intercostals space. One of the most difficult aspect in engineering such transducers is what is known as thermal management. The electronics generate heat, potentially more so at high mechanical indices (e.g. higher waveform amplitudes). These issues needed to be resolved if 3D echocardiography was to move to the operating room (Figs. 3.2–3.4).

3D TEE depends on micro-beamforming miniaturization. By reducing the electronic substrate required to beamform onto a single chip, the transducer chip is miniaturized sufficiently to pass into the human esophagus. It also significantly reduces the power requirement and hence amount of heat generated by live circuitry.

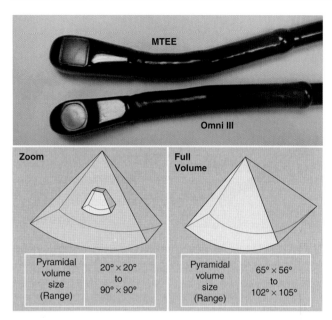

Fig. 3.5 3D scanning volumes for 3D TEE (Courtesy of the University of Chicago Medical Center, Chicago, IL. With permission.)

As mentioned above, beamforming can be split into a coarse stage that occurs in the system and a fine steering or micro-stage that occurs in the transducer. The act of combining element signals is known as summing. Summing of per element pulses is what ultimately creates a scan line. The general sequence of events are as follows:

- Compute (direction and aperture) and fire transmit scanline.
- Listen, i.e. sense returning echoes and digitally sample and store.
- Create multiple listening (after the fact) directions and foci (receive steering and dynamic focusing) from the digital data.

- Compute radiofrequency signal strength (envelope detection).
- Scan convert 3D spherical to Cartesian (cubic) voxel system.

The most important aspect of a 3D beamformer is the ability to steer both azimuthally (laterally) and elevationally. This creates a spherical coordinate system. The limits of resolution stem from lateral or elevational line spacing. Samples within a line are more finely spaced in the radial dimension (i.e. within a scanline) and are farther apart across scanlines in the lateral or elevational directions. Therefore line spacing is a fundamental determinant of image quality.

Gating refers to the act of acquiring multiple acquisitions (timed to the ECG) in order to combine them at some later point. Historic 3D acquisitions in the 1990s entailed acquiring 60–180 2D slices and interpolating them to create a 3D reconstructed volume. Since this process took several minutes it was prone to misalignment and inferior resolution. Gating is still used today to overcome limitations in the speed of sound by combining only a few 3D slabs (e.g. 4–8) to create a larger volume. This process takes only seconds. Moreover, color Doppler techniques depend on analyzing multiple transmit events fired along a single line. The multiple returning pulses are compared or cross correlates to infer velocity. Nevertheless, gating is prone to error in patients with irregular rhythms such as atrial fibrillation or multiple ventricular premature contractions (Fig. 3.6).

3D ultrasound imaging is still subject to the laws of acoustic physics. First, aperture is an important determinant of image quality. Larger apertures allow better beamforming from a focus point of view. Unlike abdominal imaging, transthoracic imaging is limited by the ultrasound aperture that can fit between a rib space. In TEE, the aperture is limited by dimensions that can be accommodated within an adult esophagus. TEE generally employs higher frequencies than

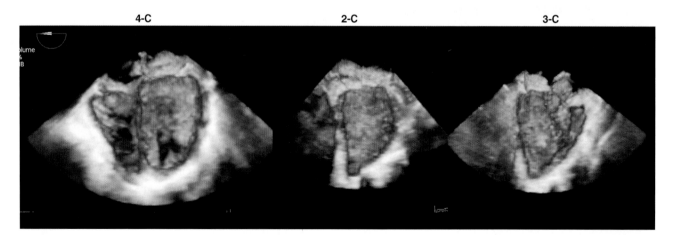

Fig. 3.6 Full volume 3D TEE acquisition encompassing the left ventricle. Depth-dependent dynamic colorization has been used to code hue according to depth perspective from the viewer. This adds visual cues to increase the "3D sense." Four-, two- and three-chamber perspectives are shown by cropping different aspects of the 3D olume away (Courtesy of the University of Chicago Medical Center, Chicago, IL. With permission.)

its transthoracic counterparts. This allows better image resolution for a given aperture size. (The higher the frequency, the better the ultrasound beam can focus but this comes at the loss of penetration.) Since TEE is not limited by significant chest wall acoustic aberration, the higher frequencies and better acoustic substrate allow higher resolution than for transthoracic imaging.

Next, artifacts such as shadowing, reverberations, multipath transmission and aberration play a role in degrading the ultrasound image. As with 2D echocardiography, 3D ultrasound cannot image through metallic or highly calcified objects. Moreover, TEE has a "blind-spot" in visualizing the aortic arch due to limitations from the airway. One of the most significant issues pertains to the image quality as seen through chest wall windows versus the esophagus. This is due mainly to two phenomena: aberration and multipath reflection. Aberration stems from wavefronts traveling through different media with different velocities of sound. Fascial tissue layers create a distortion of the traveling wavefronts. This can be corrected for, in a limited way, by accounting for the varying speeds of sound. The layers of the chest wall contain varying degrees of adipose and connective tissue. This creates aberration but also multipath degradation. As an ultrasound waves get diverted to altering paths of propagation, the superposition of transmitted and returning echo signals consists of wavefronts of both desired and nondesired targets. Unwanted but real signals are termed clutter. Since the esophagus represents a thin wall consisting of a stratified squamous epithelium and smooth muscle, these ultrasound effects do not occur in 3D TEE. Hence the image quality is higher and the clutter, lower (Fig. 3.7).

3.4 Quantification for 3D TEE

The significant advantage of 3D TEE in acquiring high resolution ultrasound images of the beating heart make it especially useful for cardiac quantification. While visualization of anatomy in its true three-dimensional state is important, many physicians believe that the single most significant value 3D echocardiography has for adult echocardiography is the ability to quantify. Myocardial and valvular motion occurs in three spatial dimensions but traditional 2D scanning planes do not capture the entire motion or else "slip" during scanning. Quantifying implies *segmenting* structures of interest from the 3D voxel set. Whereas voxels themselves can be tagged, for example coloring RV voxels separately from LV, computer vision techniques frequently employ methods that define an interface, for example an LV endocardial border. This interface is typically constructed as a mesh of points and lines and displayed by a process known as *surface rendering*.

New 3D electronically steered transesophageal transducers are yielding ultrasound images never before seen on the beating mitral valve[1-3]. (Figure. 3.8) This also allows the mitral apparatus to be segmented at end-systole with great accuracy. The true three dimensional nature of the mitral annulus, leaflets and chordal apparatus can be measured[1-9]. This further allows sophisticated analyses of the nonplanar shape of the mitral annulus. These 3D measurements include:

- Annular diameters
- Annular nonplanarity
- Commissural lengths

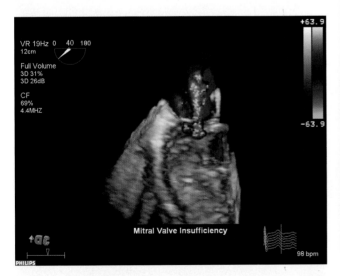

Fig. 3.7 Gated 3D TEE color acquisition. A 3D jet of mitral regurgitation is shown. The classic 2D color map has been adapted to render color voxels showing the 3D nature of the jet (Courtesy of the University of Chicago Medical Center, Chicago, IL. With permission.)

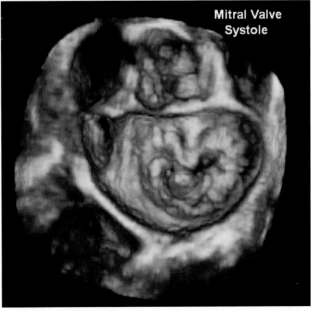

Fig. 3.8 3D TEE of the mitral valve. Note anterior and posterior leaflets. The middle scallop of the posterior leaflet is prolapsing significantly

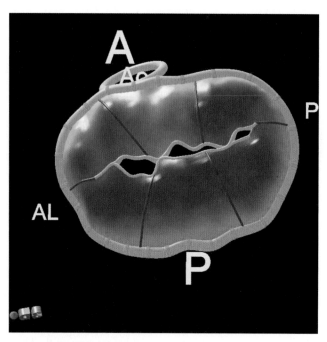

Fig. 3.9 3D quantification of the mitral leaflets (Barlow's disease). Parametric imaging demonstrates leaflet surface prolapsed. Leaflet height been computed numerically. This assessment allows quantifying the degree and extent of leaflet abnormalities such as multi-segmental leaflet prolapse (Barlow's disease)

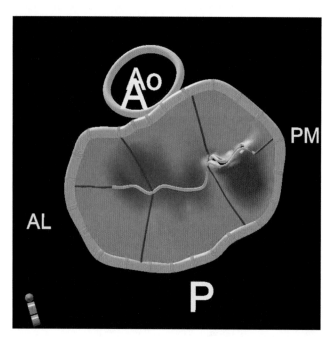

Fig. 3.10 3D quantification of fibroelastic deficiency. Note the isolated areas of leaflet prolapse

- Leaflet surface areas
- Aortic to mitral annular orientation (Figs. 3.9 and 3.10)

3D quantification of the left ventricle classically employs a surface rendered mesh. This allows accurate computation of

volume, regional wall motion and regional synchrony. Since the entire extent of the LV is taken into account, no foreshortening errors or assumption of LV volume are generated. Technically, a 3D deformable is used to find the LV endocardial surface in three dimensions. This is the most accurate way to quantify LV volumes. Moreover, 3D LV remodeling can be parametrically displayed using differential geometry techniques. Bi- and triplane methods help avoid foreshortening errors and benefit from higher frame rates than 3D live acquisitions but if an aneurysmal dilatation occurs between planes, the computed LV volumes will have some interpolation error. Quantification of LV synchrony is possible in 3D as well.[10–14] The required frame rate depends on the questions being asked. Frame rates of 30 Hz (33 ms between frames) are inadequate to quantify intramyocardial motion; these are better suited to be studied by tissue Doppler or speckle tracking techniques. However, regional synchrony *can* be measured by 3D endocardial excursion because it assesses blood ejection not tissue motion. 3D echocardiography provides advantages in providing a more complete assessment of 3D wall motion. [15,16] Frame rate limitations must be taken into account however.

3.5 Procedural Guidance for 3D TEE

Patients who undergo mitral valve repair should have intraoperative transesophageal echo as part of their care. 3D methods now allow leaflet anatomy to be displayed functionally with resolution that was not possible before. While, conventional

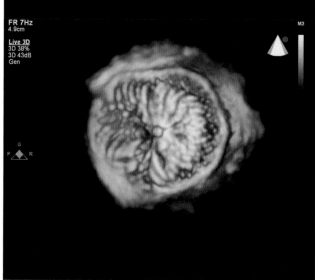

Fig. 3.11 3D TEE of Amplatzer device placement. Note the 3D nature of the device. The ability to assess tissue rim adequacy for device seating is especially useful

2D echo is likely sufficient for the detection of thrombus and vegetations, 3D echo allows visualization and quantification of the mitral and tricuspid apparatus in its living 3D state. Live 3D TEE is especially useful in delineating areas of leaflet prolapse as in patients with Barlow's disease. Moreover, 3D echo is useful is assessing the degree of leaflet restriction within the apparatus as well as annular changes. Sophisticated changes in LV remodeling can be assessed in ischemic mitral regurgitation. Changes of mitral leaflet systolic anterior motion can be assessed in hypertrophic cardiomyopathy.

3D visualization is especially useful in indentifying intracardiac problems such as atrial septal defects. This is especially useful in identifying and characterizing congenital defects for both children and the growing population of adults with congenital heart disease (Fig. 3.11).

The types of clinical applications in 3D echocardiography is still growing significantly.[3,17-29] As technologies progress, the area of image guided intervention will grow significantly. [30-38] The ability to image live structures is a key enabling aspect of creating catheter and minimally invasive rigid instrument procedures is allowing the avoidance of cardiopulmonary bypass. Current guidance applications include placement of atrial septal occluder devices but transcatheter aortic and mitral valve therapies are on the horizon. Three-dimensional imaging will be the cornerstone to many of these procedures.

The future for 3D TEE looks quite promising. Advances in technology will allow larger scanning volumes as well as more sophisticated methods of quantification. One of the most exciting areas includes the use of 3D echo to guide intracardiac procedures without the need for cardiopulmonary bypass.[31,39] Placement of ASD devices and percutaneous valve therapies will likely benefit from the live nature of 3D TEE imaging and broaden not only the diagnostic uses of 3D echocardiography but those used for therapy as well.

References

1. Kronzon I, Sugeng L, Perk G, Hirsh D, Weinert L, Garcia Fernandez MA, Lang RM. Real-time 3-dimensional transesophageal echocardiography in the evaluation of post-operative mitral annuloplasty ring and prosthetic valve dehiscence. *J Am Coll Cardiol.* 2009;53(17): 1543–1547.
2. Sugeng L, Shernan SK, Salgo IS, Weinert L, Shook D, Raman J, Jeevanandam V, DuPont F, Settlemier S, Savord B, Fox J, Mor-Avi V, Lang RM. Live 3-dimensional transesophageal echocardiography initial experience using the fully-sampled matrix array probe. *J Am Coll Cardiol.* 2008;52(6):446–449.
3. Sugeng L, Shernan SK, Weinert L, Shook D, Raman J, Jeevanandam V, DuPont F, Fox J, Mor-Avi V, Lang RM. Real-time three-dimensional transesophageal echocardiography in valve disease: comparison with surgical findings and evaluation of prosthetic valves. *J Am Soc Echocardiography.* 2008;21(12):1347–1354.
4. Salgo IS, Gorman JH, III, Gorman RC, Jackson BM, Bowen FW, Plappert T, St John Sutton MG, Edmunds LH, Jr. Effect of annular shape on leaflet curvature in reducing mitral leaflet stress. *Circulation.* 2002;106(6):711–717.
5. Watanabe N, Ogasawara Y, Yamaura Y, Kawamoto T, Toyota E, Akasaka T, Yoshida K. Quantitation of mitral valve tenting in ischemic mitral regurgitation by transthoracic real-time three-dimensional echocardiography. *J Am Coll Cardiol.* 2005; 45 (5):763–769.
6. Messas E, Yosefy C, Chaput M, Guerrero JL, Sullivan S, Menasche P, Carpentier A, Desnos M, Hagege AA, Vlahakes GJ, Levine RA. Chordal cutting does not adversely affect left ventricle contractile function. *Circulation.* 2006;114 (1):I524–I528.
7. Sugeng L, Coon P, Weinert L, Jolly N, Lammertin G, Bednarz JE, Thiele K, Lang RM. Use of real-time 3-dimensional transthoracic echocardiography in the evaluation of mitral valve disease. *J Am Soc Echocardiogr.* 2006; 19 (4):413–421.
8. Garcia-Orta R, Moreno E, Vidal M, Ruiz-Lopez F, Oyonarte JM, Lara J, Moreno T, Garcia-Fernandezd MA, Azpitarte J. Three-dimensional versus two-dimensional transesophageal echocardiography in mitral valve repair. *J Am Soc Echocardiogr.* 2007;20 (1):4–12.
9. Valocik G, Kamp O, Mannaerts HF, Visser CA. New quantitative three-dimensional echocardiographic indices of mitral valve stenosis: new 3D indices of mitral stenosis. *Int J Cardiovasc Imaging.* 2007;23 (6):707–716.
10. Kapetanakis S, Kearney MT, Siva A, Gall N, Cooklin M, Monaghan MJ. Real-time three-dimensional echocardiography a novel technique to quantify global left ventricular mechanical dyssynchrony. *Circulation.* 2005; 112:992–1000.
11. Agler DA, Adams DB, Waggoner AD. Cardiac resynchronization therapy and the emerging role of echocardiography (part 2): the comprehensive examination. [Review] [47 refs]. *J AmSoc Echocardiogr.* 2007;20(1):76–90.
12. Zamorano J, de Isla LP, Roque C, Khanhderia B. The role of echocardiography in the assessment of mechanical dyssynchrony and its importance in predicting response to prognosis after cardiac resynchronization therapy. [Review] [37 refs]. *J Am Soc Echocardiogr.* 2007;20 (1):91–99.
13. Takeuchi M, Jacobs A, Sugeng L, Nishikage T, Nakai H, Weinert L, Salgo IS, Lang RM. Assessment of left ventricular dyssynchrony with real-time 3-dimensional echocardiography: comparison with Doppler tissue imaging. *J Am Soc Echocardiogr.* 2007;20(12):1321–1329.
14. Pulerwitz T, Hirata K, Abe Y, Otsuka R, Herz S, Okajima K, Jin Z, Di Tullio MR, Homma S. Feasibility of using a real-time 3-dimensional technique for contrast dobutamine stress echocardiography. *J Am Soc Echocardiogr.* 2006;19(5):540–545.
15. Walimbe V, Garcia M, Lalude O, Thomas J, Shekhar R. Quantitative real-time 3-dimensional stress echocardiography: a preliminary investigation of feasibility and effectiveness. *J Am Soc Echocardiogr.* 2007; 20(1):13–22.
16. Takeuchi M, Otani S, Weinert L, Spencer KT, Lang RM. Comparison of contrast-enhanced real-time live 3-dimensional dobutamine stress echocardiography with contrast 2-dimensional echocardiography for detecting stress-induced wall-motion abnormalities. [see comment]. *J Am Soc Echocardiogr.* 2006;19(3):294–299.
17. Hamilton-Craig C, Boga T, Platts D, Walters DL, Burstow DJ, Scalia G. The role of 3D transesophageal echocardiography during percutaneous closure of paravalvular mitral regurgitation. *JACC: Cardiovasc Imaging.* 2009; 2 (6):771–773.
18. Caiani EG, Corsi C, Sugeng L, MacEneaney P, Weinert L, Mor-Avi V, Lang RM. Improved quantification of left ventricular mass based on endocardial and epicardial surface detection with real time three dimensional echocardiography. *Heart.* 2006; 92(2):213–219.
19. Watanabe N, Ogasawara Y, Yamaura Y, Wada N, Kawamoto T, Toyota E, Akasaka T, Yoshida K. Mitral annulus flattens in ischemic mitral regurgitation: geometric differences between inferior and anterior myocardial infarction: a real-time 3-dimensional echocardiographic study. *Circulation.* 2005; 112(9 Suppl):I458–I462.

20. Malagoli A, Bursi F, Modena MG. Failure of mitral valve repair: partial detachment of valvular ring by 3D transesophageal echocardiography reconstruction. *Echocardiography*. 2009;26(1): 111–112.

21. Yang HS, Pellikka PA, McCully RB, Oh JK, Kukuzke JA, Khandheria BK, Chandrasekaran K. Role of biplane and biplane echocardiographically guided 3-dimensional echocardiography during dobutamine stress echocardiography. *J. Am Soc Echocardiogr* 2006;19(9):1136–1143.

22. Muller S, Feuchtner G, Bonatti J, Muller L, Laufer G, Hiemetzberger R, Pachinger O, Barbieri V, Bartel T. Value of transesophageal 3D echocardiography as an adjunct to conventional 2D imaging in preoperative evaluation of cardiac masses. *Echocardiography*. 2008;25(6):624–631.

23. Ton-Nu TT, Levine RA, Handschumacher MD, Dorer DJ, Yosefy C, Fan D, Hua L, Jiang L, Hung J. Geometric determinants of functional tricuspid regurgitation: insights from 3-dimensional echocardiography. *Circulation*. 2006;114(2):143–149.

24. Jacobs LD, Salgo IS, Goonewardena S, Weinert L, Coon P, Bardo D, Gerard O, Allain P, Zamorano JL, de Isla LP, Mor-Avi V, Lang RM. Rapid online quantification of left ventricular volume from real-time three-dimensional echocardiographic data. *Eur Heart J*. 2006;27(4):460–468.

25. Jenkins C, Chan J, Hanekom L, Marwick TH. Accuracy and feasibility of online 3-dimensional echocardiography for measurement of left ventricular parameters. *J Am Soc Echocardiogr*. 2006; 19(9):1119–1128.

26. Marsan NA, Bleeker GB, Ypenburg C, Ghio S, Van De Veire NR, Holman ER, van der Wall E, Tavazzi L, Schalij MJ, Bax JJ. Real-time three dimensional echocardiography permits quantification of left ventricular mechanical dyssynchrony and predicts acute response to cardiac resynchrononization therapy. *J Cardiovasc Electrophysiol*. 2008;19:392–399.

27. Abraham T, Kass D, Tonti G, Tomassoni GF, Abraham W, Bax JJ, Marwick TH. Imaging cardiac resynchronization therapy. *J Am Coll Cardiol Imaging* 2009;2(4):486–497.

28. Marsan NA. Real-time three-dimensional echocardiography as a novel approach to quantify left ventricular dyssynchrony: a comparison study with phase analysis of gated myocardial perfusion single photon emission computed tomography. *J Am Soc Echocardiogr*. 2008;21(7):801–807.

29. Fischer GW, Salgo IS, Adams DH. Real-time three-dimensional transesophageal echocardiography: the matrix revolution. *J Cardiothor Vasc An*. 2008;22(6):904–912.

30. Hung J, Guerrero JL, Handschumacher MD, Supple G, Sullivan S, Levine RA. Reverse ventricular remodeling reduces ischemic mitral regurgitation: echo-guided device application in the beating heart. *Circulation*. 2002;106(20):2594–2600.

31. Cannon JW, Stoll JA, Salgo IS, Knowles HB, Howe RD, DuPont PE, Marx GR, del Nido PJ. Real-time three-dimensional ultrasound for guiding surgical tasks. *ComputAided Surg*. 2003;8(2):82–90.

32. Suematsu Y, Marx GR, Stoll JA, DuPont PE, Cleveland RO, Howe RD, Triedman JK, Mihaljevic T, Mora BN, Savord BJ, Salgo IS, del Nido PJ. Three-dimensional echocardiography-guided beating-heart surgery without cardiopulmonary bypass: a feasibility study. *J Thorac Cardiovasc Surg*. 2004;128(4):579–587.

33. Salgo IS. 3D echocardiographic visualization for intracardiac beating heart surgery and intervention. [Review] [16 refs]. *Semin Thorac Cardiovasc Surg*. 2007;19(4):325–329.

34. Vasilyev NV, Novotny PM, Martinez JF, Loyola H, Salgo IS, Howe RD, del Nido PJ. Stereoscopic vision display technology in real-time three-dimensional echocardiography-guided intracardiac beating-heart surgery. *J Thorac Cardiovasc Surg*. 2008; 135(6): 1334–1341.

35. Vasilyev NV, Melnychenko I, Kitahori K, Freudenthal FP, Phillips A, Kozlik-Feldmann R, Salgo IS, del Nido PJ, Bacha EA. Beating-heart patch closure of muscular ventricular septal defects under real-time three-dimensional echocardiographic guidance: a preclinical study. *J Thorac Cardiovasc Surg*. 2008;135(3):603–609.

36. Kim SS, Hijazi ZM, Lang RM, Knight BP. The use of intracardiac echocardiography and other intracardiac imaging tools to guide noncoronary cardiac interventions. [Review] [40 refs]. *J Am Coll Cardiol*. 2009;53(23):2117–2128.

37. Lodato JA, Cao QL, Weinert L, Sugeng L, Lopez J, Lang RM, Hijazi ZM. Feasibility of real-time three-dimensional transoesophageal echocardiography for guidance of percutaneous atrial septal defect closure. *Eur J Echocardiogr*. 2009;10(4):543–548.

38. Perrin DP, Vasilyev NV, Novotny P, Stoll J, Howe RD, DuPont PE, Salgo IS, del Nido PJ. Image guided surgical interventions. [Review] [58 refs]. *Curr Prob Surg*. 2009;46 (9):730–766.

39. Suematsu Y, Takamoto S, Kaneko Y, Ohtsuka T, Takayama H, Kotsuka Y, Murakami A. Beating atrial septal defect closure monitored by epicardial real-time three-dimensional echocardiography without cardiopulmonary bypass. *Circulation*. 2003; 107(5): 785–790.

Three-Dimensional Echocardiography in Clinical Practice

4

Luigi P. Badano and Denisa Muraru

4.1 The Incremental Value of the Third Dimension

The heart has a complex anatomy and it is in constant motion. Conventional two-dimensional (2D) echocardiography can only provide partial information about the spatial and temporal relationship of cardiac structures during the cardiac cycle (Fig. 4.1). Furthermore, conventional 2D echocardiography requires a difficult mental process by the operator to reconstruct a stereoscopic image of the heart based on the interpretation of multiple tomographic slices. Sometimes, the mental exercise of reconstruction may be inadequate to obtain a precise diagnosis even for an experienced observer, especially when dealing with complex congenital abnormalities of the heart. In addition, it can be difficult to convey or demonstrate a meaningful representation of cardiac pathology to those not fully conversant with 2D echocardiographic views and appearances.

Over the last decade, 3D echocardiography has transitioned from a research tool to an imaging technique useful in everyday clinical practice thus expanding the diagnostic capabilities of cardiac ultrasound. 3D echocardiography may allow a more readily appreciated, intuitive, objective and quantitative evaluation of cardiac anatomy and physiology that would reduce the subjectivity in image interpretation.[1-3]

At present there is enough scientific evidence to endorse the use of 3D echocardiography as the modality of choice to: (1) measure cardiac chamber volumes without the need for geometrical modelling; (2) visualization of detailed in vivo anatomy of cardiac valves and congenital abnormalities; (3) monitor and assess effectiveness of surgical or percutaneous transcatheter interventions. However, despite these documented advantages, the technique has not reached a widespread use yet. In this paragraph, we will try to identify and discuss the main reason that have limited the penetration of 3D echocardiography among clinical echocardiographers (Table 4.1).

Apart the obvious skepticism that surrounds any new technology when it appears in the clinical arena, there are objective facts that may explain the resistance of echocardiographers in adopting the 3D technique. 3D echocardiography sounds easy but it is not. For effective application of the technique, echocardiographers need specific education and training. They have to learn how to acquire volumetric data sets without artifacts (Fig. 4.2), and navigate within the data set to obtain the desired view (Fig. 4.3). New tools like cropping, slicing and thresholding are available to manipulate the data sets in order to visualize the cardiac structure of interest. Various ways to display the information are available. Finally, the 3D probe and software are costly and using 3D echo acquisition may impact negatively in echo lab work flow. In the next paragraph we will try to address all these issues in a practical way.

4.2 Acquisition Modes

Transthoracic 3D echocardiography has four acquisition modes: (1) real-time (live) 3D; (2) stitched 3D; (3) zoom 3D; and (4) 3D color Doppler.

Real-time 3D refers to volumes of information acquired in a single heart beat and displayed in a volume rendered manner in real-time, and it would be the ideal mode of 3D acquisition since there are no limitations related to arrhythmias, motion or need of breath holding. This acquisition mode has significant advantages: (1) No stitching artifacts in the 3D data set; (2) It's "true" real-time and allows the operator to follow interventional procedures; (3) By steering the volume using the trackball, the operator can observe the cardiac structure in 3D from different perspectives without moving the probe. For example: to obtain a sagittal view of a mitral valve stenosis in order to visualize the full mitral valve apparatus and, afterwards, to steer the probe to obtain an "en face" view of the mitral orifice to display the shape, size and dynamic changes of the residual orifice. However, since 3D

L.P. Badano (✉)
Head of Noninvasive Imaging Lab, Department
of Cardiology, Vascular and Thoracic Sciences,
University of Padua, Padua, Italy
e-mail: lpbadano@gmail.com

L.P. Badano et al. (eds.), *Textbook of Real-Time Three Dimensional Echocardiography*,
DOI: 10.1007/978-1-84996-495-1_4, © Springer-Verlag London Limited 2011

Fig. 4.1 Standard long-axis parasternal view obtained with 2D echocardiography (*left panel*, video) and the same view obtained cropping a full volume data set of the left ventricle obtained from parasternal approach (*right panel*, video). Note the depth perception and visualization of structures in their spatial orientation which is not possible with 2D imaging

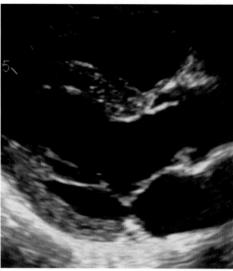 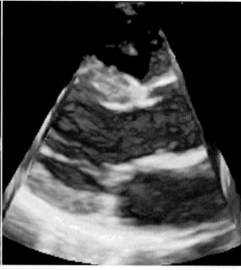

Table 4.1 Main reasons which have limited the expansion of 3D echocardiography in clinical practice

Need of specific education and training, skepticism
Present transducer technology
Bulky size and weight
Need to switch from 2D to 3D transducer for a complete study
Feasibility and present technology limitation
Limited temporal and spatial resolution
Limited acquisition volume
Data management
Time constrain to perform echo studies
No DICOM tool to manage 3D data sets
Need of automatic display of standard 2D and 3D views
Need of semi- or automatic quantification
Costs

echocardiography is an ultrasound based technique it faces spatial and temporal compromises. The key trade-off in real time 3D echocardiography is between temporal (i.e. volume rate) and spatial resolution. Spatial resolution can be improved by increasing the scan line density (the number of scan lines per volume), however it will prolong both the acquisition and process time and in the end it will reduce the temporal resolution (volume rate). A possible compromise is to reduce the acquired volume size to increase spatial resolution while maintaining the temporal resolution (zoom mode, Fig. 4.4). There are few suggestions for adequate real-time 3D echocardiography acquisitions: (1) Start with 2DE to localize the cardiac structure of interest, then switch to live 3DE or zoom mode; (2) Optimize the 2D image –"*suboptimal 2DE images produce suboptimal 3DE data sets*" [2]; (3) Select the highest resolution option that accommodates the volume of interest.

Stitched 3D mode refers to the acquisition of narrow volumes of information over several consecutive cardiac cycles (generally ranging from two to seven heart beats) that are combined to produce a single volumetric data set. This acquisition mode compensates for the poor temporal resolution of the real-time large volumes and it is very useful when a large volumes need to be acquired with an adequate temporal resolution (i.e. acquisition of right or left ventricular data sets for quantitation purposes). Furthermore, despite being called "real-time," this acquisition mode provides images that are not truly real-time, since the images are not available until the last recorded cardiac cycle is acquired. Some technical details are needed to acquire stitched 3D data sets adequate for postprocessing and image rendering. The ECG trace should be optimized in order to obtain a distinct R wave voltage. Since the most frequent artifact of gated 3DE acquisitions is the stitching artifact due to arrhythmias and patient and/or respiratory motion, the number of acquisition beats should be adjusted according to patient's needs, taking into account that the larger number of beats are acquired, the higher will be the temporal resolution and the wider the volume obtained. If the patient is unable to hold his/her respiration during multibeat acquisition or if there are significant rhythm disturbances (irregular atrial fibrillation or frequent ectopic beats) one should try to use the single beat full-volume acquisition (if available) or to stick to the live 3D mode. Then, the volume size should be optimized in order to acquire the smaller volume able to encompass the cardiac structure of interest in order to improve spatial resolution (i.e. the number of scan lines per volume) while maintaining adequate temporal resolution since the two are inversely related. Before 3DE acquisition, the 2DE image should be optimized. Finally, appropriate gain and compression should be set before acquisition, since there are limits on how much gain and/or compression can be added or removed by postprocessing once a 3DE data set is acquired. In addition, low gain settings can artificially eliminate certain structures, while high gain settings can mask structures (both leading to significant misdiagnosis). As a general rule, both gain and compression should be set in

Fig. 4.2 Examples of pitfalls (*arrows*) in 3D data set acquisition: stitching artifacts (*panel A, arrow* video); dropout artifact (*panel B, arrow* video); attenuation artifact: the large vegetation (*asterisk*) entirely visualized in diastole in *panel C* (*left*) seems to be fragmented in systole (*panel C, right,* video) when it crosses the attenuation area (*arrow*) due to calcified mitral annulus

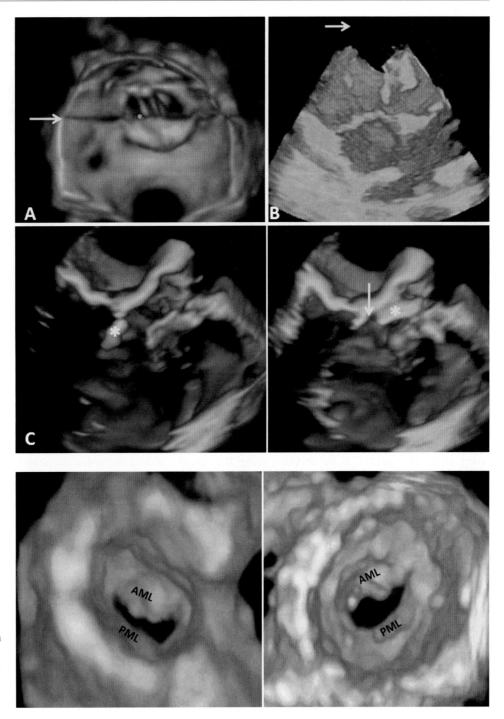

Fig. 4.3 Mitral valve viewed from the left atrium ("surgical view," *left panel*, video) and from the left ventricle (*right panel*, video). *AML* anterior mitral leaflet, *PML* posterior mitral leaflet

the mid-range and the time-gain compensation should be used to overcompensate for the brightness of the image to allow the maximum flexibility with postprocessing.

3D color Doppler is an important acquisition mode in 3D echocardiography since both anterograde or regurgitant jets may be quite variable in shape, size and extension, and therefore they may be better assessed with a 3D visualization.

Before starting to acquire a 3D data set, one need to pay attention to the image resolution issue. The resolution of images varies according to the dimension employed. For current 3D transducers it is around 0.5–1 mm in the axial (y) dimension, around 1.5–2.0 mm in the lateral (x) dimension, and around 2.5–3 mm in the elevation (z) dimension. As a result, we will obtain the best images (less degree of spreading, i.e. distortion) when using the axial dimension and the worst (greatest degree of spreading) when we use the elevation dimension. These concepts have an immediate practical application in the choice of the best approach to image a particular cardiac structure. If the goal is to obtain an *en-face* view of the mitral valve from the left atrium (the socalled

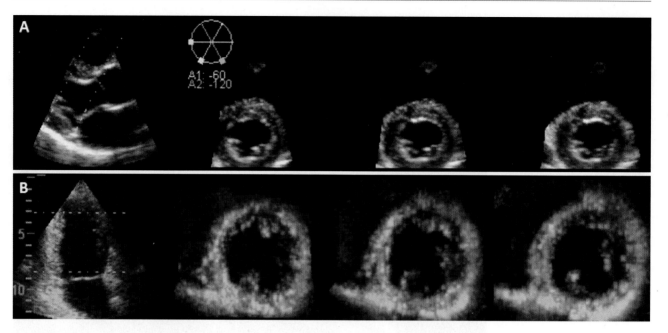

Fig. 4.4 Different image resolutions are obtained using the parasternal (lateral and axial resolution, *panel A*, video) and the apical (lateral and elevation resolution, *panel B*, video) approaches

"surgical view") or an *en-face* view of the aortic valve, the best results are expected to be obtained by using the parasternal short axis approach, because structures are imaged using the axial and lateral dimensions (Fig. 4.4). Conversely, the worst result is expected to be obtained using the apical approach which uses the lateral and elevation dimensions.

The inverse relation between frame rate, volume size and spatial resolution has been described in Chapter 2. The practical implications for the echocardiographer are straightforward: acquisitions with high temporal and spatial resolution can be obtained only at the expense of reducing the size of the acquired volume (zoom mode); large volumes can maintain adequate temporal resolution only if scan line density is reduced (reduced spatial resolution); conversely in order to maintain adequate spatial resolution of large volumes, the temporal resolution (i.e. the volume rate) should be also reduced. Therefore: to assess valve anatomy, the zoom mode acquisition is preferred; to assess spatial relationship among different cardiac structures, large volumes with reduced volume rate should be used; whereas to assess heart chamber size and function, large volumes with reduced spatial resolution are required.

4.3 How to Navigate Within the 3D Data Set and Visualize the Desired Cardiac Structure?

Acquisition of volumetric images in real-time generates the problem of how to visualize the moving structures contained within the volume on a flat, 2D monitor.

Viewing a volume rendered 3D data set of the heart is analogous to standing outside a museum and being unable to see in without taking some or part of the walls away (Fig. 4.5). Once cropped away a part of the data set, one is able to see inside the heart but necessarily, the image that is presented to the observer for interpretation is only part of all the information contained within the 3D volume (Fig. 4.6). To understand this concept, imagine yourself standing in the middle of a room: at any given point in time, you can only see the part of the room that is in front of you. To add information from what is behind you need to rotate or change your position in space in relation to rest of the room. In other words, despite the fact that the 3D structure of the room and its contents are available to be examined, only part of it can be visualized at any given point in time from any given fixed position.

Since the volume rendered 3D data set of the heart can be opened to display intracardiac structures by choosing a cutting plane and the image beyond this plane reconstructed as if the heart is cut by a surgeon, the word "view" (referred to heart's orientation to the body axis) will be no longer used, being replaced by the word "anatomical planes" or simply "planes" (referring to the heart itself) to describe orientation of the images.[3] The most frequently used planes in dissection are: (1) *the sagittal plane*, a vertical plane which divides the heart into right and left portions (Fig. 4.7); (2) the *coronal plane*, a vertical plane which divides the heart into anterior and posterior portions (Fig. 4.8); and (3) the *transverse plane*, an horizontal plane which runs parallel to the ground and divides the heart into superior and inferior portions (Fig. 4.9). The use of anatomic planes to display the cardiac

Fig. 4.5 Uncropped full-volume 3D data set acquired from the apical approach. Despite the fact that all cardiac structures are present within the pyramid of data, they cannot be viewed. This is similar to the impossibility to see the paintings and statues collected in a museum standing outside the main entrance

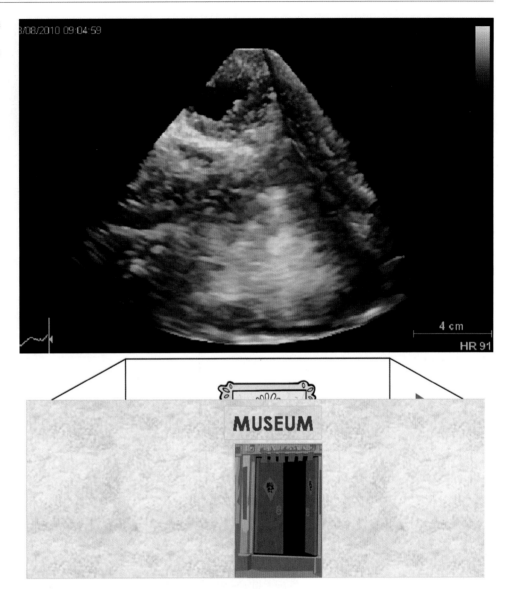

structures allows a parallelism between anatomic specimens and 3DE images and facilitates the communication with surgeons and anatomists.

The action of entering the museum/heart to visualize the cardiac structures is called cropping. Cropping the volumetric data set means to partially remove volumetric data in order to enter the data set and visualize the structure of interest. Usually there are two cropping modalities: the cropping box and the single arbitrary cropping plane (Fig. 4.10).

After cropping the 3D data set, in order to display a specific cardiac structure one should rotate it to reorient the data set until the desired structure is in front of you.

After having removed the undesired volumetric data, the adequate display of cardiac structures requires some thresholding. Thresholding allows the echocardiographer to determine how much of the volumetric data is part of the cardiac structure of interest, deemed noise or part of the cavity (Fig. 4.11). This is mainly controlled using the gain settings.

The last action to perform is to decide from which point of view you need/want to look at the desired structure, i.e. mitral valve can be viewed from the atrial side (i.e. the so-called "surgical view") or from the ventricular side (Fig. 4.3).

Once the cardiac structure of interest has been localized within the volumetric dataset, one can choose among different ways to display it on a 2D monitor. There are three broad classes of techniques for displaying 3D images: volume rendering, surface rendering, and 2D tomographic slices. The choice of the display technique is generally determined by the clinical application and it is under user's control.

Volume rendering is a technique used to display 3D images onto a 2D plane to closely resemble the true anatomy of the heart.[4] The techniques commonly used to obtain this display mode are reported in Chapter 2, but they essentially cast a

Fig. 4.6 Cropped full volume data set to show an equivalent of a 4-chamber view. Once entered into the museum/heart part of the content is visualized

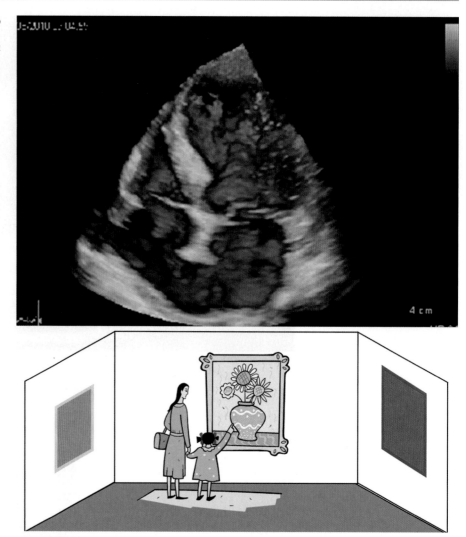

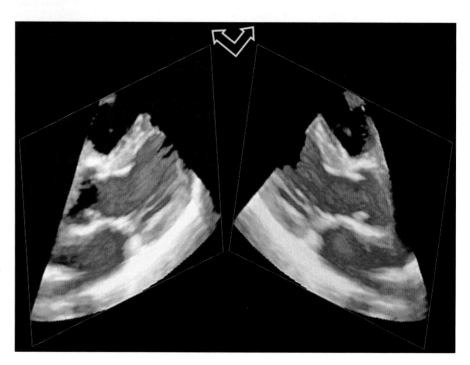

Fig. 4.7 The 3D data set of the heart can be dissected using anatomically sound section planes: a sagittal plane (long axis or longitudinal) is a vertical plane that divides an organ into right (video) and left (video) portions

Fig. 4.8 The coronal section plane (frontal) is a vertical plane (video) that divides an organ into anterior and posterior (video) portions

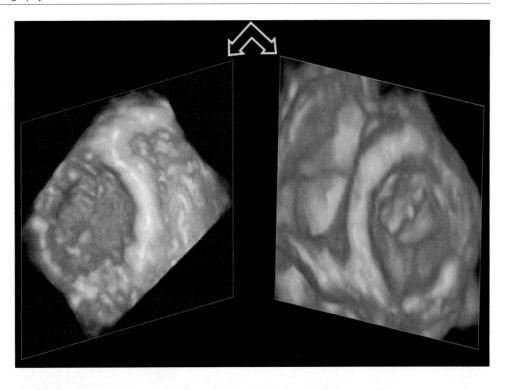

Fig. 4.9 A four-chamber view is the result of cutting the heart using a transverse plane which runs parallel to the ground and divides the organ into superior (video) and inferior (video) portions

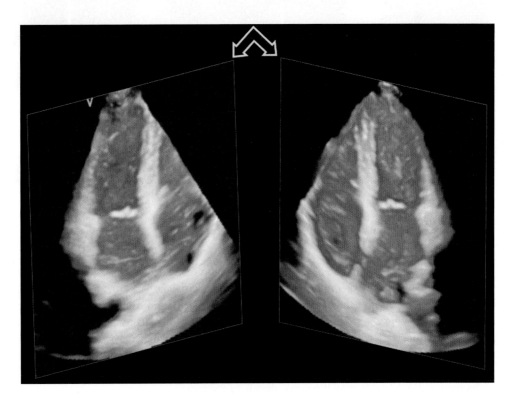

light beam through the collected voxels. Then, the voxels along each light beam are weighted to obtain a gradient of voxel values intensity that integrated with levels of opacification, shading and lighting allows a structure to appear either solid (e.g., tissue) or transparent (e.g., blood pool).[5,6] Finally, shading and/or depth encoded colorization techniques are usually used to generate a 3D display of the depths and textures of the cardiac structures (Fig. 4.12). This kind of display mode enables the assessment of the anatomy of cardiac structures and the complex spatial relationships among them.

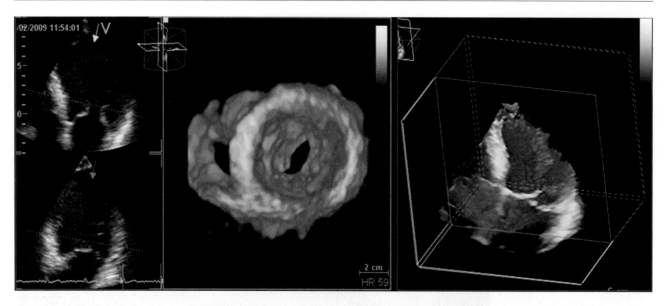

Fig. 4.10 Modalities used to crop the 3D data set: the single arbitrary cropping plane (*left panel*, video) is showed as a yellow dotted line on the 2D images; and the cropping box (*right panel*, video)

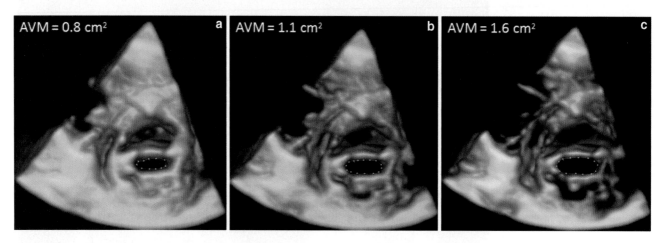

Fig. 4.11 Examples of how thresholding regulations affect the planimetry of the mitral valve orifice area in a patient with mitral stenosis. Low thresholding leads to valve area underestimation (*panel A*); optimal thresholding results (*panel B*); and low thresholding leads to valve area overestimation (*panel C*)

Surface rendering technique is based on visualization of the surfaces of structures or organs in a solid appearance (Fig. 4.13, panel A). Once the organ boundaries have been identified, shadowing algorithms can be used to create a 3D perspective.[7] Information of the tissue beneath the surface is missing. Wire frame is another way to display surface rendering in a cage-like picture (Fig. 4.13, panel B). This modes of displaying 3D data sets cannot provide details of the cardiac structure or texture of the cardiac tissue, but they are mainly used to visualize size, shape and function of cardiac chambers.

Finally, the last way to visualize the content of the data set is to slice it. Slicing is the tool that allows the echocardiographer to obtain several tomographic (i.e., 2D) views from the volumetric data set. A 2D display of a 3D data set can be obtained from any individually selected cut plane (anyplane analysis, usually used to select cutting planes aligned to the cardiac structures, which are difficult or impossible to obtain from conventional 2D imaging) (Fig. 4.14, panel A), from parallel, coronal or transverse cuts along a defined long axis (paraplane analysis) (Fig. 4.14, panel B), or from sagittal cuts with different angulations (omniplane analysis) (Fig. 4.14, panel C)

4.4 How to Handle the Present 3D Transducers Technology and the Impact of 3D on Lab Work Flow

Currently available 3D transducers are larger and heavier than conventional 2D ones, holding them all day long for routine scanning may injure sonographer's harm, joint and

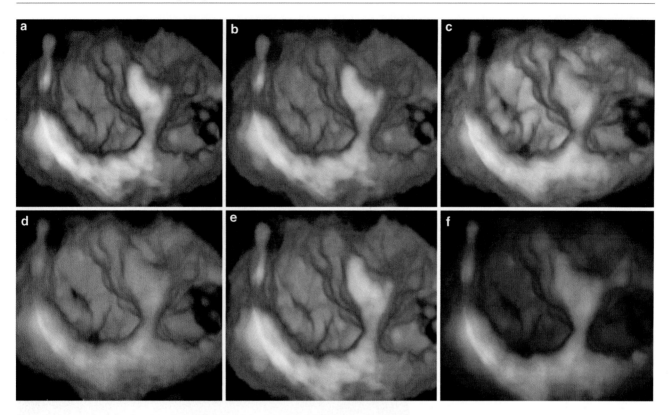

Fig. 4.12 Examples of volume rendering of the mitral valve using different depth-encoding colorizations: gray (*panel A*), bronze (*panel B*), stereo (*panel C*), bronze-gray (*panel D*), bronze-blue (*panel E*), and bronze-red (*panel F*)

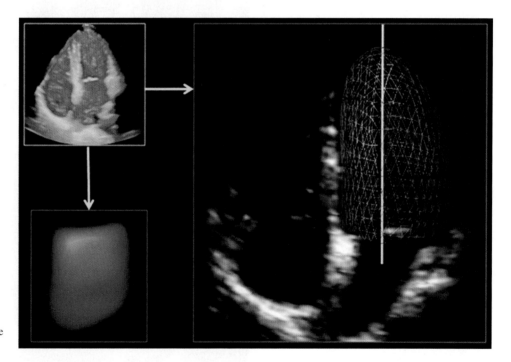

Fig. 4.13 Surface rendering of the left atrium (*left lower panel*) and the left ventricle (*Right panel*). The latter has been rendered in wire frame mode (see video)

muscles. In addition, they do not allow a 2D image quality comparable to that obtained with conventional 2D transducers, therefore it forces the echocardiographers who want to obtain 3D data sets to switch from one transducer to another in order to complete the echo study. This problem is even more exacerbated when only a limited number of echo systems in the lab have the 3D module and patients need to be moved from a scanning room to another to have the 3D acquisition. This increases the time spent for each 3D echo studie and affects the whole lab productivity.

Fig. 4.14 The 3D data set can be sliced to obtain 2D views: anyplane analysis, to obtain unique 2D visualization of cardiac structures which is difficult or impossible to obtain from conventional 2D imaging (*panel A*, video); paraplane analysis, parallel transverse cuts along a defined long axis (*panel B*, video); and omniplane analysis, multiple sagittal cuts with different angulations (*panel C*, video)

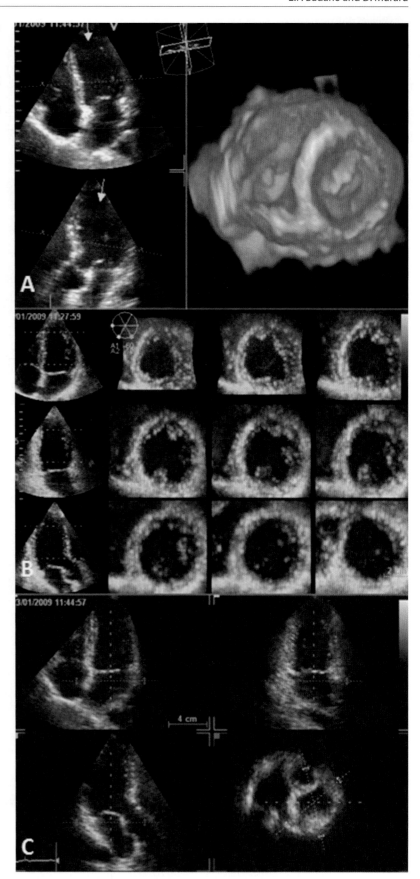

Table 4.2 Main indications to a 3D echocardiographic study in order to address suitable patients at the scanning room equipped with the 3D scanner and to limit the impact on the lab work flow

Pts with left ventricular dysfunction candidates at device implantation or complex surgical procedures
Pts with heart failure, or right heart diseases that may affect right ventricular size and function
Pts. who are candidates to mitral valve surgery
Pts. with mitral stenosis
Pts with bicuspid aortic valve who are candidates to surgery
Pts with congenital heart disease
Pts with unclear anatomy at 2D

Table 4.3 Recommended complete 3D echocardiographic acquisition protocol

From the parasternal window
Gated full-volume of the sagittal plane
Real-time zoom transversal planes of the mitral, aortic and tricuspid valves
Gated 3D color full volume of the mitral, aortic and tricuspid valves
Real-time modified parasternal transversal plane (color) of the pulmonary valve
From the apical window
Gated full-volume of the coronal plane of the left ventricle and left atrium
Gated full-volume of the coronal plane of the right ventricle and right atrium
Real-time zoom transversal planes of the mitral, aortic and tricuspid valves
Gated 3D color full volume of the mitral, aortic and tricuspid valves
From the subcostal window
Gated full-volume of the coronal plane of the right and left atrium
Gated 3D color full volume of the interatrial septum
From the suprasternal notch window
Gated full-volume of aortic arch and thoracic aorta
Gated 3D color full volume of aortic arch and thoracic aorta

Future technological improvements will provide smaller transducers capable of obtaining equally good quality 2D and 3D images as it has happened with the 3D transesophageal probe. However, at the moment we use 3D transducers to perform focused examinations by obtaining specific 3D data sets to address specific issues (i.e. anatomy of mitral valve prolapse or assessment of left or right ventricular function) at the end of a complete M-mode, 2D and Doppler study. To facilitate sonographer work, and to reduce the impact of 3D acquisitions on lab work flow we have set a specific procedure in the lab predefining which patient will benefit of a 3D study (Table 4.2).

Finally, the problem of costs of 3D technology should be viewed in perspective and not just as the cost of the probe and related software only. Technology cost should be balanced against the possibility to avoid preoperative transesophageal echocardiography to assess a sizable number of patients who are candidate to mitral valve surgery[8,9]; better selection of heart failure patients candidates to ICD and/or CRT implants, or ACE-inhibitor treatment[10]; monitoring of interventional procedures without the use of ionizing energies or costly intravascular catheters.[11] All these savings well justify the cost/effectiveness of 3D technology.

4.5 Acquisition Protocols and Imaging Views

Transthoracic 3D echocardiography full-volume acquisition mode is expected to accommodate the whole heart structures within a single 3D data set. However, with existing technology, the decrease in both spatio-temporal resolution and penetration that would result from enlarging the volume angle to acquire the whole heart from a single acoustic window makes it practically unfeasible. Therefore, to overcome such technological limitations, 3DE data sets should be acquired from multiple transthoracic acoustic windows.

In current clinical practice, two different acquisition protocols have been used: a focused examination and a complete one.[1,2]

A focused 3DE examination is usually represented by one or few anatomically oriented 3DE data sets acquired to complement an otherwise complete 2DE study. Some examples of focused 3DE examinations are: (1) the acquisition of a gated 3DE full-volume data set from the apical window in order to assess LV volumes, ejection fraction, shape and dyssynchrony in an heart failure patient; (2) two full-volume data sets from both parasternal and apical windows to visualize mitral apparatus and to quantitate residual orifice area in a patients with mitral stenosis; (3) a live 3DE zoom mode with as high a density as possible from the parasternal window to visualize the aortic valve in a patient with aortic valve disease.

A complete 3DE transthoracic examination requires multiple acquisitions from 4 acoustic windows: parasternal, apical, subcostal and suprasternal (Table 4.3). Finally, a suggested workflow about how to acquire a 3D data set is listed in Table 4.4.

Table 4.4 Suggested workflow for effective acquisition of 3D data sets

1. Identify the clinical question
2. Select the cardiovascular structure of interest
3. Position the probe to obtain the best resolution
4. Preposition the probe in 2D to the desired 3D view
5. Use real-time 3D first (higher resolution, preview of results)
6. Probe frequency as high as possible
7. Depth as minimal as possible

References

1. Hung J, Lang RM, Flackskampf F, Shernan SK, McCullogh M, Adams DB, et al. 3D echocardiography: a review of the current status and future directions. *J Am Soc Echocardiogr.* 2007; 20: 213–233.
2. Yang HS, Bansal RC, Mookadam F, Khanderia BK, Tajik J, Chandrasekaran K. Practical guide for three-dimensional transthoracic echocardiography using a fully sampled matrix array transducer. *J Am Soc Echocardiogr.* 2008;21:979–989.
3. Nanda NC, Kisslo J, Lang R, Pandian N, Marwick T, Shirali G, Kelly G. Examination protocol for three-dimensional echocardiography. *Echocardiography.* 2004;21:763–768.
4. Fenster A, Downey DB. Three-dimensional ultrasound imaging. *Annu Rev Biomed Eng.* 2000;2:457–475.
5. Rankin RN, Fenster A, Downey DB, Munk PL, Levin MF, Vellet AD. Three-dimensional sonographic reconstruction: techniques and diagnostic applications. *Am J Roentgenol.* 1992; 161:695–702.
6. Cao QL, Pandian NG, Azevedo J, et al. Enhanced comprehension of dynamic cardiovascular anatomy by three-dimensional echocardiography with the use of mixed shading techniques. *Echocardiography* 1994;11:627–633.
7. Pandian NG, Roelandt J, Nanda NC, Sugeng L, Cao QL, Azevedo J, Schwartz SL, Vannan MA, Ludomirski A, Marx G, Vogel M. Dynamic three-dimensional echocardiography: methods and clinical potential. *Echocardiography* 1994;11:237–259.
8. Pepi M, Tamborini G, Maltagliati A, Galli CA, Sisillo E, Salvi L, Naliato M, Porqueddu M, Parolari A, Zanobini M, Alamanni F. Head-to-head comparison of two- and three-dimensional transthoracic and transesophageal echocardiography in the localization of mitral valve prolapse. *J Am Coll Cardiol.* 2006;48: 2524–2530.
9. Gutiérrez-Chico JL, Zamorano Gómez JL, Rodrigo-López JL, Mataix L, Pérez de Isla L, Almería-Valera C, Aubele A, Macaya-Miguel C. Accuracy of real-time 3-dimensional echocardiography in the assessment of mitral prolapse. Is transesophageal echocardiography still mandatory? *Am Heart J.* 2008;154:694–698.
10. Hare JL, Jenkins C, Nakatani S, Ogawa A, Yu CM, Marwick TH. Feasibility and clinical decision-making with 3D echocardiography in routine practice. *Heart.* 2008;94(4):440–445.
11. Balzer J, van Hall S, Rassaf T, Böring YC, Franke A, Lang RM, Kelm M, Kühl HP. Feasibility, safety, and efficacy of real-time three-dimensional transesophageal echocardiography for guiding device closure of interatrial communications: initial clinical experience and impact on radiation exposure. *Eur J Echocardiogr.* 2009; 11:1–8.

Advanced Evaluation of LV Function with 3D Echocardiography

James N. Kirkpatrick, Victor Mor-Avi, and Roberto M. Lang

Two-dimensional echocardiography (2DE) revolutionized the assessment of left ventricular size and function. The inherent limitations of single plane imaging, however, have led investigators to develop 3D methods to image the left ventricle. Early techniques based on reconstruction of multiple, ECG-gated 2D acquisitions were extremely cumbersome but did improve the accuracy of calculations of ventricular volumes and ejection fraction and mass. In recent years, advances in ultrasound image acquisition, processing and analysis have brought real time 3D echocardiography (3DE) into the clinical realm. In addition to increased accuracy in the measurement of left ventricular volumes, ejection fraction and mass, 3DE has improved the analysis of wall motion, with applications for the detection of ischemic heart disease and dyssynchrony.

5.1 Left Ventricular Volumes and Ejection Fraction

Accurate, objective, quantitative and reproducible measures of left ventricular size and function are playing an increasingly crucial role in establishing prognosis and in guiding interventions for patients with structural heart disease. Though left ventricular dimensions and ejection fraction do not correlate well with symptoms, exercise capacity or myocardial oxygen consumption they do provide prognostic information in a variety of clinical scenarios. Cavity size, ejection fraction and spherical shape are powerful predictors of morbidity and mortality in both clinical trials and population studies. Prognosis after myocardial infarction, though influenced by a myriad of demographic and clinical factors, is most powerfully predicted by left ventricular size and ejection fraction. In early studies of acute myocardial infarction,

increased left ventricular volumes and ejection fraction <40% by cineangiography and radionuclide ventriculography predicted cardiovascular mortality and sudden death.[1] Echocardiographic left ventricular volumes and ejection fraction in patients with myocardial infarction are also powerful prognosticators for major adverse cardiac events. The size of myocardial infarction by echocardiography predicts cardiogenic shock (if >40% of the myocardium is involved), development of chronic heart failure, and mortality.[2] Both ACE-inhibitors/angiotensin receptor blockers and beta blockers are beneficial for patients with reduced left ventricular ejection fraction. Aldosterone antagonists reduce mortality in symptomatic patients hospitalized for heart failure with left ventricular ejection fraction ≤35%, and in post-myocardial infarction patients with LVEF<40%. Echocardiographic improvements in left ventricular volumes and ejection fraction are standard measures of therapeutic effect in many clinical trials. A reduction in left ventricular ejection fraction constitutes an indication to discontinue cardiotoxic medications such as anthracycline chemotherapeutic agents.

Multiple studies have established the benefit of prophylactic implantable cardioverter defibrillators for the primary prevention of sudden death in patients with severely reduced left ventricular ejection fraction.[3] Studies have demonstrated no benefit of implantable cardioverter defibrillator placement within 40 days post myocardial infarction,[4] and showed that a patient's left ventricular ejection fraction can rise above 30–35% cutoff after a month of appropriate medical therapy. Cardiac resynchronization therapy devices have traditionally been reserved for patients with severely reduced left ventricular ejection fraction. Clinical (and reimbursement) decisions about implantable cardioverter defibrillator and cardiac resynchronization therapy device placement have, until relatively recently, relied on accurate and reproducible measures of left ventricular ejection fraction. Furthermore, echocardiographic improvements in left ventricular ejection fraction and reduction of end systolic volumes serve as the main imaging marker of response to cardiac resynchronization therapy in research trials and clinical practice.

Despite the importance of these clinical indices, traditional echocardiographic methods used to assess left ventricular volumes and ejection fraction are inherently flawed.

R.M. Lang (✉)
Professor of Medicine, Section of Cardiology Director, Noninvasive Cardiac Imaging, University of Chicago
e-mail: rlang@medicine.bsd.uchicago.edu

L.P. Badano et al. (eds.), *Textbook of Real-Time Three Dimensional Echocardiography*,
DOI: 10.1007/978-1-84996-495-1_5, © Springer-Verlag London Limited 2011

Left ventricular size is extrapolated from single-plane mea-surements of end diastolic diameters performed at the base of the ventricle. The influence of atypically-shaped regions of the ventricle (such as apical aneurysms) is ignored by this method. Left ventricular ejection fraction is most often deter-mined by visual estimation, which is dependent on experi-ence and is highly sensitive to intra- and inter-observer variability. Several objective methods for left ventricular ejection fraction estimation from 2D data exist. The 2005 chamber quantification guidelines from the American Society of Echocardiography and European Association of Echo-cardiography advocate the biplane method of discs for volu-metric and ejection fraction quantification.[5] When the endocardium is not well defined, the area-length method pro-vides an acceptable alternative. Both methods, however, rely heavily on geometric models which are inaccurate in patients with hearts that depart from the idealized, bullet-shaped left ventricular morphology. Furthermore, 2D methods are easily compromised by foreshortening from plane positioning errors, leading to volume underestimation. Not surprisingly, 2D quantification of left ventricular volumes and ejection fraction lacks accuracy compared with the gold standards of magnetic resonance imaging (MRI) or radionuclide ventric-ulography for quantification,[6] and is associated with rela-tively poor inter and intraobserver variability.

3DE overcomes many of these limitations. Studies have established that 3DE is more accurate than 2DE compared to the reference standards of radionuclide ventriculography and MRI.[7,8] 3DE measurements are more reproducible than 2DE[9] and perhaps even as reproducible as MRI.[10] This methodology has proven reproducible, accurate and quantifiable in a wide range of cardiac phenotypes, including normal hearts,[11] isch-emic and non-ischemic cardiomyopathy,[12] and congenital heart disease.[13] Sugeng et al. demonstrated 3-D imaging to be superior to cardiac computed tomography in the assessment of left ventricular ejection fraction and volumes.[14] In a separate study comparing 3DE and single photon emission computed tomography in the measurement of left ventricular volumes (using MRI as the reference), 3DE was more accurate and reproducible in patients post myocardial infarction.[15] A recent study in patients post myocardial infarction demonstrated that serial 3DE measurements had low variability between initial and follow up scans, suggesting that subtle changes in LV vol-umes over time could be reliably identified by 3DE.[16] Mannaerts et al. developed a 3DE sphericity index that accu-rately predicted left ventricular remodeling post myocardial infarction patients.[17] Application of new endocardial border detection techniques to 3D images may allow direct calcula-tion of left ventricular volumes and ejection fraction, leading to improved reproducibility.[18]

These studies of RT3DE use two main techniques for measuring left ventricular volumes (Fig. 5.1). Although both have demonstrated improved accuracy over 2D techniques,

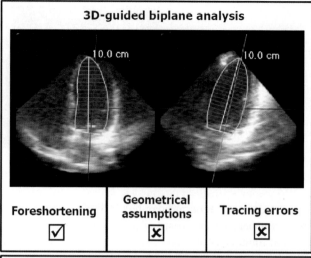

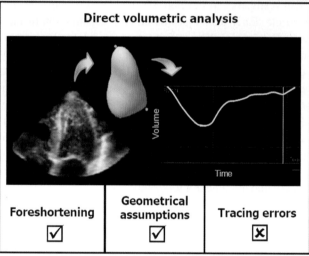

Fig. 5.1 Methods for left ventricular volume quantification using 3DE datasets. Conventional 2D volume calculations use potentially fore-shortened apical views and rely on geometric modeling of the ventricle. Chamber volumes can be measured from 3DE datasets either by guided biplane or direct volume analysis. The 3D-guided biplane technique is based on geometric modeling, but solves the problem of foreshortening (*top*). Direct volumetric analysis involves endocardial surface detection and calculation of left ventricular volumes from this surface and does not rely on geometric modeling, but does depend on accurate endocar-dial definition and is thus subject to tracing errors (*bottom*)

the limitations of each should be kept in mind. The first method involves selecting 2D imaging planes from 3DE datasets, then measuring volumes by use of the biplane method of discs, as in traditional 2D volume calculation. This 3D guided biplane approach avoids foreshortening but still relies on geometric assumptions. The second method uses the 3D dataset to make a cast of the endocardium, from which direct cavity volumes can be measured. This tech-nique can involve automated or semi-automated tracking of the endocardium over time to yield dynamic volumes throughout the cardiac cycle. While this endocardial recon-struction method does not involve geometric assumptions and is theoretically more accurate in abnormally-shaped ventricles, it is highly dependent on the definition of the endocardial-cavity border. Thus, in patients with poor acoustic windows and poor border definition, accuracy may be significantly reduced (Fig. 5.2).

A new 3DE technique for measurement of left ventricular volumes involves 3D speckle tracking. Although 2D speckle tracking has been used to describe myocardial strain[19] and rotational motion (twist/untwist) patterns,[20] it has also been used to quantify left ventricular volumes.[21] However, 2D speckle tracking left ventricular volume calculation is subject to geometric assumptions and foreshortening. In addition, speckles can move outside the plane of analysis during translational motion, leading to drop out. New software using 3DE datasets can now track speckle movement in three dimensions (Fig. 5.3), allowing measurement of true 3D tissue velocity, strain, strain rate, torsion, and endocardial-

blood interface. A study by Nesser et al. demonstrated the advantage of 3D speckle tracking calculation of left ventricular volumes over 2D speckle tracking, using MRI as the gold standard.[22] Similar to both 3D guided biplane and 3D endocardial reconstruction, the 3D speckle tracking measurements demonstrated better correlations, smaller biases and more narrow limits of agreement, as well as lower inter and intra-observer variability.

5.2 Left Ventricular Mass

Left ventricular mass is an important prognostic marker independent of the presence of coronary artery disease and ejection fraction[23] and appears to be an especially important prognostic marker in patients with hypertension.[24] Accurate measurement

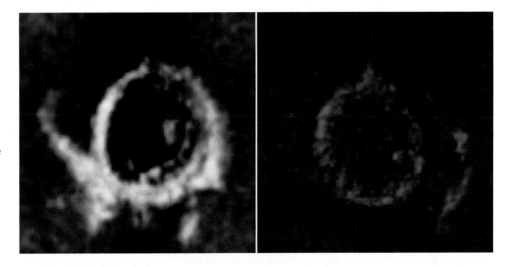

Fig. 5.2 Spatial resolution as a main source of error in 3DE endocardial tracing. Example of short-axis cut-planes extracted from 3DE datasets: while in one patient (*left*), trabeculae can be well visualized and clearly differentiated from the myocardium, in another patient (*right*), the spatial resolution of the 3DE image is not sufficient to provide this kind of detail

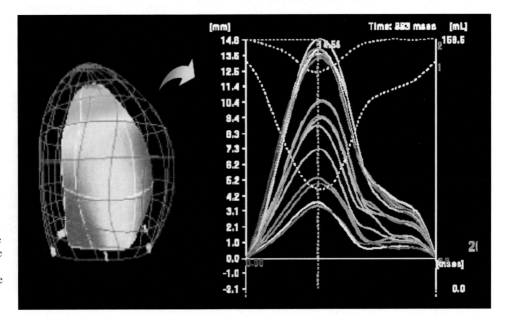

Fig. 5.3 Speckle tracking analysis of 3DE datasets. Displacement of speckles can be tracked throughout the cardiac cycle: end diastole shown as blue wire-frame and end systole as the smaller, color-coded cast (*left*). Curves of displacement over time are generated for each myocardial segment (*right*)

of left ventricular mass may facilitate its use as a surrogate outcome marker in trials of antihypertensive medications.

However, left ventricular mass assessment by 2DE is subject to the same limitations in reproducibility and accuracy affecting left ventricular dimensions and ejection fraction calculations. While the currently recommended method of left ventricular mass calculation, the cubed formula (most commonly applied to 2D-targeted M-mode images), has been validated against post-mortem pathology findings, it relies on the geometric assumption that the left ventricular is a prolated ellipsoid.[5] This assumption is inaccurate in both remodeled and non-symmetrically contracting ventricles. The two other 2D-based methods (the truncated ellipsoid and the area-length formula) also rely on geometric assumptions and are subject to errors due to foreshortening, though they may be less invalid for distorted ventricles with regional wall motion abnormalities.

Several studies using off-line analysis of reconstructed 3D echocardiographic images demonstrated improved accuracy for left ventricular mass calculation compared with 2D techniques. Inter-observer variability is reduced. Mor-Avi et al. demonstrated that, as with volumetric measurements, left ventricular mass by 3DE had greater accuracy and better reproducibility than 2D techniques, compared with the gold standard of MRI.[25] 3DE bias was minimal (3%). The results of this early study were confirmed in a large number of patients with concentric LV hypertrophy,[26] in patients with wall motion abnormalities[10] and in others with congenital heart disease.[27] A recent study compared two methods for left ventricular mass measurement by 3DE. One technique identifies non-foreshortened 2D images planes from 3DE datasets and uses them to calculate left ventricular mass (3DE-guided biplane measurement). The other one involves the semiautomatic identification of endocardial and epicardial surfaces at end diastole from the 3D dataset, calculates the volume between them and converts it into mass. The two techniques correlated well with each other and better with MRI than standard 2D methods.[28]

5.3 Left Ventricular Wall Motion

Diagnosis of regional wall motion abnormalities is an important component of transthoracic echocardiography. Wall motion at rest and during stress echocardiography is an important marker for epicardial coronary artery disease, microvascular disease, myocarditis, stress-induced cardiomyopathy, toxic cardiomyopathy, pericardial disease and cardiac involvement by sarcoidosis. Wall motion analysis by echocardiography has become the central component of defining mechanical dyssynchrony potentially amendable to cardiac resynchronization therapy in patients with heart failure. While not all patients with a wide QRS (>120 ms) and symptom criteria (NYHA class III and IV heart failure) will respond to cardiac resynchronization therapy, a subgroup of patients who lack these criteria do benefit from cardiac resynchronization therapy.[29]

Wall motion analysis requires the visual integration of regional endocardial motion and wall thickening. It is complicated by a number of factors, including inadequate endocardial definition, foreshortening, translational motion, ventricular pacing, post-sternotomy septal dyssynchrony, plane-positioning and compression from extra-cardiac structures (such as diaphragmatic impingement on the inferior surface of the heart). Furthermore, the time required to acquire multiple views with a single-plane transducer becomes problematic when trying to capture wall motion at peak stress in exercise testing. By the time the heart has been adequately imaged, as many as 13–40% of wall motion abnormalities present at peak stress may have resolved.[30] This drawback reduces either diagnostic sensitivity or specificity or both. As in the visual assessment of left ventricular ejection fraction, the reproducibility of visual wall motion assessment is inherently limited by subjectivity and reader experience.

The use of transthoracic 3DE datasets overcomes many of these limitations. The contraction of the entire left ventricle can be captured in true real-time. By cropping the 3D dataset, one can obtain all 2D views. 3DE analysis software allows quantification of regional wall motion (Fig. 5.4),

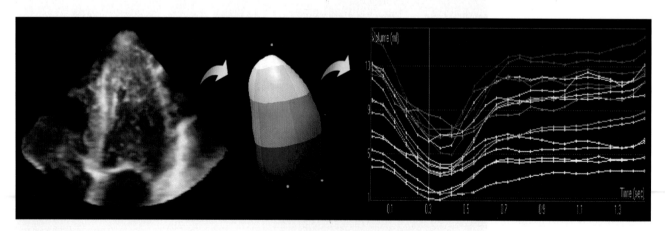

Fig. 5.4 3DE analysis of regional LV wall motion. 3DE datasets (*left*) can be used to detect 3D endocardial surface that can be segmented using standard segmentation (*middle*) and used to calculate regional left ventricular volumes over the course of a cardiac cycle (*right*)

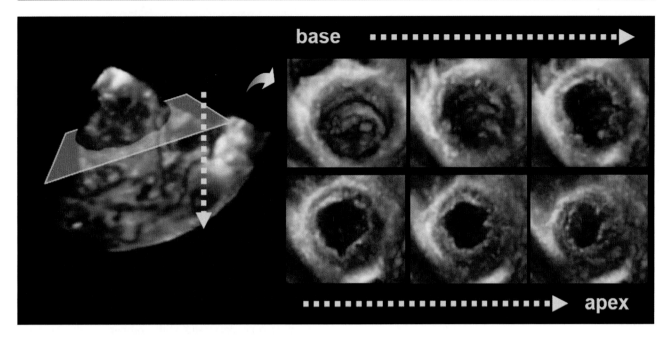

Fig. 5.5 3D stress echocardiography. Navigating through a 3DE dataset allows selecting arbitrary 2D slices for viewing. For example, moving the view plane from base to apex (*left*) provides short axis views at different levels of the left ventricle (*right panels*), thus allowing simultaneous assessment of all segments

reducing inter-measurement variability. A recent study validated 3DE regional ejection fraction against MRI, with sensitivity of 85% and specificity of 81%.[31] Studies comparing wall motion assessment during stress testing using 3DE techniques with standard 2D wall motion methods have shown high levels of agreement and similar accuracy compared to scintigraphic myocardial perfusion imaging.[32] Importantly, with 3DE, complete data for wall motion assessment (Fig. 5.5) can be collected in less time after peak stress.[33]

Although the majority of studies investigating echocardiographic assessment of mechanical dyssynchrony have used Doppler or speckle tracking techniques, 3DE has several theoretical advantages and has shown promise in recent studies. 3DE can quickly capture the dynamics of the entire ventricle, while simultaneously assessing regional wall motion. The index of systolic dyssynchrony used in most 3DE dyssynchrony studies has been the standard deviation of the interval between the R wave and minimum systolic left ventricular volume in different left ventricular segments (regional ejection time). To date, there is fair to poor correlation with tissue Doppler imaging techniques, probably due to the fact that these two techniques measure different parameters (timing of longitudinal velocity only for tissue Doppler vs. timing of combined endocardial motion in longitudinal, radial and circumferential directions for 3DE).

Studies have demonstrated the ability of 3DE to predict acute response in patients with cardiac resynchronization therapy devices. A study by Kapetenakis et al. used regional ejection times to calculate a systolic dyssynchrony index and found it to be predictive of response to cardiac resynchronization therapy in patients with low left ventricular ejection fraction and heart failure symptoms but narrow QRS.[34] In a separate trial of 56 patients, a cut off value of 5.6% for the systolic dyssynchrony index demonstrated an 88% sensitivity and 86% specificity to predict improvement in left ventricular end systolic volume.[35] 3DE has been used to identify the latest contracting segments to guide placement of the left ventricular pacing catheter through the coronary sinus at the time of implant.[36]

5.4 Uses of Contrast with Real-Time 3D Echocardiography

5.4.1 Chamber Opacification

Poor 2D echocardiographic windows prevent adequate detection of endocardial borders in 15–30% of patients. Multiple factors contribute to this difficulty, including concurrent lung disease, obesity and recent thoracic or abdominal surgery.[37] In these settings, the use of echocardiographic contrast for left ventricular opacification has become standard practice. Mechanical reverberation of contrast microbubbles by the ultrasonic beam enhances visualization of the blood pool itself, thereby improving the definition of the blood-tissue interface. This improved definition results in improved assessment of regional and global myocardial function, translating into more accurate quantification of left ventricular size and overall systolic contractile function. Application of contrast techniques increases the ability to obtain clinically significant information in up to 94% of patients.[37]

Nevertheless, 2D imaging with contrast is still limited, particularly by foreshortening. The use of contrast with 3DE has become a clinical reality in recent years. In addition to requirements for cumbersome off-line reconstruction in the past, 3DE with contrast has to overcome the problem of increased microbubble destruction from the increased ultrasound energy transmitted into the entire ventricle, rather than a thin slide (as in 2D imaging). Both low mechanical index imaging and selected triggering to image only at end systole and end diastole have been used with success. Alternative contrast imaging modes, such as pulse inversion and power modulation, may also be useful.

A number of studies have validated 3DE contrast techniques. Left ventricular triplane imaging with contrast enhancement was found to be accurate and reproducible compared with MRI imaging for left ventricular ejection fraction. Feasibility of interpreting contrast images was 100%, and underestimation of left ventricular volumes reduced with contrast, with improvement in intra- and interobserver variability.[38] Assessment of resting regional wall motion is also substantially improved with the addition of contrast enhancement to 3DE compared to MRI, particularly in patients with inadequate endocardial definition.

3DE with contrast was recently used in dobutamine stress testing. Pulerwitz et al. [39] found that contrast enhancement significantly increased the proportion of adequately visualized segments at both rest and peak stress stages (91–98% and 87–99%, respectively) with improved agreement between observers over non-contrast images (96.9% vs. 84.4% at rest and 98.2% vs. 79.9% at peak stress). Time of acquisition both with and without contrast was <90 seconds.[39] Nevertheless, Takeuchi et al. (40), demonstrated in a larger patient sample with known or suspected coronary artery disease that a substantially greater number of segments could not be assessed at both baseline and peak stress with contrast-enhanced 3D imaging versus contrast-enhanced 2D imaging (out of 1278 segments, 88 (7%) at baseline and 39 (3%) at peak stress for 3D vs. 1 (<1%) and 5 (<1%) for 2D). Concordance rate of positive or negative findings per patient was 69%. The anterior and lateral walls, in particular, were less adequately visualized with 3D imaging.[40] A very recent study compared contrast-enhanced 3DE with coronary angiography and found a sensitivity of 61% and specificity of 88% for the detection of significant coronary artery disease.[41]

5.5 Myocardial Perfusion

In addition to improving wall motion assessment, echocardiographic contrast agents can be used to evaluate microcirculatory perfusion. The degree of contrast enhancement increases in proportion to the extent of blood flow. Failure to enhance signifies destruction of the coronary microcirculation. Of note, enhancement can occur in the setting of reduced perfusion, signaling viability with preserved microvascular integrity.

Although 2D contrast perfusion allows visual assessment of perfusion defects and even quantification of defect size, actual quantification of tissue blood flow requires repeated bolus injections of contrast for each imaging plane. 3DE allows imaging of the entire ventricle during a single contrast injection. Toledo et al.[42] investigated 3DE based volumetric analysis of myocardial contrast flow in rabbits, pigs and normal volunteers using interruptions in continuous infusion of contrast and video-intensity detection software. Peak contrast inflow rate decreased with coronary occlusions and increased with adenosine infusion in humans.[42] A separate study compared contrast-enhanced 2D and 3DE low mechanical index perfusion imaging during dobutamine stress testing. Perfusion could be assessed in 98% of 2D and 95.2% of 3D segments with good agreement between the two techniques.[43] An initial investigation using custom software to semi-quantify myocardial perfusion from contrast-enhanced 3DE datasets suggested that automated assessment of 3D perfusion is feasible.[44] Larger studies investigating the use of contrast-enhanced 3DE stress testing to detect angiographically-proven coronary stenoses and predict cardiovascular outcomes are pending and may improve the moderate sensitivity of 3D wall motion analysis alone in detecting angiographically significant coronary artery disease.

5.6 Limitations of 3DE Evaluation of the Left Ventricle

Current 3D echocardiographic images are acquired at a lower frame rate than most 2D imaging, resulting in reduced image quality. 3DE transducers are large and often do not fit well into intercostal spaces. Four-beat full volume 3D data sets involve the "stitching" together of data from multiple cardiac cycles and are thus prone to motion artifacts, sometimes severely compromising anatomic quality and impeding volume and mass calculations. Both acquisition and interpretation of 3D images requires significant training and expertise.

Notwithstanding high correlation with the MRI reference values and generally excellent reproducibility, studies have reported that left ventricular volumes by 3DE were significantly underestimated.[14] The amount of underestimation in single center studies varied from a few milliliters to 30% of the measurements. A multicenter study investigating the sources of this error found that the spatial resolution of 3DE is not high enough to differentiate between myocardium and endocardial trabeculae which are more frequently than not incorporated into the myocardial wall (Fig. 5.2), leading to an underestimation of cavity size.[45] This study underscored the need for unified standards in performing 3DE volumetric analysis. Inadequate spatial resolution is an even larger problem in the assessment of left ventricular mass, since mass measurements require identification of both the endocardial and the epicardial borders.

The ability to visualize all wall segments simultaneously during stress may improve the sensitivity and specificity for detection of wall motion abnormalities at high workloads. At present, however, the relatively low frame rate and the size of the transducer footprint often prevent adequate endocardial definition, especially during tachycardia. Furthermore, translational motion, arrhythmias and respiration introduce artifacts into full-volume datasets, thus complicating wall motion assessment, even with the addition of contrast. 3D border tracking of regional endocardial motion has shown promise in characterizing LV dyssynchrony but is also limited by low frame rate.

5.7 Future Developments

Advances in transducer and processing technology have already made single-beat full volume acquisition available for clinical use. This development shortens the time required to produce a 3DE dataset and eliminates stitching artifacts. Future developments in transducer technology will result in reduced footprint size and improvements in both spatial and temporal resolution. Newer 3D transducers will combine 2D and 3D capabilities with comparable image quality, similar to the recently-developed 3D transesophageal probe. These multitasking transducers will shorten the time required to acquire a full 2D and 3D study.

These advances will enable 3DE to become an integral part of standard echocardiographic examinations, providing enhanced reproducibly and accuracy in quantification of ventricular size, morphology and function. Increased frame rates for 3DE speckle tracking will result in improved measures of ventricular volumes, strain, strain rate, and torsion. 3DE speckle tracking will also overcome the major limitation of 2D speckle tracking wherein speckles move out of the imaging plane. Improvements in quantification will, in turn, provide a better basis for determining candidacy for heart failure medications and implantable cardioverter defibrillator and cardiac resynchronization therapy devices, and will improve the ability to detect response to these interventions. Patients receiving cardiotoxic chemotherapy will benefit from better accuracy in detecting subtle decrements in left ventricular ejection fraction which may indicate the need to stop treatments. Future software developments will make analysis of RT3DE datasets increasingly automated, available and user-friendly, and will allow fusion of RT3DE data with CMR, computed tomography (figure 6), and electrophysiological mapping data. Such fusion of 3DE datasets with data from other imaging modalities will significantly advance the integration of anatomic and physiological information to improve the understanding of cardiac structure and function in both normal and pathologic states. In particular, fusion of 3DE automated wall motion analysis with computerized tomographic venography will enable the positioning of the LV lead into the proper coronary veins during biventricular pacemaker implantation.

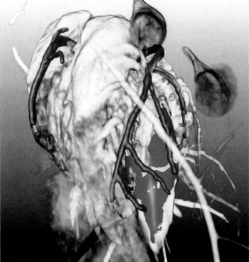 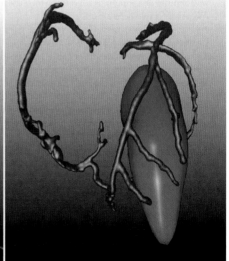

Fig. 5.6 Fusion of multimodality images. An endocardial cast of the left ventricle obtained from a 3DE dataset (*purple*) is merged with a computed tomographic image, wherein coronary arteries are displayed in red (*left*). After removing irrelevant structures, the resultant composite image of the left ventricular cavity and the coronary arteries can provide clinically valuable information, such as stenosis in a specific coronary artery as an underlying cause of a wall motion abnormality

5.8 Disclosure

There are no potential conflicts of interest relevant to this chapter.

References

1. Multicenter Postinfarction Research Group. Risk stratification and survival after myocardial infarction. *N Engl J Med.* 1983;309: 331–336.
2. Burns RJ, Gibbons RJ, Yi Q, Roberts RS, Miller TD, Schaer GL, Anderson JL, Yusuf S; CORE Study Investigators. CORE Study Investigators. The relationship of left ventricular ejection fraction, end-systolic volume index and infarct size to six-month mortality after hospital discharge following myocardial infarction treated by thrombolysis. *J Am Coll Cardiol* 2002;39:30–36.
3. Bardy GH, Lee KL, Mark DB, Poole JE, Packer DL, Boineau R, Domanski M, Troutman C, Anderson J, Johnson G, McNulty SE, Clapp-Channing N, Davidson-Ray LD, Fraulo ES, Fishbein DP, Luceri RM, Ip JH; Sudden Cardiac Death in Heart Failure Trial (SCD-HeFT) Investigators. Amiodarone or an implantable cardioverter-defibrillator for congestive heart failure. *N Engl J Med* 2005;352:225–237.
4. Hohnloser SH, Kuck KH, Dorian P, Roberts RS, Hampton JR, Hatala R, Fain E, Gent M, Connolly SJ; DINAMIT Investigators. Prophylactic use of an implantable cardioverter-defibrillator after myocardial infarction. *N Engl J Med.* 2004;351(24):2481–2488.
5. Lang RM, Bierig M, Devereux RB, Flachskampf FA, Foster E, Pellikka PA, Picard MH, Roman MJ, Seward J, Shanewise JS, Solomon SD, Spencer KT, Sutton MS, Stewart WJ; Chamber Quantification Writing Group; American Society of Echocardiography's Guidelines and Standards Committee; European Association of Echocardiography. Recommendations for chamber quantification. *J Am Soc Echocardiogr.* 2005;18:1440–1463.
6. Bellenger NG, Burgess MI, Ray SG, Lahiri A, Coats AJ, Cleland JG, Pennell DJ. Comparison of left ventricular ejection fraction and volumes in heart failure by echocardiography, radionuclide ventriculography and cardiovascular magnetic resonance. Are they interchangeable? *Eur Heart J.* 2000;21(16):1387–1396.
7. Arai K, Hozumi T, Matsumura Y, Sugioka K, Takemoto Y, Yamagishi H, Yoshiyama M, Kasanuki H, Yoshikawa J. Accuracy of measurement of left ventricular volume and ejection fraction by new real-time three-dimensional echocardiography in patients with wall motion abnormalities secondary to myocardial infarction. *Am J Cardiol.* 2004;94:552–558.
8. Nikitin NP, Constantin C, Loh PH, Ghosh J, Lukaschuk EI, Bennett A, Hurren S, Alamgir F, Clark AL, Cleland JG. New generation 3-dimensional echocardiography for left ventricular volumetric and functional measurements: comparison with cardiac magnetic resonance. *Eur J Echocardiogr.* 2006;7:365–372.
9. Jenkins C, Bricknell K, Hanekom L, Marwick TH. Reproducibility and accuracy of echocardiographic measurements of left ventricular parameters using real-time three dimensional echocardiography. *J Am Coll Cardiol.* 2004;44:878–886.
10. Pouleur AC, le Polain de Waroux JB, Pasquet A, Gerber BL, Gerard O, Allain P, Vanoverschelde JL. Assessment of left ventricular mass and volumes by three dimensional echocardiography in patients with or without wall motion abnormalities: comparison against cine magnetic resonance imaging. *Heart.* 2008;94(8):1050–1057.
11. Gopal AS, Keller AM, Rigling R, King DL Jr., King DL. Left ventricular volume and endocardial surface area by three-dimensional echocardiography: comparison with two-dimensional echocardiography and nuclear magnetic resonance imaging in normal subjects. *J Am Coll Cardiol.* 1993;22:258–270.
12. Shiota T, McCarthy PM, White RD, Qin JX, Greenberg NL, Flamm SD, Wong J, Thomas JD. Initial clinical experience of real-time three dimensional echocardiography in patients with ischemic and idiopathic dilated cardiomyopathy. *Am J Cardiol.* 1999;84:1068–1073.
13. van den Bosch AE, Robbers-Visser D, Krenning BJ, Voormolen MM, McGhie JS, Helbing WA, Roos-Hesselink JW, Simoons ML, Meijboom FJ. Real-time transthoracic three-dimensional echocardiographic assessment of left ventricular volume and ejection fraction in congenital heart disease. *J Am Soc Echocardiogr.* 2006;19:1–6.
14. Sugeng L, Mor-Avi V, Weinert L, Niel J, Ebner C, Steringer-Mascherbauer R, Schmidt F, Galuschky C, Schummers G, Lang RM, Nesser HJ. Quantitative assessment of left ventricular size and function: side-by-side comparison of real-time three-dimensional echocardiography and computed tomography with magnetic resonance reference. *Circulation.* 2006;114(7):654–661.
15. Chan J, Jenkins C, Khafagi F, Du L, Marwick TH. What is the optimal clinical technique for measurement of left ventricular volume after myocardial infarction? A comparative study of 3-dimensional echocardiography, single photon emission computed tomography, and cardiac magnetic resonance imaging. *J Am Soc Echocardiogr.* 2006;19:192–201.
16. Jenkins C, Bricknell K, Chan J, Hanekom L, Marwick TH. Comparison of two- and three dimensional echocardiography with sequential magnetic resonance imaging for evaluating left ventricular volume and ejection fraction over time in patients with healed myocardial infarction. *Am J Cardiol.* 2007;99:300–306.
17. Mannaerts HF, van der Heide JA, Kamp O, Stoel MG, Twisk J, Visser CA. Early identification of left ventricular remodelling after myocardial infarction, assessed by transthoracic 3D echocardiography. *Eur Heart J.* 2004;25:680–687.
18. Corsi C, Lang RM, Veronesi F, Weinert L, Caiani EG, MacEneaney P, Lamberti C, Mor-Avi V. Volumetric quantification of global and regional left ventricular function from real-time three-dimensional echocardiographic images. *Circulation.* 2005;112(8):1161–1170.
19. Amundsen BH, Helle-Valle T, Edvardsen T, Torp H, Crosby J, Lyseggen E, Stoylen A, Ihlen H, Lima JA, Smiseth OA, Slordahl SA. Noninvasive myocardial strain measurement by speckle tracking echocardiography: validation against sonomicrometry and tagged magnetic resonance imaging. *J Am Coll Cardiol.* 2006; 47:789–793.
20. Helle-Valle T, Crosby J, Edvardsen T, Lyseggen E, Amundsen BH, Smith HJ, Rosen BD, Lima JA, Torp H, Ihlen H, Smiseth OA. New noninvasive method for assessment of left ventricular rotation: speckle tracking echocardiography. *Circulation.* 2005;112:3149–3156.
21. Nishikage T, Nakai H, Mor-Avi V, Lang RM, Salgo IS, Settlemier SH, Husson S, Takeuchi M. Quantitative assessment of left ventricular volume and ejection fraction using two-dimensional speckle tracking echocardiography. *Eur J Echocardiogr.* 2009;10(1): 82–88.
22. Nesser HJ, Mor-Avi V, Gorissen W, Weinert L, Steringer-Mascherbauer R, Niel J, Sugeng L, Lang RM. Quantification of left ventricular volumes using three-dimensional echocardiographic speckle tracking: comparison with MRI. *Eur Heart J.* 2009;30(13): 1565–1573.
23. Quiñones MA, Greenberg BH, Kopelen HA, Koilpillai C, Limacher MC, Shindler DM, Shelton BJ, Weiner DH, for the SOLVD investigators. Echocardiographic predictors of clinical outcomes in patients with left ventricular dysfunction enrolled in the SOLVD registry and trials: significance of left ventricular hypertrophy. *J Am Coll Cardiol.* 2005;35(5):1237–1244.
24. Ghali JK, Liao Y, Simmons B, Castaner A, Cao G, Cooper RS. The prognostic role of LV mass measurements. LV hypertrophy in patients with or without coronary artery disease. *Ann Intern Med* 1992;117:831–836.
25. Mor-Avi V, Sugeng L, Weinert L, MacEneaney P, Caiani EG, Koch R, Salgo IS, Lang RM. Fast measurement of left ventricular mass with real-time three-dimensional echocardiography: comparison with magnetic resonance imaging. *Circulation.* 2004;110(13):1814–1818.

26. Yap SC, van Geuns RJ, Nemes A, Meijboom FJ, McGhie JS, Geleijnse ML, Simoons ML, Roos-Hesselink JW. Rapid and accurate measurement of LV mass by biplane real-time 3D echocardiography in patients with concentric LV hypertrophy: Comparison to CMR. *Eur J Echocardiogr.* 2008;9(2):255–260.

27. van den Bosch AE, Robbers-Visser D, Krenning BJ, McGhie JS, Helbing WA, Meijboom FJ, Roos-Hesselink JW. Comparison of real-time three-dimensional echocardiography to magnetic resonance imaging for assessment of left ventricular mass. *Am J Cardiol.* 2006;97:113–117.

28. Takeuchi M, Nishikage T, Mor-Avi V, Sugeng L, Weinert L, Nakai H, Salgo IS, Gerard O, Lang RM. Measurement of left ventricular mass by real-time three-dimentional echocardiography: validation against magnetic resonance and comparison with two-dimensional and m-mode measurements. *J Am Soc Echcardiogr.* 2008;21 (9): 1001–1005.

29. Achilli A, Sassara M, Ficili S, Pontillo D, Achilli P, Alessi C, De Spirito S, Guerra R, Patruno N, Serra F. Long-term effectiveness of cardiac resynchronization therapy in patients with refractory heart failure and "narrow" QRS. *J Am Coll Cardiol.* 2003;42(12): 2117–2124.

30. Hecht HS, DeBord L, Sotomayor N, Shaw R, Dunlap R, Ryan C. Supine bicycle stress echocardiography: peak exercise imaging is superior to postexercise imaging. *J Am Soc Echocardiogr.* 1993; 6:265–271.

31. Nesser HJ, Sugeng L, Corsi C, Weinert L, Niel J, Ebner C, Steringer-Mascherbauer R, Schmidt F, Schummers G, Lang RM, Mor-Avi V. Volumetric analysis of regional left ventricular function with real-time three-dimensional echocardiography: validation by magnetic resonance and clinical utility testing. *Heart.* 2007;93:572–578.

32. Yang HS, Pellikka PA, McCully RB, Oh JK, Kukuzke JA, Khandheria BK, Chandrasekaran K. Role of biplane and biplane echocardiographically guided 3-dimensional echocardiography during dobutamine stress echocardiography. *J Am Soc Echocardiogr.* 2006;19:1136–1143.

33. Sugeng L, Kirkpatrick J, Lang RM, Bednarz JE, DeCara JM, Lammertin G, Spencer KT. Biplane stress echocardiography using a prototype matrix-array transducer. *J Am Soc Echocardiogr.* 2003;16:937–941.

34. Kapetanakis S, Kearney MT, Siva A, Gall N, Cooklin M, Monaghan MJ. Real-time three dimensional echocardiography: a novel technique to quantify global left ventricular mechanical dyssynchrony. *Circulation.* 2005;112:992–1000.

35. Marsan NA, Bleeker GB, Ypenburg C, Ghio S, van de Veire NR, Holman ER, van der Wall EE, Tavazzi L, Schalij MJ, Bax JJ. Real-time three-dimensional echocardiography permits quantification of left ventricular mechanical dyssynchrony and predicts acute response to cardiac resynchronization therapy. *J Cardiovasc Electrophysiol.* 2008;19:392–399.

36. Becker M, Hoffmann R, Schmitz F, Hundemer A, Kuhl H, Schauerte P, Kelm M, Franke A. Relation of optimal lead positioning as defined by three-dimensional echocardiography to long-term benefit of cardiac resynchronization. *Am J Cardiol.* 2007;100: 1671–1676.

37. Kaufmann BA, Wei K, Lindner JR. Contrast echocardiography. *Curr Prob Cardiology.* 2007;32:51–96.

38. Malm S, Frigstad S, Sagberg E, Steen PA, Skjarpe T. Real-time simultaneous triplane contrast echocardiography gives rapid, accurate, and reproducible assessment of left ventricular volumes and ejection fraction: a comparison with magnetic resonance imaging. *J Am Soc Echocardiogr.* 2006;19:1494–1501.

39. Pulerwitz T, Hirata K, Abe Y, Otsuka R, Herz S, Okajima K, Jin Z, Di Tullio MR, Homma S. Feasibility of using a real-time 3-dimensional technique for contrast dobutamine stress echocardiography. *J Am Soc Echocardiogr.* 2006;19:540–545.

40. Takeuchi M, Otani S, Weinert L, Spencer KT, Lang RM. Comparison of contrast enhanced real-time live 3-dimensional dobutamine stress echocardiography with contrast 2-dimensional echocardiography for detecting stress-induced wall-motion abnormalities. *J Am Soc Echocardiogr.* 2006;19:294–299.

41. Krenning BJ, Nemes A, Soliman OI, Vletter WB, Voormolen MM, Bosch JG, Ten Cate FJ, Roelandt JR, Geleijnse ML. Contrast-enhanced three-dimensional dobutamine stress echocardiography: between Scylla and Charybdis? *Eur J Echocardiogr.* 2008; 9(6):757–760.

42. Toledo E, Lang RM, Collins KA, Lammertin G, Williams U, Weinert L, Bolotin G, Coon PD, Raman J, Jacobs LD, Mor-Avi V. Imaging and quantification of myocardial perfusion using real-time three-dimensional echocardiography. *J Am Coll Cardiol.* 2006; 47:146–154.

43. Bhan A, Kapetanakis S, Rana BS, Ho E, Wilson K, Pearson P, Mushemi S, Deguzman J, Reiken J, Harden MD, Walker N, Rafter PG, Monaghan MJ. Real-time three-dimensional myocardial contrast echocardiography: is it clinically feasible? *Eur J Echocardiogr.* 2008;9(6):715–716.

44. Veronesi F, Caiani EG, Toledo E, Corsi C, Collins KA, Lammertin G, Lamberti C, Lang RM, Mor-Avi V. Semi-automated analysis of dynamic changes in myocardial contrast from real-time three-dimensional echocardiographic images as a basis for volumetric quantification of myocardial perfusion. *Eur J Echocardiogr.* 2009;10(4):485–490.

45. Mor-Avi V, Jenkins C, Kuhl HP, Nesser HJ, Marwick TH, Franke A, Ebner C, Freed BH, Steringer-Mascherbauer R, Pollard H, Weinert L, Niel J, Sugeng L, Lang RM. Real-time 3D echocardiographic quantification of left ventricular volumes: Multicenter study for validation with magnetic resonance imaging and investigation of sources of error. *J Am Coll Cardiol Imaging.* 2008; 1:413–423.

Three-Dimensional Echocardiographic Evaluation of the Mitral Valve

6

José Luis Zamorano and Jose Alberto de Agustín

The mitral valve apparatus is a complex structure that can be affected by a multitude of acquired and congenital disorders. An optimal interaction of the different anatomic elements comprising the annulus, the leaflets, the chordae tendinae, the papillary muscles and the left atrial and left ventricular walls is necessary for its functional integrity. The interpretation of two-dimensional echocardiographic (2DE) images requires a complex mental integration of multiple image planes for a true understanding of anatomic and pathologic structures. One of the most significant developments of the last decade, particularly in the field of cardiac imaging, has been three dimensional echocardiography (3DE). The display of cardiac anatomy in three dimensions from any perspective has clear advantages over conventional 2D imaging and provides an insight into the functional and anatomic properties of cardiac structures. The benefits of 3DE are particularly well suited to the study of the mitral valve apparatus given its complex morphology and the importance of delineating its anatomy precisely in various pathological states. Comparing with 2DE, 3DE offers advantages for the morphologic and quantitative assessment of mitral valve stenosis, prolapse and regurgitation. The 3DE data sets can be acquired with the transthoracic or transesophageal approach. The development of a fully sampled matrix array transducer has enabled easy and fast acquisition of real-time 3DE volumetric imaging of the mitral valve from the transthoracic approach. It has sparked an emerging interest in using this methodology in clinical practice.

views of the mitral valve apparatus can easily be obtained, as can surgical and "en face" views from either the left atrium or the left ventricle. 3DE by viewing the mitral valve from the left atrium shows that the anterior and posterior mitral leaflets have indentations dividing them into segments or scallops[1]. The anterior leaflet is divided into three segments: A1 (anterolateral), A2 (middle), and A3 (posteromedial), and the posterior leaflet is composed of three scallops: P1 (anterolateral), P2 (middle), and P3 (posteromedial). The anterior and posterior leaflets are fused medially and laterally forming the commissures (anterolateral and posteromedial). The anterior leaflet comprises two thirds of the valve area and is somewhat triangular. It is attached to the septum and fibrous annulus of the heart, and it is relatively nondistensible. The posterior leaflet is more elongated and it is attached to the posterior two thirds of the mitral annulus, which is primarily muscular explaining its tendency to distend. Mitral annulus and leaflets have a non-planar saddle shape configuration. There are two high points near the aortic root and near the posterior left ventricular wall and two low points located medially and laterally at the commissures. The leaflet annular nonplanarity shape provides a configuration capable of withstanding the stresses imposed by left ventricular pressure during systole. The mitral annular area can decrease by lowering of the distance between the high and lower points of the annulus[2].

6.1 Three-Dimensional Echocardiographic Anatomy of the Normal Mitral Valve

The assessment of the morphology and function of the mitral valve apparatus by 3DE became more accurate. For 3DE a parasternal or apical view is generally used. Stereoscopic

6.2 Mitral Valve Regurgitation

The assessment of patients with mitral regurgitation is one of the most promising clinical applications of 3DE. Dynamic 3D reconstruction of mitral valve structure en face from either a left atrial or left ventricular perspective, including detailed visualisation of the mitral leaflets, commissures, and mitral valve orifice, are helpful in a comprehensive analysis of the underlying valve anomaly and pre-operative assessment. The use of colour Doppler flow mapping, combined with 3D morphologic data, provides clinically relevant supplementary information for the assessment of this pathology.

J. Zamorano (✉)
Unidad de Imagen Cardiovascular, Hospital Clínico San Carlos, Madrid, Spain
e-mail: jzamorano.hcsc@salud.madrid.org

L.P. Badano et al. (eds.), *Textbook of Real-Time Three Dimensional Echocardiography*,
DOI: 10.1007/978-1-84996-495-1_6, © Springer-Verlag London Limited 2011

6.2.1 Organic Mitral Valve Regurgitation

Mitral valve prolapse is a frequently encountered problem in clinical cardiology and the most common cause of isolated mitral regurgitation. An integrated assessment of mitral morphology and regurgitant severity is used in deciding the repairability of the mitral valve and the optimal timing of surgery. The mitral valve apparatus has a complex 3D structure, especially in the presence of myxomatous degeneration with leaflet prolapse, and it makes interpretation of conventional 2D images difficult. 3DE has the potential to overcome these difficulties. Dynamic volume rendered 3DE of the mitral valve displays both leaflets entirely from any desired perspective. This allows clear visualisation of the location and extent of the prolapsing leaflet (see Fig. 6.1). Looking down in the left atrium, mitral valve prolapse is viewed as a bulge, whereas looking up in the left ventricle mitral valve prolapse appears as a spoon-like depression. In patients with mitral valve prolapse and regurgitation, a leak due to noncoaptation can be visualized (see Video 6.1). 3DE is helpful in the preoperative planning of mitral valve repair because it provides a view of the valve similar to that seen intraoperatively by the surgeon, with the major advantage of displaying the dynamic motion of the valve (see Video 6.2). In contrast to 2DE, 3DE allows measurements of the area of the prolapsed portion (see Fig. 6.2). This information assists

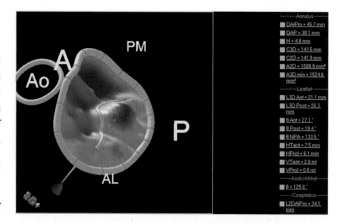

Fig. 6.2 Volume renderings of the mitral valve obtained with quantitative analysis software showing posterior mitral valve leaflet

the surgeon in deciding the extent of valvular tissue resection. Several works[3, 4] have showed that transthoracic or transesophageal 3DE are feasible and useful methods in identifying the location of mitral valve prolapse, and superior in the description of pathology in comparison with the corresponding 2DE techniques. An excellent correspondence between the localization and volume of the prolapse and surgically resected tissue has also been demonstrated[5]. Transesophageal 3DE approach allows more accurate identification of all mitral valve lesions in comparison to transthoracic approach[4].

6.2.2 Functional Mitral Valve Regurgitation

Functional mitral regurgitation is defined as an insufficiency of the structurally normal mitral valve, developing as a consequence of regional or global left ventricular dysfunction. It is a complication of either chronic ischemic heart disease, dilated or hypertrophic cardiomyopathy. The presence of significant functional mitral regurgitation is a major determinant for the outcome of left ventricular dysfunction, and this is known to be a marker of a poor long-term prognosis independent on left ventricular dysfunction. Mitral annulus dilatation, tethering of mitral leaflets secondary to left ventricular dilatation with outward displacement of papillary muscles, and reduced transmitral pressure to coapt the leaflets have been implicated as mechanisms for functional mitral regurgitation. Characterization of the mitral valve apparatus using 3DE have played a crucial role in describing the geometry of the mitral annulus, leaflet surface, tethering distances, tenting volumes, and the relationship between the mitral apparatus and the position of the papillary muscles, providing new light on the pathophysiology of functional mitral regurgitation. 3DE techniques have showed that

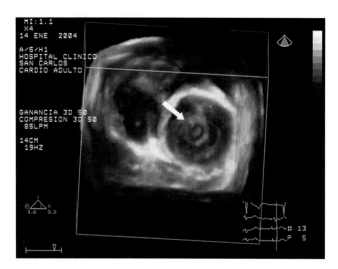

Fig. 6.1 RT3DE reconstruction of the mitral valve from ventricular perspective showing the depression on the ventricular side in correspondence of a prolapsed (A2) scallop (arrow)

Video 6.1 The display of mitral valve in three dimensions from any perspective provides superior evaluation of the mitral valve prolapse

Video 6.2 3DE stereoscopic "en face" views of the mitral valve from the left atrium showing posterior mitral valve leaflet

tethering due to displacement of the papillary muscle is the main mechanism of functional mitral regurgitation. Watanabe et al. investigated 3D geometric deformity of the mitral leaflets and annulus in ischemic mitral regurgitation with 3DE[6], showing a flattened annulus with apparent tenting of the leaflets. Maximum and mean tenting length were longer and tenting volume was larger in ischemic mitral regurgitation than control subjects. They also compared geometric deformity of the mitral annulus in inferior and anterior myocardial infarction. Annulus was further deformed in anterior myocardial infarction than with inferior myocardial infarction[7]. Kwan et al. studied the difference of mitral valve deformation between ischemic and dilated cardiomyopathy with significant functional mitral regurgitation[8]. The pattern of mitral valve deformation was symmetrical in dilated cardiomyopathy, whereas it was asymmetrical in ischemic heart disease. Medial and posterior shift of the medial papillary muscle is a fundamental cause of functional mitral regurgitation for the patients with ischemic cardiomyopathy particularly for the patients without severe left ventricular dilatation[9].

6.2.3 Assessment of the Degree of Regurgitation

Assessment of the severity of mitral regurgitation is an important issue. The use of colour Doppler flow mapping, combined with 3D morphologic data of the surrounding cardiac anatomy, provides clinically relevant supplementary information for the assessment of mitral regurgitation. This mode may enable exact definition of jet origin, direction, length and relationship to adjacent structures (see Fig. 6.3). It became possible to measure regurgitant orifice areas, estimate regurgitant volumes, as

Video 6.3 Three-dimensional echocardiography improves the assessment of eccentric regurgitant jets with "coanda" effect

well as improve the delineation of valvular leaks, paravalvular leaks and multiple jets. 3D colour flow imaging improves the assessment of eccentric regurgitant jets because the full extent of these jets is better appreciated, and it recognizes different patterns of eccentric regurgitant jets, such as cylinder, spiral and spoon-like patterns (see Video 6.3). In addition dynamic changes in phases of valvular regurgitant jets flows may be rapidly and stereoscopically visualized.

The flow convergence or proximal isovelocity surface area method is based on the phenomenon that flow accelerates towards the regurgitant orifice and forms a series of concentric hemispheric shells of increasing velocity. Conventional 2D methods rely on assumptions that the isovelocity surface is hemispheric. However, the flow convergence zone is a complex 3D shape dependent on the shape of the regurgitant orifice[10]. 3DE can address the real geometry and area of the isovelocity surface (see Fig. 6.4). 3DE displays the entire flow convergence region en face viewing it from the left atrium, and a more accurate assessment of its area can be done without the need to make geometric assumptions[11].

Up to now, measurement of the regurgitant orifice area was based on 2D Doppler methods. High-resolution 3DE allows direct visualisation and planimetry of the regurgitant orifice in the optimal plane. By cropping from the top of the data set, the image plane is placed at the level of the vena contracta in a parallel plane to the orifice. It has been shown that the anatomic regurgitant orifice area measured directly by planimetry from 3D volume rendered images correlates well with effective regurgitant orifice area calculated by the 2D proximal isovelocity surface area method[12, 13]. 3DE can overcome the limitations of the 2D proximal isovelocity

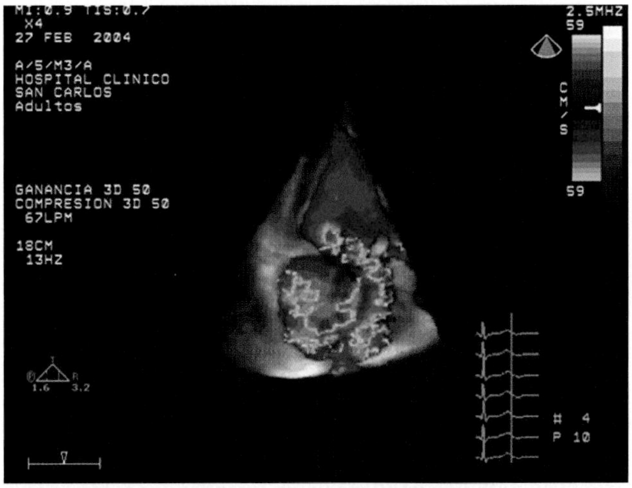

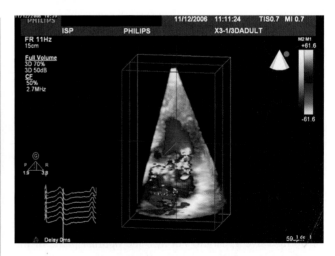

Fig. 6.3 Example of image of valvular regurgitant jet

Fig. 6.4 Example of proximal isovelocity surface area (PISA) assessment by RT3DE

surface area method in cases of mitral regurgitation with elliptic orifice shapes. Iwakura et al. examined the feasibility of measuring the mitral regurgitant orifice area using 3DE compared with effective regurgitant orifice area calculated using the 2D proximal isovelocity surface area method or quantitative Doppler echocardiography[14]. In the cases of mitral regurgitation with elliptic regurgitant orifice shapes, the 2D proximal isovelocity surface area method underestimated the area compared with quantitative Doppler echocardiography. In contrast, the 3D method and the quantitative Doppler method showed an almost identical coincidence regardless of orifice shape.

6.2.4 Postoperative Assessment of Mitral Valve Repair

Accurate postoperative assessment of mitral valve repairs is essential to document operative success. Hoole et al. compared transthoracic 3DE and 2DE assessment of mitral valves following mitral valve repair at 3 months into the postoperative period[15]. 3DE was better than 2DE in correctly identifying the site of repair, in particular in identifying the commissures where visualization is poor by 2DE. Furthermore the mitral valve area measured by 3DE planimetry had a stronger correlation to pressure half-time derived mitral valve area than 2DE planimetry. Armen et al. evaluated the mechanisms underlying mitral valve competency after the implantation of an annuloplasty ring using 3DE[16]. Mitral annuloplasty significantly diminished mitral regurgitation, which was associated with the decrease in mitral valve annulus area. The intercommissural distance decreased by 20% whereas the septolateral distance decreased by 38% following annuloplasty. The maximum reduction in the diameter occurred at the level of A2–P2. The tethering of the mitral leaflets into the left ventricle also disappeared after annuloplasty.

6.3 Mitral Valve Stenosis

To assess patients with rheumatic mitral valve stenosis, clinical data, morphologic evaluation and accurate measurements of the mitral valve orifice area are necessary. Classic methods to determine mitral valve area have several limitations. 3DE allows a different and superior evaluation of the mitral valve apparatus. It provides not only the anatomic structure of mitral valve apparatus but also the optimal plane of the smallest mitral valve orifice, and allows a more accurate measurement of mitral valve area.

6.3.1 Morphological Assessment

Mitral valve stenosis is a progressive disease associated with progressive morphologic changes of the valve leaflets and the subvalvular structures. Percutaneous mitral valvuloplasty is the treatment of choice for selected patients with favourable valve anatomy. The echocardiographic Wilkins score is a significant predictor for success or failure of the percutaneous mitral valvuloplasty procedure[17]. Choosing the patients who are the most favourable for percutaneous mitral valvuloplasty requires precise evaluation of mitral valve and particularly commissural anatomy. The position and degree of leaflet fusion and thickening, as well as the fused and thickened chordae tendinae can all be visualized clearly on 3DE. In a previous work of our group the inter-observer variability of Wilkins score by using 2DE and 3DE was evaluated[18]. The 3DE assessment showed better inter- and intraobserver agreement for the morphologic evaluation of the rheumatic mitral valve.

6.3.2 Functional Assessment

Until now the gold standard method to determine mitral valve area has been invasive hemodynamic evaluation, using the catheter-based data and the Gorlin's equation. Gorlin's equation, however, uses hemodynamics obtained from fluid-filled catheters. It is invasive, uses numerous assumptions, and clearly can result in complications and has numerous limitations. Most notably, it is inaccurate when significant valvular regurgitation is present. 2DE has been the usual method to determine mitral valve area in routine clinical practice. Mitral valve area is assessed indirectly by the pressure-half-time method, or by direct planimetry. All these methods have their advantages and limitations. Pressure-half-time-derived mitral valve area can be obtained easily, but may be influenced by hemodynamic factors (heart rate, cardiac index, cardiac rhythm, left ventricular systolic and diastolic dysfunction, left ventricular and atrium compliance, left ventricular hypertrophy and concomitant valvular disease)[19, 20]. The main advantage of planimetry is that it provides a relatively hemodynamic-independent assessment of the anatomical mitral valve area although one might imagine that the orifice could be larger when left atrial pressure is high. Until now, direct measurements of the mitral valve area only could be performed using planimetry traced on 2DE images but this method has several limitations; the greatest is that there is no controlled sectioning of the mitral funnel orifice. Measurements of the mitral valve area are made in the short axis view with no simultaneous independent imaging to verify that the imaging plane corresponds to the smallest and most perpendicular view of the mitral orifice (see Fig. 6.5). Because of it, this method requires significant experience and operator skill to obtain the correct imaging plane that displays the true mitral valve orifice. In addition, 2D planimetry is limited to patients with favorable image quality from a parasternal window.

The assessment of patients with mitral valve stenosis is one of the most promising clinical applications of 3DE. 3DE can provide not only the anatomic structure of mitral valve (commissural splitting and leaflet tears), but also the optimal plane of the smallest mitral valve orifice, consequently it accurately measures the mitral valve area. 3DE provides unique orientations of the cardiac structures not obtainable by routine 2DE (see Video 6.4). Short-axis cut plane is further positioned at the mitral valve cusp tips, which is selected for area measurement by planimetry, and errors due to malpositioning can be obviated (see Fig. 6.6). In addition, planimetry using 3DE is not limited to the parasternal window and permits mitral valve area measurement from an apical window. The introduction of a full matrix-array transducer has enabled online real-time 3DE and rendering. It became possible to rapidly evaluate the mitral valve structure and mitral valve area. The utility of 3DE in the evaluation of mitral stenosis and accuracy of mitral valve area measurements have been established by multiple studies. Our group conducted a study where 3DE

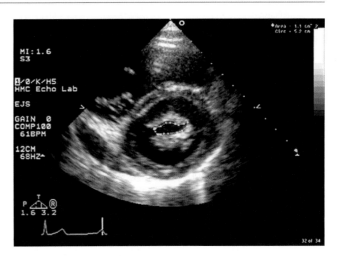

Fig. 6.5 Example of planimetry of a stenotic mitral valve using standard 2DE. There is no verification from an orthogonal plane that the measurement is at the mitral leaflet tips

Video 6.4 The display of mitral valve in three dimensions from any perspective provides a superior evaluation of the mitral valve apparatus and allows a more accurate measurement of mitral valve area

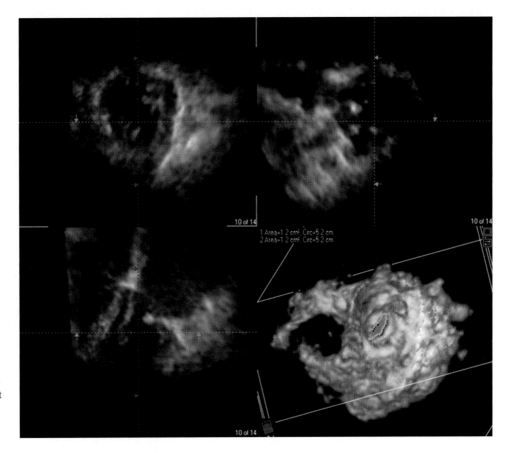

Fig. 6.6 The 3D transducer allows simultaneous display of more than one 2D view. The advantage of this is the ability to confirm that the parasternal short axis view of the mitral orifice is in fact at the tip of the mitral leaflets

was compared with current 2DE methods for the assessment of mitral valve area in patients with rheumatic mitral stenosis (2D planimetry, pressure-half-time method and proximal isovelocity surface area method)[18]. The gold standard method was the mitral valve area invasively determined using the Gorlin's equation. 3DE planimetry was performed "enface" at the ideal cross section of the mitral valve during its greatest diastolic opening. The ideal cross section was defined as the most perpendicular view on the plane with the smallest mitral valve orifice. Analysis showed a better agreement when comparing the invasively determined mitral valve area with 3DE determined mitral valve area than when comparing it with the current 2DE methods. Similar results have been reported in other works[21–23]. Kasliwal et al. compared the mitral valve area by 3DE with the true mitral orifice measured directly at operation. The comparison achieved a high degree of agreement[24].

Presently there is sufficient evidence that 3DE is superior to 2DE and may be routinely used in the quantification of the mitral valve area in mitral stenosis. The exceptional quality of the images of the mitral valve suggests that this modality could become the new "gold standard" for the mitral valve area quantification. Gorlin's method has several pitfalls, such as using the assumption that a properly confirmed wedge pressure accurately reflects left atrial pressure, the misalignment of the pulmonary capillary wedge and left ventricular pressure tracings and the calibration errors. Furthermore significant mitral regurgitation and the presence of an atrial septal defect may confound measurements of trans-mitral volume flow. A recent work has evaluated if 3DE planimetry is more accurate than the Gorlin method to measure the mitral valve area[25]. A median value of the mitral valve area, obtained from the measurements of three classical non-invasive methods (2D planimetry, pressure-half-time and proximal isovelocity surface area method), was used as the gold-standard. This value was compared with 3DE planimetry and Gorlin method. The analysis showed that the accuracy of 3DE planimetry is superior to the accuracy of the invasive Gorlin's method for assessing mitral valve area in rheumatic mitral stenosis, when the median (or composite data set) was used as the standard. Thus, taking that into account, we should keep in mind the fact that 3DE planimetry may be a better reference method than the Gorlin method to assess the severity of rheumatic mitral stenosis. In addition Gorlin is an invasive method that may result in complications and inaccuracies for the patient. In future 3DE might replace Gorlin's method as the gold standard for the quantification of the mitral valve area, and may eventually make routine preoperative cardiac catheterization unnecessary. In Table 6.1 there is a detailed comparison of the different methods to evaluate a rheumatic mitral stenosis.

Table 6.1 Comparison of the different methods to evaluate a rheumatic mitral stenosis

Method	Influence of hemodynamic conditions	Acoustic window needed	Useful after PMV	Invasive technique
2D planimetry	-	++	+	-
PHT	++	++	-	-
PISA	+	++	+	-
RT3DE	-	++	++	-
Gorlin	++	-	++	++

PMV percutaneous mitral valvuloplasty, *2D* 2D echocardiography, *PHT* half pressure time, *PISA* proximal isovelocity surface area, *RT3DE* real-time 3D echocardiography.

6.3.3 Monitoring Percutaneous Mitral Valvuloplasty

3DE can provide additional information to 2DE in patients with mitral stenosis, pre- and post-percutaneous mitral valvuloplasty. Many studies have demonstrated large discrepancies in the immediate post-percutaneous mitral valvuloplasty period, between mitral valve area measurements obtained using the pressure-half-time-method and those derived invasively in the catheterization laboratory[26, 27]. There are various reasons for this inaccuracy including: (1) the development of an atrial septal defect in many patients after percutaneous mitral valvuloplasty and (2) the pressure-half-time-method assumes that the left atrial and left ventricular compliances remain stable; this assumption is not valid in the immediate period following percutaneous mitral valvuloplasty because rapid changes in the left atrial pressure and left ventricular filling occur in this setting, affecting the compliance of both the left atrium and ventricle[28]. 2D planimetry of mitral valve area is not as dependent on hemodynamic variables[29]; and theoretically should be more accurate than pressure-half-time after percutaneous mitral valvuloplasty, but it is not exempt of limitations because following valvuloplasty the mitral orifice becomes irregular and is technically difficult to trace, particularly if calcium is present. Due to the variable geometry of the stenotic mitral valve orifice, correct plane orientation frequently becomes difficult. By means of 3DE it is possible to assess the morphology of the mitral valve also in percutaneous mitral valvuloplasty which is important in the evaluation of the mechanism and success of the procedure. By volume-rendered 3DE, dynamic 3D reconstructions can be performed of the mitral valve structure en face of either a left atrial or a left ventricular perspective, including detailed visualization of the commissures, leaflets, and subvalvular structures not seen with 2DE. The ease of acquisition and on-line review of 3DE facilitates immediate assessment of the mitral valve commissural splitting, stretching or tearing after percutaneous mitral valvuloplasty in the cardiac catheterization laboratory. In a study of our group was examined the problem of the mitral valve area evaluation immediately after a percutaneous mitral valvuloplasty[30]. The gold standard method was the mitral valve area invasively determined. The main findings were that 3DE was the most accurate ultrasound technique for measuring mitral valve area, with a better pre- and post-procedural agreement with the invasively (Gorlin) derived mitral valve area. Post-percutaneous mitral valvuloplasty the agreement with the Gorlin-derived mitral valve area was much better than 2D planimetry and pressure-half-time-derived mitral valve area. In conclusion, 3DE is also a very suitable technique for monitoring the efficacy of the percutaneous mitral valvuloplasty, with a better accuracy compared to 2D planimetry and pressure-half-time derived-mitral valve area.

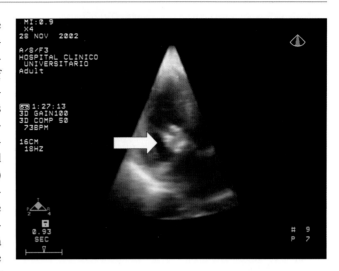

Fig. 6.7 3DE imaging showing a vegetation attached to the mitral valve

6.4 3D Echocardiography in the Evaluation of Prosthetic Valves

Entire views and motions of prosthetic heart valves may be well displayed by 3DE for anatomic detail and function. 3DE is able to delineate the site, size, and shape of the paravalvular leaks (see Video 6.5), and it can be applied for accurate prosthetic valvular planimetry. Mannaerts et al. studied the feasibility of prosthetic orifice area measurement by transesophageal 3DE in patients with normally functioning valve prostheses in the mitral and aortic positions, compared with Doppler methods[31]. Orifice area-3D correlated better than orifice area-Doppler with orifice area manufacturer. The orifice area-3D method may also provide better insight into the extent and mechanisms of valvular obstruction and may be able to better differentiate pathologic obstruction from severe patient valve mismatch.

6.5 Mitral Valve Endocarditis

Echocardiography, is considered mandatory in the clinical diagnosis and treatment of mitral valve endocarditis because of its high sensitivity for valvular vegetations and complications. 3DE could be helpful in endocarditis by its ability to display valvular and other cardiac structures[32]. 3DE shows

Video 6.5 Example of paravalvular leak assessment by transesophageal three-dimensional echocardiography

the stereoscopic configuration, attachment, and mobility of vegetations (see Fig. 6.7). In addition the 3D dataset can be cropped accurately to correctly characterize valvular perforations, and it is useful in excluding abscess formation. Ongoing refinements of this technology are likely to make 3DE a useful tool in mitral valve endocarditis.

6.6 Disclosure

There is no conflict of interest concerning this manuscript.

References

1. Valocik G, Kamp O, Visser CA. Three-dimensional echocardiography in mitral valve disease. *Eur J Echocardiogr*. 2005;6:443–454.
2. Kaplan SR, Bashein G, Sheehan FH, Legget ME, Munt B, Li XN, et al. Three-dimensional echocardiographic assessment of annular shape changes in the normal and regurgitant mitral valve. *Am Heart J*. 2000;139:378–387.
3. Gutiérrez-Chico JL, Zamorano Gómez JL, Rodrigo-López JL, Mataix L, Pérez de Isla L, Almería-Valera C, Aubele A, Macaya-Miguel C. Accuracy of real-time 3-dimensional echocardiography in the assessment of mitral prolapse. Is transesophageal echocardiography still mandatory? *Am Heart J*. 2008;155:694–698.
4. Pepi M, Tamborini G, Maltagliati A, Galli CA, Sisillo E, Salvi L, et al. Head-to-head comparison of two- and three-dimensional transthoracic and transesophageal echocardiography in the localization of mitral valve prolapse. *J Am Coll Cardiol*. 2006;48:2524–2530.
5. Delabays A, Jeanrenaud X, Chassot PG, Von Segesser LK, Kappenberger L. Localization and quantification of mitral valve prolapse using three-dimensional echocardiography. *Eur J Echocardiogr*. 2004;5:422–429.

6. Watanabe N, Ogasawara Y, Yamaura Y, Kawamoto T, Toyota E, Akasaka T, et al. Quantitation of mitral valve tenting in ischemic mitral regurgitation by transthoracic real-time three-dimensional echocardiography. *J Am Coll Cardiol.* 2005;45:763–769.

7. Watanabe N, Ogasawara Y, Yamaura Y, Wada N, Kawamoto T, Toyota E, et al. Mitral annulus flattens in ischemic mitral regurgitation: geometric differences between inferior and anterior myocardial infarction: a real-time 3-dimensional echocardiographic study. *Circulation.* 2005;112:458–462.

8. Kwan J, Shiota T, Agler DA, Popovic ZB, Qin JX, Gillinov MA, et al. Geometric differences of the mitral apparatus between ischemic and dilated cardiomyopathy with significant mitral regurgitation. Real-time three-dimensional echocardiography study. *Circulation.* 2002;107:1135–1140.

9. Liel-Cohen N, Guerrero JL, Otsuji Y, Handschumacher MD, Rudski LG, Hunziker PR, et al. Design of a new surgical approach for ventricular remodeling to relieve ischemic mitral regurgitation. Insights from 3-dimensional echocardiography. *Circulation.* 2000; 101:2756–2763.

10. Li X, Shiota T, Delabays A, Teien D, Zhou XD, Sinclair B, et al. Flow convergence flow rates 3-dimensional reconstruction of color Doppler flow maps for computing transvalvular regurgitant flows without geometric assumptions: an in vitro quantitative flow study. *J Am Soc Echocardiogr.* 1999;12:1035–1044.

11. Sitges M, Jones M, Shiota T, Qin JX, Tsujino H, Bauer F, et al. Real-time three-dimensional color Doppler evaluation of the flow convergence zone for quantification of mitral regurgitation: validation experimental study and initial clinical experience. *J Am Soc Echocardiogr.* 2002;16:38–45.

12. Breburda ChS, Griffin BP, Pu M, Rodriguez L, Cosgrove DM, Thomas JD. Three-dimensional echocardiographic planimetry of maximal regurgitant orifice area in myxomatous mitral regurgitation: intraoperative comparison with proximal flow convergence. *J Am Coll Cardiol.* 1998;32:432–437.

13. Lange A, Palka P, Donnelly E, Burstow DJ. Quantification of mitral regurgitation orifice area by 3-dimensional echocardiography: comparison with effective regurgitant orifice area by PISA method and proximal regurgitant jet diameter. *Int J Cardiol.* 2002;86:87–98.

14. Iwakura K, Ito H, Kawano S, Okamura A, Kurotobi T, Date M, Inoue K, Fujii K. Comparison of orifice area by transthoracic three-dimensional Doppler echocardiography versus proximal isovelocity surface area (PISA) method for assessment of mitral regurgitation. *Am J Cardiol.* 2006;97:1630–1637.

15. Hoole SP, Liew TV, Boyd J, Wells FC, Rusk RA. Transthoracic real-time three-dimensional echocardiography offers additional value in the assessment of mitral valve morphology and area following mitral valve repair. *Eur J Echocardiogr.* 2008;9:625–630.

16. Armen TA, Vandse R, Crestanello JA, Raman SV, Bickle KM, Nathan NS. Mechanisms of valve competency after mitral valve annuloplasty for ischaemic mitral regurgitation using the Geoform ring: insights from three-dimensional echocardiography. *Eur J Echocardiogr.* 2008 May 13 [Epub ahead of print].

17. Wilkins GT, Weyman AE, Abascal VM, Block PC, Palacios IF. Percutaneous balloon dilatation of the mitral valve: an analysis of echocardiographic variables related to outcome and the mechanism of dilatation. *Br Heart J.* 1988;60:299–308.

18. Zamorano J, Cordeiro P, Sugeng L, Perez de Isla L, Weinert L, Macaya C, Rodríguez E, Lang RM. Real-time three-dimensional

19. Hatle L, Angelsen B, Tromsdal A. Noninvasive assessment of atrioventricular pressure half-time by Doppler ultrasound. *Circulation.* 1979;60:1096–1104.

20. Rodriguez L, Thomas JD, Monterroso V, et al. Validation of the proximal flow convergence method: calculation of orifice area in patients with mitral stenosis. *Circulation.* 1993;88:1157–1165.

21. Binder TM, Rosenhek R, Porenta G, Maurer G, Baumgartner H. Improved assessment of mitral valve stenosis by volumetric real-time three-dimensional echocardiography. *J Am Coll Cardiol.* 2000; 36:1355–1361.

22. Xie MX, Wang XF, Cheng TO, Wang J, Lu Q. Comparison of accuracy of mitral valve area in mitral stenosis by real-time, three-dimensional echocardiography versus two-dimensional echocardiography versus Doppler pressure half-time. *Am J Cardiol.* 2005;95:1496–1499.

23. Sebag IA, Morgan JG, Handschumacher MD, Marshall JE, Nesta F, Hung J, Picard MH, Levine RA. Usefulness of three-dimensionally guided assessment of mitral stenosis using matrix-array ultrasound. *Am J Cardiol.* 2005;96:1151–1156.

24. Kasliwal R, Trehan N, Mittal S. A new "gold standard" for the measurement of mitral valve area? Surgical validation of volume rendered three-dimensional echocardiography. *Circulation.* 1996;94 (Suppl.):355.

25. Perez de Isla L, Casanova C, Almeria C, Rodrigo JL, Cordeiro P, Mataix L, Aubele AL, Lang R, Zamorano J. Which method should be the reference method to evaluate the severity of rheumatic mitral stenosis? Gorlin's method versus 3D-echo. *Eur J Echocardiogr.* 2007;8:470–473.

26. Reid CL, Rahimtoola SH: The role of echocardiography/Doppler in catheter balloon treatment of adults with aortic and mitral stenosis. *Circulation.* 1991;84(Suppl.):240–249.

27. Vahanian A, Michel PL, Cormier B, et al. Results of percutaneous mitral commissurotomy in 200 patients. *Am J Cardiol.* 1989; 63:847–852.

28. Thomas JD, Wilkins GT, Choong CY, et al. Inaccuracy of mitral pressure-halftime immediately after percutaneous mitral valvotomy: dependence on mitral gradient and left atrial and ventricular compliance. *Circulation.* 1988;78:980–993.

29. Faletra F, Pezzano A Jr, Fusco R, et al. Measurement of mitral valve area in mitral stenosis: four echocardiographic methods compared with direct measurement of anatomic orifices. *J Am Coll Cardiol.* 1996;28:1190–1197.

30. Zamorano J, Pérez de Isla L, Sugeng L, Cordeiro P, Rodrigo JL, Almería C, Weinert L, Feldman T, Macaya C, Lang RM, Hernandez Antolín R. Non invasive assessment of mitral valve area during percutaneous balloon mitral valvuloplasty: role of real time 3D echocardiography. *Eur Heart J.* 2004;25:2086–2091.

31. Mannaerts H, Li Y, Kamp O, Valocik G, Hrudova J, Ripa S, Visser CA. Quantitative assessment of mechanical prosthetic valve area by 3-dimensional transesophageal echocardiography. *J Am Soc Echocardiogr.* 2001;14:723–731.

32. Pérez De Isla L, Zamorano J, Malangatana G, Almería C, Rodrigo JL, Cordeiro P, et al. Usefulness of real-time 3-dimensional echocardiography in the assessment of infective endocarditis: initial experience. *J Ultrasound Med.* 2005;4:231–233.

Three Dimensional Echocardiographic Evaluation of LV Dyssynchrony and Stress Testing

7

Vasileios Sachpekidis, Amit Bhan, and Mark J. Monaghan

7.1 Assessment of Intraventricular Dyssynchrony

7.1.1 Do We Really Need 3D Echocardiography?

Cardiac dyssynchrony refers to an uncoordinated pattern of electrical activation, mechanical contraction and relaxation of the heart. When present it adversely affects ventricular function and may lead or worsen left ventricular (LV) remodeling and heart failure.[1] Traditionally, prolonged QRS duration (most commonly LBBB) has been considered to be the hallmark of dyssynchrony because it is associated with an abnormal LV contraction pattern and therefore is considered a possible surrogate marker for LV mechanical dyssynchrony.[2,3] This makes intuitive sense and thus it is not surprising that all major studies that demonstrated benefit from cardiac resynchronization therapy (CRT) defined QRS prolongation as one of the major inclusion criteria.[4–9]

This approach however has not proved entirely successful. Repeatedly, the percentage of patients not responding to CRT, as assessed by clinical criteria or objective evidence of the absence of reverse LV remodeling is between 25% and 30% of participants.[10] This may be at least partially due to the fact that patients with heart failure and LBBB are a heterogeneous group. Interestingly there are patients with LBBB and absence of significant mechanical dyssynchrony and conversely patients with normal QRS duration and pronounced regional contractile heterogeneity.[11,12,13] Based on the currently recommended criteria for CRT therapy the former patients would have received a device and likely not benefit from it, while the latter would have be considered inappropriate candidates for CRT despite having high probability of functional improvement with the device. It is

obvious that the great deal of the problem with QRS duration is that does not consistently identify mechanical dyssynchrony which is the goal of treatment with CRT.

In the pursuit of identifying the group of patients who will derive the greatest benefit from CRT, echocardiography has emerged as a very promising technique due to its ability to directly assess mechanical dyssynchrony via a number of different rapidly evolving methods. Although strictly speaking dyssynchrony can be divided into atrioventricular (delay in atrioventricular conduction), interventricular (delay between right ventricular and LV contraction) and intraventricular (regional delay within the LV)[14], it is the latter form of dyssynchrony that is thought to be most important and has received most of the attention in echocardiographic studies, resulting in a large variety of methods for its assessment. Although both traditional M-Mode[15] and 2D echocardiographic parameters[16,17] were originally used towards this end, Tissue Doppler Imaging (TDI) has been the most investigated modality for the assessment of mechanical dyssynchrony and response to CRT. Single center preliminary data with the use of TDI technology were very promising for predicting a favorable or unfavorable response to CRT[18–21]. However a recently prospective, multicenter study demonstrated modest sensitivity and specificity of TDI parameters to measure dyssynchrony and predict the result of CRT[22]. This has further confused the field of interventricular dyssynchrony assessment. Thus the optimal echocardiographic method for assessing dyssynchrony continues to be sought. Slowly accumulating data now exist that support the use of 3D echocardiography for the assessment of LV dyssynchrony making it a potential useful, reproducible, easily performed and robust technique for this cause. A detailed analysis of the 3D technique used to assess dyssynchrony combined with the weight of evidence favoring its use follows.

7.1.2 How to Assess Mechanical LV Dyssynchrony with 3D Echocardiography

A dataset that includes the whole LV is required to assess dyssynchrony. With the current commercially available

M.J. Monaghan (✉)
Department of Non-Invasive Cardiology, King's College Hospital,
London, United Kingdom
e-mail: mark.monaghan@nhs.net

L.P. Badano et al. (eds.), *Textbook of Real-Time Three Dimensional Echocardiography*,
DOI: 10.1007/978-1-84996-495-1_7, © Springer-Verlag London Limited 2011

machines, this is usually achieved by electronically "stitching" together smaller real time datasets (usually over –four to seven consecutive cardiac cycles), while the patient briefly holds their respiration. The dataset is acquired with the transducer positioned over the apical region and particular attention should be paid to be focused on the LV. A pyramidal 3D dataset is obtained this way at a frame rate of 20–40 Hz. Irregular heart rate (as it occurs with atrial fibrillation or multiple extra-systolic atrial and ventricular beats) and inability of the patient to hold his breath may decrease the quality of obtained images and create significant problems in subsequent analysis, due to stitching artifacts. Moreover it must be emphasized that 3D technology is limited by the laws of physics, just as every other echocardiographic technique. Poor apical windows with 2D acquisition will remain poor with 3D technology. Considering all the above, it is not a surprise that a significant proportion of patients with heart failure (which was reported to be as high as 13.9% in earlier studies)[23] have inadequate 3D images for dyssynchrony analysis. Contrast enhancement of 3D datasets is possible and improves the success rate of image acquisition and analysis in difficult subjects. Other technology advances will likely overcome many of the above problems very soon. The latest generation echocardiographic machines are able to capture a full volume LV dataset in just one beat, although the spatial and temporal resolution is not as optimal as with the stitching sub-volume technique. In addition, experience is still limited with these new systems but definitely they represent the future of 3D technology.

7.1.2.1 The Systolic Dyssynchrony Index

Kapetanakis et al.[23] developed a method for quantifying LV mechanical dyssynchrony using 3D echocardiography. This requires obtaining a full volume LV dataset and setting some endocardial definition landmarks for both end diastole and end systole using three 2D planes (apical four-, two- and three-chamber views). An edge-detection algorithm allows the extrapolation of these points to define the endocardial border accurately in each frame. A mathematical cast of the LV is then automatically created which in turn is divided into the standard 16 or 17 segments recommended by the American Society of Echocardiography.[24] The centre of gravity of each cast can also be calculated and the volume of each segment relative to the centre of gravity measured. Subsequently the volume of each segment is calculated and plotted throughout the cardiac cycle. In this way, time–volumes curves are derived for each segment of the LV and can be used to assess the time to minimum volume in each segment (Fig. 7.1). The standard deviation of the times to peak segmental contraction (minimum regional volume) corrected for the R–R interval is used as a measure of the degree of dispersion and has been termed as the Systolic Dyssynchrony Index (SDI). In the

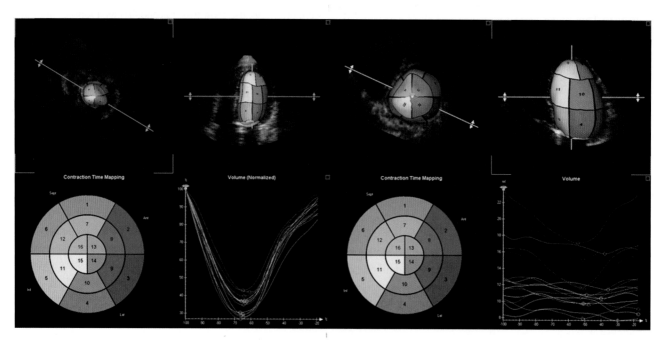

Fig. 7.1 Two examples of left ventricular dyssynchrony analysis using 3-D echocardiography. Each analysis is presented using a long axis and short axis view of the derived mathematical LV cast (*top*). The bottom left hand areas show a color coded schematic of the 16 LV segments. The areas in the bottom right of each picture show the time-volume curves for each LV segment, with their time to minimum highlighted. Note the segments in the left hand picture all reach their minimum volume close to each other demonstrating synchronous contraction. The picture on the right is from a patient with a history of myocardial infarctions and the segments reach their minimum volume at very different times

original report by Kapetanakis et al.[23] a 16 segment model was applied (SDI-16) and the software used for analysis was from TomTec (TomTec Imaging Systems GmbH, Germany).

Since then many other investigators have used the SDI index making it the most widely studied 3D echocardiographic tool for assessment of dyssynchrony. Differences between studies related to the number of segments used (16 or 17 segment model) and software (QLab, Phillips Medical Systems) utilized for the analysis exist. Although the main concept remains the same, the above differences, particularly in software may account for the variation in SDI values obtained between investigators. QLab software calculates the SDI index using a left ventricular model derived using two 2D orthogonal planes representing the standard apical four- and two-chamber views as guides. Five anatomical landmarks are set that include the septal, lateral, anterior, inferior mitral annulus and the LV apical endocardium in both end diastole and end systole. The software then recreates a 3D model using automated border detection algorithm for these two phases of the cardiac cycle. Manual correction can be done if deemed necessary. The software then performs a volumetric analysis creating a cast of the LV cavity throughout the cardiac cycle. Finally it divides the left ventricular cast into 17 segments and excludes the apical segment to give a value that is also termed SDI-16 but is actually 17 segments − 1. It is obvious that although both software aim to calculate the same index, there are differences in the segmentation, definition of centre of gravity and edge-detection algorithms of the LV endocardium. Therefore, the generated SDI values obtained are not necessarily directly comparable.

As with every new technique the questions that immediately aroused after the first description of SDI were: what are its normal values? Is it reproducible? Is it able to predict the results of CRT and if yes is there a cut-off point for this? And how it competes with other modalities used for dyssynchrony assessment?

7.1.2.2 Normal Values and Reproducibility of SDI

Since SDI is a relatively new measurement of dyssynchrony there has been great interest by various researchers[23,25–39] to define the normal values for this parameter. All reported values are summarized in Table 7.1. Four of these studies are worth mentioning because they involved a large number (over 100) of healthy volunteers. In three[28,34,38] of them TomTec analysis software was used and the reported mean SDI (± SD) for the 16th segment LV model ranged from 2.22 ± 0.91% (Sonne et al.[38]) to 2.74 ± 1.08% (Conca et al.[34]). In one of these studies[38] the mean SDI for the 17th segment (SDI-17) model was also estimated and was found to be very similar, although a bit higher compared to SDI-16 (2.29 ± 1.12% vs. 2.22 ± 0.91%). In the fourth study (Gimenes et al.[30]) where QLab software was used for the analysis similar mean SDI (± SD) values were obtained (1.59 ± 0.99%, with a range of 0.29–4.88%) for a 16th segment model.

Table 7.1 Normal values for SDI as reported in various studies

First author	Number of normal volunteers	Age (±SD) (years)	EF (±SD) (%)	Software	Number of LV segments used for SDI	SDI (±SD) (%)
Kapetanakis[23]	78	44 ± 17	61.0 ± 6.4	TomTec	16	3.50 ± 1.60
Zeng[25]	25	66 ± 6	66.2 ± 6.0	QLab	17	1.10 ± 0.60
Brunekreeft[26]	23	57 ± 19	62.7 ± 6.7	TomTec	16	2.50 ± 1.30
Baker[27]	9	4–17 (range)	44.3–72.1 (range)	QLab	16	0.71–2.78 (range)
De Castro[28]	116	45 ± 16	59.2 ± 4.5	TomTec	16	2.37 ± 0.81
Delgado[29]	10	25 ± 6	62.0 ± 4.0	QLab	17	1.50 ± 0.70
Gimenes[30]	120	46 ± 14	66.1 ± 7.1	QLab	16	1.59 ± 0.99
Liu[31]	9	68 ± 15	58.9 ± 5.5	TomTec	17	5.28 ± 1.64
Migrino[32]	10	60 ± 3	62.4 ± 0.6	QLab	16	1.67 ± 0.87
van Dijk[33]	16	58 ± 5	54.0 ± 5.0	TomTec	16	5.60 ± 3.60
Conca[34]	120	44 ± 13	64.7 ± 6.4	TomTec	16	2.74 ± 1.08
Liodakis[35]	35	55 ± 10	55.0 ± 5.0	TomTec	16	9.80 ± 2.00
Raedle-Hurst[36]	30	15 ± 6	NA	TomTec	16	3.10 ± 1.20
					17	3.70 ± 1.20
Soliman[37]	60	41 ± 15	60.0 ± 8.0	Qlab	16	4.1 ± 2.2
Sonne[38]	135	3–88 (range)	57.0 ± 5.0	TomTec	16	2.22 ± 0.91
					17	2.29 ± 1.12
Ten Harkel[39]	67	15 ± 2	60 ± 8	QLab	16	1.26 ± 0.53

Although better standardization of the method will allow more definite normal values to be created, in the majority of studies (irrespective of the software used) there is agreement that normal individuals very rarely have SDI values over 6%. In our laboratory the upper limit of normal is considered to be 5%. It must be underlined that the majority of studies have used the 16th segment model for calculation of the SDI and until more data accumulate for the 17th model we recommend using the former for everyday clinical practise. In agreement with this are preliminary data stating that SDI-16 can better separate normal individuals from patients with dyssynchrony compared to SDI-17.[38] It is important to note that normal SDI values appear not to be significantly affected by sex, weight, body surface area and age, with perhaps the exception of children in the first decade of life who have slightly less dyssynchrony compared to older subjects.[27,29,36,38,39] Finally, in one study comparing SDI-16 measurements with 4 or 7 beats acquisition mode (higher number of beats acquired results in higher frame rate) no significant difference between the two options was found, provided that endocardial border definition is adequate.[39]

A special subset of patients is those who have normal LV systolic function (as assessed by ejection fraction) and LBBB. Two studies both involving a small group of patients estimated SDI in these patients.[33,38] They both concluded that SDI-16 derived values were slightly higher compared to normal individuals without LBBB (although in one of the studies this difference did not reach statistical significance).[33] Interestingly however when compared to heart failure patients with and without LBBB the SDI-16 was still significantly lower, suggesting that SDI may be a useful tool for assessing dyssynchrony in this group of patients as well. Further studies addressing this issue are needed for estimating reference SDI values in these patients.

The intra- and inter-observer variation of SDI measurement was assessed in numerous single centre studies. All investigators have reported results ranging from good[30,32,33,43] to excellent[23,26,28,29,31,34,37,38–42,44–46] intra- and inter-observer reproducibility. Having in mind however the recent results of the multicenter PROSPECT study[22] where a significant variability in the analysis of various dyssynchrony parameters (other than 3D) between centres was documented, it is crucial to plan a multicenter study testing the reproducibility of SDI as a reliable index of dyssynchrony assessment.

7.1.3 Usefulness of SDI in Predicting the Results of CRT

The aim of every measure of dyssynchrony is to be able to identify reliably not only patients who will respond to CRT (sensitivity), but also the patients who will not benefit from it

(specificity). The ideal test should have both high sensitivity and specificity. This is particularly truth for CRT because it is a very expensive therapy and the economic burden of applying it indiscriminatingly in all heart failure patients with wide QRS will likely be very high. As already stated with the current criteria for CRT up to 30% of patients will not respond.

The role of SDI in separating responders from non-responders has been studied in various studies involving small number of patients, but the results appear to be very promising.[23,29,35,37,40,42,44,45,47] Kapetanakis et al.[23] in their original report studied 26 patients who fulfilled traditional criteria for CRT and found out that responders (defined as persistent symptomatic improvement at a mean of 10 months) had a significant higher SDI index before implantation of the device compared to non-responders. Interestingly all of the rest pre-implantation characteristics between the two groups (including ejection fraction, end diastolic LV volumes and NYHA class) were similar. In addition responders demonstrated a significant decrease in SDI after biventricular pacing, while at the same time non-responders had an actual increase of the same index.

Marsan et al.[40] evaluated the ability of SDI to predict the acute response to CRT in 56 patients who had device implantation based on the usual clinical and electrocardiographic criteria. Acute response to CRT was defined as a reduction of $\geq 15\%$ in LV end-systolic volume immediately after device insertion. Thirty-five (63%) patients were classified as acute responders. The investigators found that baseline characteristics were similar between responders and non-responders, except for the SDI which was significantly higher in responders. Consistent with previous findings, responders demonstrated a significant reduction of SDI immediately after CRT whereas SDI did not change in non-responders. The authors found that a cut-off SDI value of 5.6% yielded a very good sensitivity (88%) and specificity (86%) to predict acute echocardiographic response to CRT.

The same group went a step further and assessed the importance of SDI in predicting mid-term response (at 6 months) after CRT therapy.[42] They studied 51 heart failure patients with wide QRS who had a biventricular pacemaker put in and followed them for 6 months. They used the same definition as above to define responders. Thirty-four patients (67%) were classified as responders and again the only baseline characteristic that differentiated this group from non-responders was the SDI. Using receiver operating characteristic (ROC) curve analysis they reported a cut-off SDI value of 6.4% that had a sensitivity of 88% and a specificity of 85% for predicting mid-term response to CRT. Similarly to their previous study SDI in responders decreased significantly after CRT, while this was not the case in non-responders.

Interestingly, very recently Kleijn et al.[44] tested the above cut-off point (6.4%) in a cohort of 27 patients eligible for CRT therapy. They defined response to CRT clinical improvement of ≥1 NYHA functional class and a reduction of ≥15% in LV end-systolic volume (reverse remodeling) at 6 months. Clinical response was observed in 70% of patients, whereas reverse remodeling occurred in 63% of patients. By applying the SDI cut-off value of 6.4% in their study population they reported a sensitivity of 95% and 88% and a specificity of 87% and 60% for predicting clinical response and reverse remodeling respectively. Using ROC curve analysis they found that a slightly higher cut off-point of 6.7% yielded better sensitivity (90% and 88%) and specificity (87% and 70%) for predicting respectively clinical and LV remodeling response to CRT.

Finally, Soliman et al.[45] addressed the same issue prospectively in a larger cohort of 90 heart failure patients that received CRT based on the currently accepted criteria. They evaluated the patients before device implantation and 12 months after, using clinical and echocardiographic criteria. Sixty-eight (76%) patients were classified as responders based on ≥15% decrease in LV end-systolic volume. Consistent with all previous studies the only characteristic at baseline that was different between responders and non-responders was the SDI. Moreover, at 12 months responders demonstrated a significant decrease in SDI accompanied by improvement of clinical (as assessed by NYHA class and 6-min walking test) and echocardiographic (LV end-diastolic volume, ejection fraction and severity of mitral regurgitation) variables. On the other hand non-responders demonstrated an increase in SDI and less significant changes in all other variables. The authors reported a cut-off SDI point of 10% (higher than previous studies) that could predict CRT response with good sensitivity (96%) and specificity (88%).

Other studies involving small number of patients eligible for CRT based on traditional criteria, have reported similar results with the above mentioned studies.[29,35,37,47] Of note that although they have been reports stating that heart failure patients with narrow QRS have significantly higher SDI values than normal individuals,[23,28,29,38] to the best of our knowledge no study has been conducted so far aiming to determine a cut-off SDI value that can predict response to CRT in this subgroup of patients.

In conclusion, these findings together suggest that SDI-16 may be a useful predictor of symptomatic benefit from CRT, and also that SDI-16 is a better predictor than QRS duration in determining acute response to CRT and long-term clinical outcomes. A potential problem is that the cut-off value that best determines CRT response varies between studies from 5.5% to 10%. This difference between investigators may be attributed to the small number of patients studied, different versions of software used, as well as to lack of standardization of this new technique. It is likely that as experience accumulates more agreement will be achieved in the reported results. Until then, although a widely accepted cut-off value is the ideal goal, we suggest each institution to use locally derived cut-off values. In our centre baseline values over 10% are considered to be able to predict a positive response to CRT. On the other hand values than 5% are associated with lack of improvement with CRT even if traditional criteria are fulfilled. Although based on current guidelines it is unethical to deprive these patients from CRT it is our practise to give a word of caution to the treating physicians that the chances of improvement are small. Finally SDI values between 5% and 10% are the most difficult to interpret. If all other criteria for CRT are fulfilled we usually keep a neutral position as far as the ability of 3D analysis to predict response is concerned. It is obvious that further multicenter studies, involving large number of patients, are warranted to clarify all these issues and give a definite answer in the ability of SDI to predict response to CRT.

7.1.4 Comparison of SDI with Other Methods of Assessing Dyssynchrony

Many techniques (mainly echocardiographic) have been developed to assess dyssynchrony. Although initial reports for all of them have been promising, the goal is to find a technique that reliably and reproducibly will identify patients who will respond or not to CRT. In the lines that follow we will try briefly to provide existing evidence from studies comparing 3D derived SDI with other measures of dyssynchrony, both in terms of agreement as well as for predicting a favourable or not response to CRT.

7.1.4.1 Gated Myocardial Perfusion Single Photon Emission Computed Tomography (GMPS)

GMPS is a scintigraphic technique that has proved to have reasonable ability to predict response to CRT.[48] Based on these findings Marsan et al.[41] tested the correlation between GMPS and 3D SDI in a cohort of 40 heart failure patients and demonstrated a good correlation between the two. Since GMPS involves radiation the authors concluded that SDI is a reasonable alternative for assessing dyssynchrony.

7.1.4.2 Magnetic Resonance Imaging (MRI)

Recent data support that MRI assessment of dyssynchrony and myocardial scar predicts function class improvement following CRT.[49] Although direct comparison between MRI and 3D SDI for predicting the response to CRT has never been done, De Castro et al.[28] performed both 3D and MRI dyssynchrony analysis in 20 healthy patients and demonstrated high agreement between the two techniques. More studies however are needed to further evaluate the merits and weaknesses of each technique.

7.1.4.3 Tissue Doppler Imaging (TDI)

TDI is the echocardiographic technique that has been more widely studied for assessing dyssynchrony. Although early data were very promising[20,21] the recent PROSPECT[22] study revealed that this technique is far from being considered the gold standard for dyssynchrony. Few authors have compared 3D SDI with TDI for assessing dyssynchrony. Takeuchi et al.[50] were the only investigators that reported relatively good correlation between 3D derived time to minimum systolic volumes using a 17th segment model and TDI derived time to peak systolic velocities from the traditionally used 12 LV segments. Kapetanakis et al.[23] and Burgess et al.[51] on the other hand reported that 3D SDI and TDI measurements had at most moderate correlation. Since there is no widely accepted gold standard for dyssynchrony the above studies were unable to demonstrate clearly the superiority of one method over the other. Kleijn et al.[44] addressed this issue very recently. They studied 120 patients (30 normal individuals and 90 patients with heart failure) with both TDI using the standard deviation of time to peak systolic tissue velocity and 3D SDI. Consistent with the findings of previous studies they reported moderate correlation between TDI and SDI. Interestingly although no significant difference in the overall presence of mechanical dyssynchrony was detected between the two methods when they applied previously reported cut-off points for each one of the techniques (that is 32 ms for TDI-SDI[21] and 6.4% for 3D-SDI[42]), there was up to 30% non agreement depending on the severity of LV dysfunction. The authors went a step further and examined a subgroup of 27 patients that fulfilled traditional criteria and had a CRT device implanted. They estimated TDI-SDI and 3D-SDI in this subgroup at baseline and after 6 months of device implantation. Indicators of response to CRT were a clinical improvement of ≥1 NYHA class and reverse remodeling defined as a reduction of ≥15% in LV end-systolic volume at 6 months. Seventeen (63%) patients were classified as responders. All baseline characteristics were similar between responders and non-responders, except for mechanical dyssynchrony assessed by 3D, which was significantly higher in responders compared to non-responders. By applying previously defined cut-off values, ROC curve analysis demonstrated a sensitivity of 58% with a specificity of 50% for TDI and a sensitivity of 95% with a specificity of 87% for 3D-SDI to predict clinical response to CRT. For prediction of reverse remodeling after CRT, sensitivity and specificity were 59% and 50% for TDI, and 88% and 60% for 3D-SDI, respectively. It is obvious that in this small subgroup of patients, 3D-SDI performed better than TDI for predicting the result of CRT. This result

was explained by the authors by the fact that 3D analysis of dyssynchrony is deprived by many of the limitations of TDI mainly its 2D nature, the angle dependency of the ultrasound signal, and the resulting signal noise. Consequently, TDI does not allow analysis of the LV apical segments and also provides information only of the longitudinal motion of the heart without taking into consideration radial and circumferential myocardial shortening. Since the pattern of LV contraction changes in different settings, exclusion of apex from dyssynchrony analysis may lead to erroneous results.[28] On the other hand the temporal resolution of TDI is much higher than currently acquitted 3D datasets. Further studies involving large number of patients and comparing these two modalities head to head are needed to demonstrate the superiority, if any of the one method over the other.

7.1.5 Other Applications of 3D Echocardiography in Dyssynchrony Assessment

7.1.5.1 Assessment of the Latest Contracting Segment

The identification of the latest contracting segment of the LV is reported to be of importance with reference to the success of CRT.[52,53] Three dimensional echocardiography can provide this information by means of identifying the segment with the greatest delay in achieving its minimum volume.[28,29] This information can be displayed very vividly in bulls eye views (contraction front mapping – CFM) of the heart (Fig. 7.2). Although one would expect that there would be significant agreement between techniques in identifying the latest contracting LV segment, a recently published study could not demonstrate this.[46] More specifically, TDI derived indexes identified the lateral wall as the most frequent latest contraction site, longitudinal speckle tracking showed the anterior wall as the most frequent latest contraction site and 3D echocardiogram most frequently identified the inferior and septal walls as the latest contraction sites. More studies are needed to explain these differences.

7.1.5.2 Triplane TDI

Recently, a 3D probe allowing simultaneous acquisition of TDI data in three imaging planes became available. This 3D probe allows for acquisition and analysis of the 3D data set along three major planes with a simultaneous visualization of the apical four-, two-, and three-chamber views. Sample volumes can be placed simultaneously in 12 LV segments, and time to peak systolic velocities (Ts) of any LV

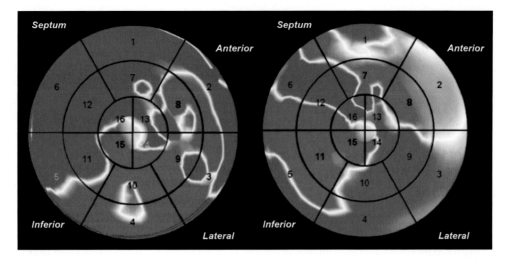

Fig. 7.2 Contraction Front Mapping (CFM) imaging demonstrating areas of delayed contraction (*red color*). On the left there is an example of a patient with LBBB where one can easily see there is a delay in con-traction of the lateral wall. On the right is an example of a patient with ischaemic heart disease, and previous myocardial infarctions, and het-erogeneous contraction pattern (delay in the anterior and inferior walls)

segment can be compared during the same heartbeat. Thus one of the disadvantages of TDI, i.e. acquisition of data through different cycles is overcome by this technique. Van de Veire[54] et al. applied this method in 60 patients undergo-ing CRT and demonstrated that the standard deviation of Ts of 12 (6 basal and 6 mid segments) LV segments with a cut-off value of 33 ms, was able to predict reverse LV remodel-ing with a sensitivity of 90% and a specificity of 83%. Data are scarce for this technique up to now and no direct com-parison of triplane TDI with 3D-SDI exists so far. Further clinical evaluation of triplane TDI is mandatory before its widespread application as a dyssynchrony assessment tool.

7.1.6 Conclusions: Future Directions

Existing data suggest that 3D echocardiography is a very promising and reliable method of dyssynchrony assessment. Advances in technology will enable to acquire a full volume 3D dataset with adequate temporal and spatial resolution in just one beat and thus will offset the majority of current limi-tations such as stitching artefacts and inability to apply the method in many patients with irregular rhythm. It is very important to have 3D images with good spatial resolution because small changes in the time–volume curves from improper tracing of the segment from the software can result in significant changes of the derived SDI and thus erroneous results.[38] Better standardization of the technique is mandatory before its widespread application. To achieve this, differences in the software used must be spotted and efforts should be made to minimize them. In addition, physicians who do the 3D dataset analysis should be well trained in centres with

expertise in 3D imaging to avoid disappointing results like the ones observed in the PROSPECT trial. If all the above conditions are fulfilled we are confident that 3D will very soon become a powerful tool for dyssynchrony assessment.

7.2 Three-Dimensional Stress Echocardiography

7.2.1 Rationale for Using 3D for Stress Echocardiography: Limitations of 2D Echocardiography

Indisputably 2D stress echocardiography has established its role as an accurate tool for detection of coronary artery dis-ease during the last two decades.[55] Traditionally four imaging planes of the LV (parasternal short axis, apical four chamber, apical two chamber and parasternal long axis or apical three chamber views) are acquired both at rest and stress. Although this set of images has been proved overall to be able to detect ischaemia with very good accuracy it is well accepted that the sensitivity of the test is reduced when a small area of the heart is involved in the ischaemic process.[56] Apical foreshortening is another common problem with 2D echocardiography even by expert sonographers, particularly during stress when there is a need for rapid acquisition of images. This may lead to reduced sensitivity for detecting apical ischaemia. In addition, it is not rare peak stress images not being identical with rest images making localization of ischaemia really difficult. Theoretically all the above issues can be overcome by 3D echocardiography which offers the ability to obtain numerous tomographic views of the heart, avoid apical foreshortening and precisely match rest and stress images. What makes 3D even more appealing is that it can potentially achieve all the above with faster image acquisition compared to 2D, which may be of importance in certain forms of stress echocardiography such as treadmill exercise echocardiography.

7.2.2 Modes of Using 3D Echocardiography in Stress Echocardiography: Pros and Cons

Currently there are two main ways of applying 3D echocardiography during stress protocols: real time biplane or triplane 3D imaging and "near" real time full volume acquisition. Each one has its advantages and disadvantages. Real time biplane or triplane 3D imaging of the whole LV can be achieved in a single beat by current 3D transducers positioned in the apex of the heart with reasonable temporal and spatial resolution for imaging interpretation (Fig. 7.3). The images acquired are apical four and two chamber for biplane and apical four, two and three chamber views for triplane mode. A big advantage of this mode is that it allows capturing of all views from every single beat negating the need for summing smaller volumes from four or more beats as required for full volume mode. While this feature may be of no significant importance at rest, during stress when the heart moves really fast and also the motion of respiratory muscles is enhanced,

real time imaging allows acquisition of 3D images without "stitching" artifacts. This is particularly true when exercise protocols are used to stress the heart, where sometimes it is really difficult to acquire even single beat 2D images. Moreover, in patients with irregular rhythms such as atrial fibrillation this specific mode is clearly advantageous, since 3D full volume is practically not feasible and also 2D acquisition of different planes is achieved in different cardiac cycles which may affect image analysis and interpretation (varying cycle lengths result in varying contractile LV patterns). The big disadvantage of real time biplane or triplane 3D imaging is that wall motion analysis is limited in the two or three apical long axis planes acquired and there is no option of "cropping" the heart through multiple planes to assess subtle wall motion abnormalities. This drawback has limited the widespread use of this 3D mode during stress echocardiography. At the time of writing this chapter certain manufacturers have developed 3D transducer technology that allows full volume LV acquisition in just one beat with adequate temporal and spatial resolution for wall motion analysis, thus making 3D biplane or triplane imaging less useful in this setting. Until the widespread application of this technology however, it is reasonable to use this mode in certain forms of stress echocardiography protocols such as exercise echocardiography protocols.

Considering all the above, it is not surprising that the majority of investigators use "near" real time 3D full volume acquisition of the LV for wall motion analysis during stress protocols. The technique for acquiring this dataset is the same as described previously for dyssynchrony. However there are

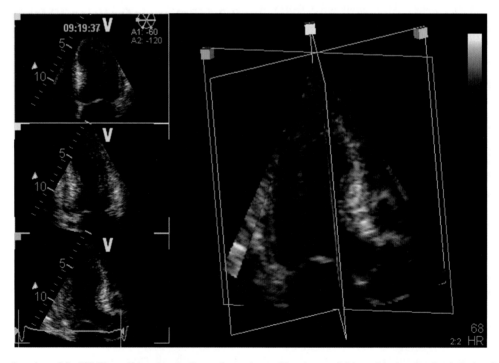

Fig. 7.3 Triplane imaging of the LV. Three dimensional echocardiography enables the acquisition of 4-chamber (top), 2-chamber (middle) and 3-chamber (bottom) views of the heart in a single beat

some important issues during 3D stress acquisition protocols that the sonographer must be aware of, otherwise the final 3D dataset may be suboptimal and sometimes even non interpretable. These issues are related to improving the spatial and temporal resolution of the acquired dataset. To optimize spatial resolution the sector angle should be narrowed, resulting in a higher line density avoiding however to exclude parts of the LV. At the same time temporal resolution as expressed by available frames per heart cycle may increase by reducing the depth size just as to include only the LV and by increasing the number of stitched volumes from 4 to 7. These actions are very important during stress protocols because available frames per heart cycle decrease with increasing heart rate and if not optimized the peak stress dataset may be insufficient for analysis due to low frame rate. Unfortunately actions taken to improve spatial resolution may worsen temporal resolution and vice versa and the best balance should be sought in each case. For example increasing the number of stitched volumes from 4 to 7 increases temporal resolution but simultaneously raises the risk of ending up with "stitching" artefacts. Similarly image-processing technique options offered by some manufacturers may improve visualization of tissue patterns, but have a negative effect on the frame rate and in general should not be used during 3D stress echocardiography analysis.[57] Some researchers also advocate acquiring a full volume 3D dataset from the parasternal long axis view in an effort to visualize better the basal segments of the LV;[58] however this increases acquisition time and it is not routine practice. Indisputably, avoidance of "stitching" artifacts is much more challenging during stress for obvious reasons and significant expertise is required by the sonographer.

Full volume 3D acquisition is deprived of many of the problems encountered with 2D (such as apical foreshortening) but its most important advantage is its unique ability to obtain unlimited views from the acquired dataset. This allows precise match of rest and stress images and also "cropping" of the LV from multiple planes enabling the physician to detect even small areas of ischaemia. Although the necessary number of planes that are required to fully assess the LV has not been defined, it has been suggested that the use of multiple (nine) short axis views of the LV from base to apex can increase the diagnostic accuracy of the method when compared to the standard practice of analysis of the three apical planes (apical two, three and four chamber views) (Fig. 7.4).[59] Moreover 3D dataset may provide additional information related to time of contraction and relaxation of various LV segments that could aid in more accurate interpretation of the stress test results.[60] The greatest problem with 3D full volume dataset which still limits its widespread use is the lower spatial and temporal resolution compared to 2D even after paying meticulous attention to all the above mentioned issues, which in part is related to the larger footprint of the 3D transducer that lowers the ability to adequately visualize all LV segment (particularly the anterior ones) due to acoustic shadowing from surrounding ribs. Good image quality is a prerequisite for stress echocardiography and thus inability to acquire adequate images with 3D may off-set all other theoretical advantages it has, compared to 2D echocardiography. It is certain that technology advances will help overcome these problems. Finally it is important to notice that there is a lack of dedicated 3D stress echocardiography analysis software which may not enable the full exploitation of 3D dataset information. Research has been recently underway towards this end and preliminary results appear promising.[61,62]

7.2.3 Feasibility of 3D Stress Echocardiography: Use of Contrast

The rate of successful visualization of LV segments with 3D compared to 2D echocardiography during stress testing has been tested in a number of studies where various stress modalities were used. As expected the majority of studies investigating feasibility of 3D stress echocardiography involved dobutamine stress protocols in order to avoid "stitching" artifacts from exercise induced hyperventilation. The three studies where a treadmill stress protocol was used demonstrated that 3D echocardiography is feasible in this setting, although not as widely applicable as 2D echocardiography.[60,63,64] Indeed, in two of these studies[60,64] 7–8% of patients were considered to have poor quality 3D images and were excluded from further analysis. In studies where dobutamine stress echocardiography protocols were used, the success visualization rate of the different LV segments was similar to that achieved by 2D, exceeding 90% in the majority of them.[65–68] In three of these studies the number of segments visualized by 2D echocardiography was higher than 3D although not statistically significant.[65–67] However in the study by Takeuchi et al[68] significant more segments were not visualized with 3D compared to 2D especially involving the anterior and lateral walls, a fact that adversely affected the diagnostic accuracy of the method as discussed subsequently in this chapter. It must be stressed that the heterogeneity noted between these studies concerning the 3D acquisition mode they used and the use or not of contrast, makes direct comparisons between them not applicable. Finally the feasibility of 3D echocardiography was tested in a small group of patients submitted to dipyridamole stress testing and the number of visualized segments was similar with both 3D and 2D echocardiography, although the authors noted that image quality was better with 2D acquisition.[69] The lower number of visualized segments with 3D imaging reported by all authors must be attributed to the lower spatial and temporal resolution of the method, the larger footprint of the 3D probe which may prevent adequate visualization of the anterior wall and to stitching artifacts during acquisition process.

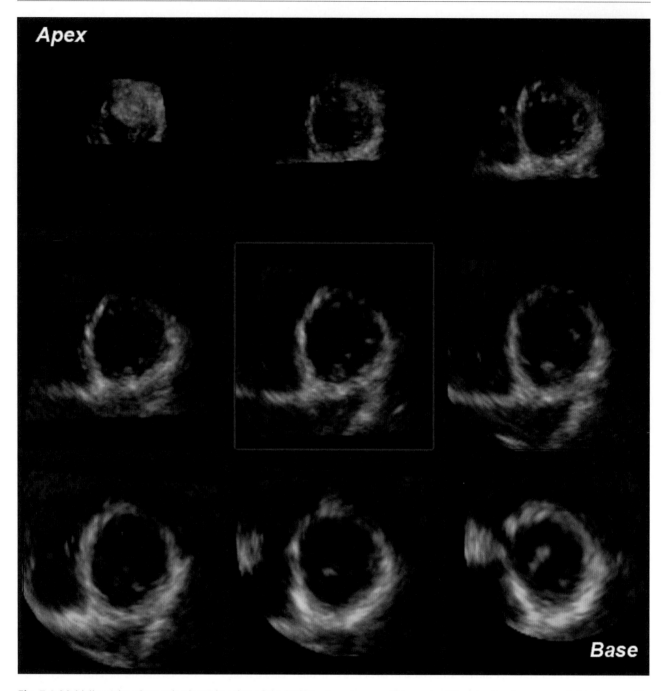

Fig. 7.4 Multislice (nine short axis views) imaging of the LV from base to apex. This mode of imaging has been suggested to increase the diagnostic accuracy of 3-D stress echocardiography when compared to the standard practice of analysis of the three apical planes

In an effort to increase the number of visualized segments with 3D stress imaging many investigators have used contrast opacification of the LV.[62,70–72] In all of these studies the number of visualized segments with 3D imaging increased significantly both at rest and stress compared to non-contrast 3D imaging. In addition, in the study by Pulerwitz et al.[70] the use of contrast during 3D imaging was able to increase the number of visualized segments to levels at or above that of 2D imaging without contrast. However, in the only study directly comparing 2D and 3D contrast stress imaging, the former performed better than the latter in terms of number of visualized segments.[68] In our opinion there are two things that are worth noting: the first one is that in the studies[62,70–72] that used contrast, the percentage of visualized segments with 3D imaging without the use of opacification was reported to be significantly lower (approximately 75%) compared to studies[65–67] that did not use contrast at all (over 90%). This finding may indicate that patients recruited in the latter studies were pre-selected to have good image quality and thus the reported success rates of LV segments visualization may not apply in everyday practice. The second thing is that although the use of contrast opacification appears very appealing it comes with the prize of further reducing the low temporal resolution of 3D imaging when the preset imaging function of power modulation (a multipulse technique whereby the acoustic amplitude of the transmitted pulses is changed) is used. Although this method improves contrast imaging quality significantly, during high heart rates it may reduce the number of frames per heart cycle to levels that are too low for diagnostic assessment. For this reason many authors recommend using only pulse inversion or second harmonic imaging with a low mechanical index when 3D contrast imaging is applied during stress echocardiography.[57] Some 3D ultrasound systems have separate LV opacification and Low MI (myocardial contrast) settings. The latter modality uses techniques like Power Modulation and consequently volume rates are significantly lower.

7.2.4 Acquisition Time

A consistent finding in all studies involving dobutamine or dipyridamole stress protocols is that 3D acquisition time from a single apical window is shorter compared to 2D acquisition of all four standard views.[65–67,69,73,74] This applies for both real time 3D biplane/triplane mode and full volume mode acquisition. In these studies mean total reported acquisition times with 3D is usually 20–40 s lower than 2D imaging. The physician has to remember however that this comes with the cost of significantly higher analysis time due to off-line generation of image planes from the acquired 3D dataset. In one study[69] estimated wall motion analysis time was 2.8 ± 0.5 min for 2D and 13 ± 7 min for 3D echocardiography. Limited data are also available for acquisition time during exercise protocols where imaging time at peak stress is of utmost importance (images must be acquired within 60 s from the end of exercise). In the study by Peteiro et al.[64] 3D volume acquisition was shorter at peak stress compared to 2D (22 ± 8 vs. 43 ± 14 s), while in the study by Jenkins et al. the superiority of 3D imaging on this specific issue was not that clear.[60]

7.2.5 Reproducibility of 3D Stress Echocardiography

Data are conflicting regarding interobserver variability in assessment of ischaemic segments when 3D stress imaging is used. In theory the precise match of rest and peak stress images and the ability to assess each segment from many different planes could result in increased interobserver

agreement on identification of ischaemic segments. Studies comparing interobserver reproducibility between 2D and 3D stress echocardiography demonstrated similar or marginally better results with 3D technology.[64,65,73,74] The reported interobserver agreement of ischaemic territories in these studies were consistently over 85% with 3D imaging. These results were not reproduced in two other studies in which the interobserver agreement of 3D imaging without the use of contrast was in the 74–76% range and increased significantly with the use of contrast (86–88%).[71,72] It must be noted that it is likely that the latter studies recruited patients with poorer echo windows and this may explain the observed difference. However since no comparison with 2D imaging was performed in these two studies direct comparison with the former ones is difficult. Irrespective of that, the results of all these studies imply that image quality is a more significant determinant of interobserver agreement of ischaemic regions compared to precise match of rest and peak stress images. Further studies are needed to examine this issue.

7.2.6 Diagnostic Accuracy of 3D Stress Echocardiography

Only a few studies involving various stress modalities and different reference standards for coronary artery disease detection have estimated the sensitivity and specificity of 3D stress echocardiography and the results are summarized in Table 7.2. In two of these studies no direct comparison with 2D stress echocardiography was performed.[59,72] In these studies specificity of 3D stress echocardiography as assessed by coronary angiogram was found to be high (95% and 88% respectively); in contrast sensitivity was found to be lower in the study by Krenning et al.[72] (61%) compared to Yoshitani et al.[59] (72%). This observed difference may be attributed to the high proportion of beta blocker therapy (60%) in the former study which adversely affects the sensitivity of dobutamine stress echocardiography. Unfortunately the absence of 2D stress echocardiography data makes impossible to evaluate this assumption.

Perhaps the most important question that must be answered before the widespread clinical application of 3D stress echocardiography is how it performs compared to 2D stress echocardiography in terms of sensitivity and specificity in detecting coronary artery disease. To our best of our knowledge seven studies have addressed this specific issue (Table 7.2). Two of them have used treadmill exercise test as the stress modality and subsequent angiogram as the reference standard (luminal narrowing >70% was considered abnormal). The results of these studies are contradictory. Peteiro et al.[64] reported reasonable sensitivity (78%) and

Table 7.2 Reported sensitivity and specificity of 3D stress echocardiography in various studies

First author	Number of patients	3D mode	Stress modality	Reference standard	3D Sensitivity (%)	3D Specificity (%)	2D Sensitivity (%)	2D Specificity (%)
Ahmad[73]	90	Full volume	Dobut	Angio (>50%)	88	88	79	81
Matsumura[66]	56	Full volume	Dobut	Exercise Tl SPECT	86	80	86	83
Eroglu[67]	36	Triplane	Dobut	Angio (>50%)	93	75	93	75
Takeuchi[68,a]	78	Full volume	Dobut	2D echo	58	75	Reference method	Reference method
Aggeli[74,a]	56	Full volume	Dobut	Angio (>50%)	78	89	73	93
Peteiro[64]	84	Full volume	Treadmill	Angio (>70%)	78	73	84	76
Krenning[72,a]	45	Full volume	Dobut	Angio (>50%)	61	88	NA	NA
Jenkins[60]	90	Full volume	Treadmill	Angio (>70%)	40	65	83	78
Yoshitani[59]	71	Full volume (multislice)	Dobut	Angio (>50%)	72	95	NA	NA

Dobut dobutamine, *Angio* angiogram.
[a]Contrast opacification was used in all patients.

specificity (73%) of 3D stress echocardiography compared to 2D stress imaging (84% and 76% respectively) while Jenkins et al.[60] found significantly lower sensitivity of 3D compared to 2D stress echocardiography (40% vs. 83%). This difference may be explained by the fact that in the latter Exercise Echo study, 3D acquisition was performed after 2D imaging and this may have allowed time for wall motion abnormalities to resolve (the mean time from the end of exercise until the end of 3D echocardiography was 109 ± 55 s). In contrast in the study by Peteiro et al.[64] exercise 2D and 3D imaging were performed on separate days within 1 week in a random order. In both of these studies however 3D could not demonstrate any additional benefit compared to 2D stress imaging, suggesting that in this setting is still insufficient for clinical use.

The remaining five studies involved patients submitted to dobutamine stress echocardiography. In three of them coronary angiography (luminal narrowing >50% was defined as abnormal) was used as a reference standard for detection of CAD[67,73,74] while in the other two exercise thallium SPECT[66] and 2D stress echocardiography[68] were used for this reason. In four of these studies, 3D reported sensitivity and specificity were similar or slightly better than 2D stress imaging.[66,67,73,74] Interestingly Aggeli et al.[74] suggested that this trend for slight superiority of 3D stress imaging is likely due to the lack of apical foreshortening compared to 2D. This is based on their finding that regional apical wall motion scores were higher with 3D imaging. In contrast, Takeuchi et al[68] reported poor apical endocardial border delineation with contrast as a result of increased bubble destruction caused by the 3D matrix transducer. In their study using 2D stress imaging results as the reference standard they found low sensitivity (58%) of 3D stress echocardiography for detection of CAD. This finding was attributed to the lower temporal and spatial

resolution of 3D imaging, as well as to the large footprint of the 3D transducer which resulted in inadequate fitting in the intercostal space in some patients and lateral wall dropout. Although data from 3D stress imaging appear more promising when dobutamine is used as the stress modality, further studies need to be undertaken that will test its additional value before it can be widely applied in clinical practice.

7.2.7 Conclusions: Future Directions

Three-dimensional stress echocardiography has the potential to overcome many of the problems encountered with 2D imaging such as apical foreshortening, limited views to analyze and qualitative assessment of wall motion and thickening. Current technology however limits its use because of problems related to inferior image quality compared to 2D echocardiography. As a result there are no data to date that demonstrate clear superiority of this new technology compared to standard practice for detection of reversible ischaemia. Moreover, there are no studies testing 3D stress imaging ability for detection of viable myocardium. Despite all these, it is our strong belief that in the near future technologic developments will result in smaller transducer size and acquisition of full volume datasets with adequate temporal and spatial resolution in just one beat. This will offset many of the problems seen today with the use of 3D stress echocardiography and will allow this new technology to be applied in more heterogeneous patient populations. Moreover the development of dedicated 3D stress analysis software and the application of quantitative analysis of 3D stress datasets will potentially increase interobserver agreement for detection of CAD and make stress echocardiography a more robust and reliable tool for this reason. 3D Stress echocardiography needs to move beyond the point of creating 2D images from 3D datasets to one where the power of 3D is harnessed in terms of assessing LV volumes, ejection fraction, dyssynchrony and contraction front mapping during stress. These approaches should make the technique more robust, and less subjective. It should also shorten the learning curve for stress echocardiography.

7.3 Three-Dimensional Speckle Tracking

7.3.1 Theoretical Advantages and Limitations of 3D Compared to 2D Speckle Tracking

Speckle Tracking (ST) is an echocardiographic method that tracks the movement of natural acoustic markers (speckles) in gray scale echocardiographic images from frame to frame. The speckles are the result of scattering, reflection and interference of the ultrasound beam in myocardial tissue.[75] Automated measurement of distance between speckles enables calculation of angle-independent strain (a measure of deformation of a specific myocardial region) which is the big advantage of this technique over TDI, which is angle dependent. This allows measurement of longitudinal strain from the apical LV areas, and circumferential and radial strain from LV short axis views.[76] These unique features of ST have attracted the attention of investigators who have applied this technique to 2D images and found it to be a useful tool for understanding of LV function,[77] measurement of LV volumes[78] and assessment of dyssynchrony.[79] Although 2D ST is devoid of many of the limitations of TDI it still is an imperfect tool for assessing LV function. This is mainly because it follows speckles in 2D planes, while in reality the myocardial regions represented by speckle patterns move in 3D space; thus only

a portion of the real motion can be detected. The ability to acquire 3D full volume datasets led to the development of 3D ST software which assess the real movement of speckles in 3D space and not just in a 2D plane (Fig. 7.5).[80] Interestingly, the high frame rate which is considered to be a prerequisite for 2D ST is not necessarily a limiting factor for 3D ST. The reason for this is that the 3D dataset encompasses the total area in which the speckles can move. The danger encountered with 2D ST that with low frame rate the speckle will move out of the 2D plane does not apply with 3D ST.[80] The main current limitation of 3D ST is that it is highly dependent on the quality of 3D dataset images and particularly the endocardial definition and therefore in patients with inadequate image quality the derived results may be misleading. Moreover, at the time of writing of this book there was only one commercial 3D ST system available with limited validation data. Obviously better validation of the new technique is needed before its application in everyday clinical practice.

7.3.2 How to Perform 3D Speckle Tracking

A full volume 3D dataset from the apical window must be acquired as already described with special attention to achieve optimal endocardial visualization. Frame rates of between 15 and 30 Hz have been used in different studies with satisfying results. With the software currently in use, endocardial and epicardial contours are manually traced in the four, two and three chamber views. The 3D and 2D images of the LV wall are automatically divided into 16 segments. Then, the 3D endocardial surface is automatically reconstructed and tracked in 3D throughout the cardiac cycle in three different vectors simultaneously to calculate each strain data. The strains are measured by calculating the mean value in each segment.

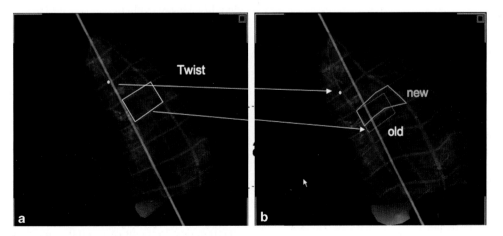

Fig. 7.5 Three-dimensional Speckle Tracking. An area of interest is shown highlighted at end-systole (**a**) and end-diastole (**b**). From this, data can simultaneously be derived on longitudinal, radial and circumferential deformation as well as left ventricular torsion. (Image courtesy of TomTec Imaging Systems GmbH, Germany)

7.3.3 Existing Data: Reproducibility of the Method

Although 3D ST appears very promising for assessment of LV function, limited data exist so far testing this new technique. Nesser et al.[81] tested the accuracy of 3D versus 2D ST for LV volume measurements in a small group of 43 patients using cardiac magnetic resonance as the reference technique. LV volumes were calculated by counting the number of voxels inside a manually traced endocardial surface during the different phases of the cardiac cycle. Although both 2D and 3D ST correlated well with cardiac magnetic resonance, the inter- and intra- observer variability was lower and also less spread in measurements were obtained with 3D ST. The authors concluded that 3D ST may be a more accurate and reproducible technique for assessment of LV volumes compared to previously used 2D ST. Two other studies have tested the ability of 3D ST to evaluate left ventricular strain by comparing it with 2D ST.[82,83] Although the reported results concerning 3D strain values were not similar, both studies agreed that 3D ST is faster than 2D ST for strain analysis (both image acquisition and offline analysis were significantly shorter with 3D ST). The inter- and intra-observer reproducibility of 3D ST strain measurements was found to be very good in these studies. Moreover, in the study by Pérez de Isla et al.[82] a greater number of segments could be analyzed with 3D compared to 2D ST. It is clear that more studies are needed to further validate this new technique, define normal values for strain measurements, evaluate its usefulness in other clinical settings (such as dyssynchrony) and test its reliability in patients with suboptimal image quality.

7.3.4 Conclusions: Future Directions

Three dimensional ST appears to be a promising tool for a more objective quantification of left ventricular volumes and function. In addition, it has the theoretical potential to offer new insights into left ventricular mechanics by providing 3D strain and dyssynchrony data. However since this technique has only just started to be evaluated, all these theoretical advantages must be proved first in practice before it can become a useful clinical tool for everyday use. It is our belief that the two main problems of 3D ST, i.e. low temporal resolution and random noise that affects the ability to track speckles will be overcome as 3D technology advances. We expect in the near future that this 3D imaging technique will grow up and ultimately become a reliable method for quantitative LV assessment.

7.4 Assessment of Myocardial Perfusion Using 3D Echocardiography

7.4.1 Theoretical Advantages of 3D Compared to 2D Echocardiography for Assessment of Myocardial Perfusion

Many authors have demonstrated the feasibility of 2D contrast echocardiography for myocardial perfusion imaging. This method utilizes gas-filled microbubbles (contrast) that have the ability to remain entirely within the vascular space just like red cells. If a contrast agent is infused at a constant rate, after a while a steady state is attained in the myocardial micro-circulation. By applying high energy ultrasound the microbubbles are destroyed and the rate of microbubble replenishment within the ultrasound beam is measured. In this way both qualitative and quantitative analysis of myocardial perfusion can be achieved.[84] With 2D imaging usually three planes (apical two, three and four chamber views) are used in an effort to assess perfusion in all LV walls. Although this technique provides important information about myocardial micro-circulation it has not become part of the routine assessment of ischemic heart disease. One of the main reasons for this is that the extent of a perfusion defect cannot be accurately assessed from a few slices of the heart. Moreover 2D perfusion imaging acquisition and interpretation requires significant experience. Indeed, slight changes of the position of the transducer during image acquisition can create erroneous results. This is because bubble destruction with high energy ultrasound occurs in just one plane which must remain the same during the whole process. In addition drop-out artifacts are commonly seen with contrast and the examiner must be able to recognize them to avoid giving false positive results. Theoretically 3D perfusion imaging is devoid of the above limitations of 2D echocardiography (except from drop-out artifacts) and could potentially become a robust technique for the assessment of myocardial perfusion.

7.4.2 Weight of Evidence for 3D Myocardial Perfusion: Limitations to Overcome

The basic conditions that have to be fulfilled before 3D echocardiography can be applied to clinical practice are: acquisition of the whole LV in a single beat with reasonable spatial and temporal resolution, a technique to destroy contrast in the myocardium during "flash imaging," finding of a proper contrast injection method for 3D perfusion imaging, development of a reliable method for volumetric quantification of myocardial perfusion and finally studies demonstrating the accuracy of this new technique when compared to other reference perfusion techniques.

Newer generation echo machines now have the ability to obtain a full LV volume 3D dataset in one cardiac cycle. However, the spatial and temporal resolution is not yet optimal, particularly in the setting of contrast infusion which as already stated can have a negative effect in the number of frame rates acquired per cardiac cycle. Although at the time of writing this chapter this limitation is a significant obstacle for application of 3D myocardial perfusion echocardiography in clinical practice, it is very likely that this will be overcome as technology progresses. It must be emphasized that the few studies testing 3D myocardial perfusion in humans have used only partial volumes of the LV for the analysis.[85,86]

Another issue that is still to be investigated is the development of the most appropriate contrast technology that should be used to assess 3D myocardial perfusion. The standard technique utilized with 2D perfusion imaging, i.e., high energy ultrasound pulses (Flash imaging) after a steady state of microbubbles in the myocardium has been achieved, is difficult to be used with 3D echocardiography because of the great amount of energy required to destroy all the bubbles in the whole heart. Furthermore, the use of stitched full volume datasets acquired over multiple cardiac cycles precludes the use of Flash Imaging techniques. The alternative option of using boluses of contrast is not ideal due to the need to guess a priori the optimal imaging settings for best visualization of myocardial perfusion.[87] In an effort to overcome all these difficulties Toledo et al.[85] proposed a transient contrast inflow maneuver that includes optimization of contrast infusion rate and imaging settings during steady state enhancement, infusion interruption to allow contrast clearance and resumption of contrast infusion, resulting in contrast inflow. With this protocol, image acquisition starts approximately five seconds before resumption of contrast infusion in order to capture the transition of non-contrast to reinstated steady–state enhancement. The authors tested this protocol in 8 normal volunteers and found that contrast replenishment occurred in all subjects within <45 s, and was captured in a single acquisition.

Regarding the issue of volumetric quantification of 3D myocardial perfusion in humans, preliminary data have been published which appear promising. These studies apply manually or semi-automated algorithms for defining 3D regions of interest from which calculation of mean myocardial video-intensity can be made.[85,86] However, these data come from analysis of small portions of the LV and it is not established that they will necessarily work for the full volume LV data set. Moreover these studies included only normal subjects and application of these volumetric techniques

in patients with perfusion defects and validation against other reference methods is mandatory.

So far validation data of 3D myocardial perfusion echocardiography against reference techniques come from animal studies. These studies using different methodologies concerning 3D data acquisition and contrast infusion have demonstrated the feasibility of 3D perfusion imaging and also found a very good correlation between the amount of underperfused myocardium estimated by 3D and the extent of underperfusion from postmortem anatomical specimens.[85,88–92] Obviously more data are needed validating the technique in humans.

7.4.3 Conclusions: Future Directions

It is evident from existing data that there is a long way before 3D myocardial perfusion imaging can become a standard tool in everyday clinical practice. The reason for this is that there are limitations not only related to technological restrictions (which will likely be overcome with 3D probe technology advances) but also to development of optimal ways of contrast infusion and 3D volumetric perfusion quantification. Slow steps have been made up to date to solve these problems. Therefore, we believe that extensive research is needed in the above mentioned fields in order to develop a robust technique that performs well against competing imaging modalities. If not, 3D myocardial perfusion imaging will end up being used by a few dedicated and highly specialized in 3D echocardiography centers and it will never get the widespread clinical application it deserves.

References

1. Leclercq C, Hare JM. Ventricular resynchronization: current state of the art. *Circulation.* 2004;109:296–299.
2. Liu L, Tockman B, Girouard S, et al. Left ventricular resynchronization therapy in a canine model of left bundle branch block. *Am J Physiol Heart Circ Physiol.* 2002;282:H2238–H2244.
3. Nelson GS, Curry CW, Wyman BT, et al. Predictors of systolic augmentation from left ventricular preexcitation in patients with dilated cardiomyopathy and intraventricular conduction delay. *Circulation.* 2000;101:2703–2709.
4. Cazeau S, Leclercq C, Lavergne T, et al; Multisite Stimulation in Cardiomyopathies (MUSTIC) Study Investigators. Effects of multisite biventricular pacing in patients with heart failure and intraventricular conduction delay. *N Engl J Med* 2001;345:293–294.
5. Abraham WT, Fisher WG, Smith AL, et al; MIRACLE Study Group. Multicenter InSync Randomized Clinical Evaluation. Cardiac resynchronization in chronic heart failure. *N Engl J Med.* 2002;346:1845–1853.

6. Auricchio A, Stellbrink C, Sack S, et al; Pacing Therapies in Congestive Heart Failure (PATH-CHF) Study Group. Long-term clinical effect of hemodynamically optimized cardiac resynchronization therapy in patients with heart failure and ventricular conduction delay. *J Am Coll Cardiol*. 2002;39:2026–2033.

7. Young JB, Abraham WT, Smith AL, et al; Multicenter InSync ICD Randomized Clinical Evaluation (MIRACLE ICD) Trial Investigators. Combined cardiac resynchronization and implantable cardioversion defibrillation in advanced chronic heart failure: the MIRACLE ICD trial. *JAMA*. 2003;289:2685–2694.

8. Bristow MR, Saxon LA, Boehmer J, et al; Comparison of Medical Therapy, Pacing, and Defibrillation in Heart Failure (COMPANION) Investigators. Cardiac-resynchronization therapy with or without an implantable defibrillator in advanced chronic heart failure. *N Engl J Med*. 2004;350:2140–2150.

9. Cleland JG, Daubert JC, Erdmann E, et al; Cardiac Resynchronization-Heart Failure (CARE-HF) Study Investigators. The effect of cardiac resynchronization on morbidity and mortality in heart failure. *N Engl J Med*. 2005;352:1539–1549.

10. Kass DA. Predicting cardiac resynchronization response by QRS duration: the long and short of it. *J Am Coll Cardiol*. 2003;42:2125–2127.

11. Auricchio A, Fantoni C, Regoli F, et al. Characterization of left ventricular activation in patients with heart failure and left bundle-branch block. *Circulation*. 2004;109:1133–1139.

12. Fung JW, Yu CM, Yip G, et al. Variable left ventricular activation pattern in patients with heart failure and left bundle branch block. *Heart*. 2004;90:17–19.

13. Achilli A, Sassara M, Ficili S, et al. Long-term effectiveness of cardiac resynchronization therapy in patients with refractory heart failure and "narrow" QRS. *J Am Coll Cardiol*. 2003;42:2117–2124.

14. Kapetanakis S, Bhan A, Monaghan MJ. Echo determinants of dyssynchrony (atrioventricular and inter- and intraventricular) and predictors of response to cardiac resynchronization therapy. *Echocardiography*. 2008;25:1020–1030.

15. Pitzalis MV, Iacoviello M, Romito R, et al. Cardiac resynchronization therapy tailored by echocardiographic evaluation of ventricular asynchrony. *J Am Coll Cardiol*. 2002;40:1615–1622.

16. Breithardt OA, Stellbrink C, Kramer AP, et al; PATH-CHF Study Group. Pacing Therapies for Congestive Heart Failure. Echocardiographic quantification of left ventricular asynchrony predicts an acute hemodynamic benefit of cardiac resynchronization therapy. *J Am Coll Cardiol*. 2002;40:536–545.

17. Cazeau S, Bordachar P, Jauvert G, et al. Echocardiographic modeling of cardiac dyssynchrony before and during multisite stimulation: a prospective study. *Pacing Clin Electrophysiol*. 2003;26: 137–143.

18. Søgaard P, Egeblad H, Kim WY, et al. Tissue Doppler imaging predicts improved systolic performance and reversed left ventricular remodeling during long-term cardiac resynchronization therapy. *J Am Coll Cardiol*. 2002;40:723–730.

19. Bax JJ, Bleeker GB, Marwick TH, et al. Left ventricular dyssynchrony predicts response and prognosis after cardiac resynchronization therapy. *J Am Coll Cardiol*. 2004;44:1834–1840.

20. Yu CM, Fung WH, Lin H, Zhang Q, Sanderson JE, Lau CP. Predictors of left ventricular reverse remodeling after cardiac resynchronization therapy for heart failure secondary to idiopathic dilated or ischemic cardiomyopathy. *Am J Cardiol*. 2003;91:684–688.

21. Yu CM, Fung JW, Zhang Q, et al. Tissue Doppler imaging is superior to strain rate imaging and postsystolic shortening on the prediction of reverse remodeling in both ischemic and nonischemic heart failure after cardiac resynchronization therapy. *Circulation*. 2004;110:66–73.

22. Chung ES, Leon AR, Tavazzi L, et al. Results of the Predictors of Response to CRT (PROSPECT) trial. *Circulation*. 2008;117: 2608–2616.

23. Kapetanakis S, Kearney MT, Siva A, Gall N, Cooklin M, Monaghan MJ. Real-time three-dimensional echocardiography: a novel technique to quantify global left ventricular mechanical dyssynchrony. *Circulation*. 2005;112:992–1000.

24. Cerqueira MD, Weissman NJ, Dilsizian V, et al. Standardized myocardial segmentation and nomenclature for tomographic imaging of the heart: a statement for healthcare professionals from the Cardiac Imaging Committee of the Council on Clinical Cardiology of the American Heart Association. *Circulation*. 2002;105:539–542.

25. Zeng X, Shu XH, Pan CZ, et al. Assessment of left ventricular systolic synchronicity by real-time three-dimensional echocardiography in patients with dilated cardiomyopathy. *Chin Med J (Engl)*. 2006;119:919–924.

26. Brunekreeft JA, Graauw M, de Milliano PA, Keijer JT. Influence of left bundle branch block on left ventricular volumes, ejection fraction and regional wall motion. *Neth Heart J*. 2007;15:89–94.

27. Baker GH, Hlavacek AM, Chessa KS, Fleming DM, Shirali GS. Left ventricular dysfunction is associated with intraventricular dyssynchrony by 3-dimensional echocardiography in children. *J Am Soc Echocardiogr*. 2008;21:230–233.

28. De Castro S, Faletra F, Di Angelantonio E, et al. Tomographic left ventricular volumetric emptying analysis by real-time 3-dimensional echocardiography: influence of left ventricular dysfunction with and without electrical dyssynchrony. *Circulation: Cardiovasc Imag*. 2008;1:40–48.

29. Delgado V, Sitges M, Vidal B, et al. Assessment of left ventricular dyssynchrony by real-time three-dimensional echocardiography. *Rev Esp Cardiol*. 2008;61:825–834.

30. Gimenes VM, Vieira ML, Andrade MM, Pinheiro J Jr, Hotta VT, Mathias W Jr. Standard values for real-time transthoracic three-dimensional echocardiographic dyssynchrony indexes in a normal population. *J Am Soc Echocardiogr*. 2008;21:1229–1235.

31. Liu WH, Chen MC, Chen YL, et al. Right ventricular apical pacing acutely impairs left ventricular function and induces mechanical dyssynchrony in patients with sick sinus syndrome: a real-time three-dimensional echocardiographic study. *J Am Soc Echocardiogr*. 2008;21:224–229.

32. Migrino R, Harmann L, Woods T, Bright M, Truran S, Hari P. Intraventricular dyssynchrony in light chain amyloidosis: a new mechanism of systolic dysfunction assessed by 3-dimensional echocardiography. *Cardiovasc Ultrasound*. 2008;6:40.

33. van Dijk J, Dijkmans PA, Götte MJ, Spreeuwenberg MD, Visser CA, Kamp O. Evaluation of global left ventricular function and mechanical dyssynchrony in patients with an asymptomatic left bundle branch block: a real-time 3D echocardiography study. *Eur J Echocardiogr*. 2008;9:40–46.

34. Conca C, Faletra FF, Miyazaki C, et al. Echocardiographic parameters of mechanical synchrony in healthy individuals. *Am J Cardiol*. 2009;103:136–142.

35. Liodakis E, Al Sharef O, Dawson D, Nihoyannopoulos P. The use of real time three dimensional echocardiography for assessing mechanical synchronicity. *Heart* 2009 May 25. [Epub ahead of print]

36. Raedle-Hurst TM, Mueller M, Rentzsch A, Schaefers HJ, Herrmann E, Abdul-Khaliq H. Assessment of left ventricular dyssynchrony and function using real-time 3-dimensional echocardiography in patients with congenital right heart disease. *Am Heart J*. 2009; 157:791–798.

37. Soliman OI, van Dalen BM, Nemes A, et al. Quantification of left ventricular systolic dyssynchrony by real-time three-dimensional echocardiography. *J Am Soc Echocardiogr*. 2009;22:232–239.

38. Sonne C, Sugeng L, Takeuchi M, et al. Real-time 3-dimensional echocardiographic assessment of left ventricular dyssynchrony: pitfalls in patients with dilated cardiomyopathy. *JACC Cardiovasc Imaging*. 2009;2:802–812.

39. Ten Harkel AD, Van Osch-Gevers M, Helbing WA. Real-time transthoracic three dimensional echocardiography: normal reference data for left ventricular dyssynchrony in adolescents. *J Am Soc Echocardiogr*. 2009;22:933–938.

40. Marsan NA, Bleeker GB, Ypenburg C, et al. Real-time three-dimensional echocardiography permits quantification of left ventricular mechanical dyssynchrony and predicts acute response to cardiac resynchronization therapy. *J Cardiovasc Electrophysiol.* 2008;19:392–399.

41. Marsan NA, Henneman MM, Chen J, et al. Real-time three-dimensional echocardiography as a novel approach to quantify left ventricular dyssynchrony: a comparison study with phase analysis of gated myocardial perfusion single photon emission computed tomography. *J Am Soc Echocardiogr.* 2008;21:801–807.

42. Marsan NA, Bleeker GB, Ypenburg C, et al. Real-time three-dimensional echocardiography as a novel approach to assess left ventricular and left atrium reverse remodeling and to predict response to cardiac resynchronization therapy. *Heart Rhythm.* 2008;5:1257–1264.

43. Vieira ML, Cury AF, Gustavo N, et al. Ventricular dyssynchrony index: comparison with two-dimensional and three-dimensional ejection fraction. *Arq Bras Cardiol.* 2008;91:142–147, 156–162.

44. Kleijn SA, van Dijk J, de Cock CC, et al. Assessment of intraventricular mechanical dyssynchrony and prediction of response to cardiac resynchronization therapy: comparison between tissue Doppler imaging and real-time three-dimensional echocardiography. *J Am Soc Echocardiogr.* 2009 Jul 30. [Epub ahead of print]

45. Soliman OI, Geleijnse ML, Theuns DA, et al. Usefulness of left ventricular systolic dyssynchrony by real-time three-dimensional echocardiography to predict long-term response to cardiac resynchronization therapy. *Am J Cardiol.* 2009;103:1586–1591.

46. Faletra FF, Conca C, Klersy C, et al. Comparison of eight echocardiographic methods for determining the prevalence of mechanical dyssynchrony and site of latest mechanical contraction in patients scheduled for cardiac resynchronization therapy. *Am J Cardiol.* 2009;103:1746–1752.

47. Deplagne A, Bordachar P, Reant P, et al. Additional value of three-dimensional echocardiography in patients with cardiac resynchronization therapy. *Arch Cardiovasc Dis.* 2009;102:497–508.

48. Henneman MM, Chen J, Dibbets P, et al. Can LV dyssynchrony as assessed with phase analysis on gated myocardial perfusion SPECT predict response to CRT? *J Nucl Med.* 2007;48:1104–1111.

49. Bilchick KC, Dimaano V, Wu KC, et al. Cardiac magnetic resonance assessment of dyssynchrony and myocardial scar predicts function class improvement following cardiac resynchronization therapy. *JACC Cardiovasc Imaging.* 2008;1:561–568.

50. Takeuchi M, Jacobs A, Sugeng L, et al. Assessment of left ventricular dyssynchrony with real-time 3-dimensional echocardiography: comparison with Doppler tissue imaging. *J Am Soc Echocardiogr.* 2007;20:1321–1329.

51. Burgess MI, Jenkins C, Chan J, Marwick TH. Measurement of left ventricular dyssynchrony in patients with ischaemic cardiomyopathy: a comparison of real-time three-dimensional and tissue Doppler echocardiography. *Heart.* 2007;93:1191–1196.

52. Ypenburg C, van Bommel RJ, Delgado V, et al. Optimal left ventricular lead position predicts reverse remodeling and survival after cardiac resynchronization therapy. *J Am Coll Cardiol.* 2008;52:1402–1409.

53. Butter C, Auricchio A, Stellbrink C, et al. Effect of resynchronization therapy stimulation site on the systolic function of heart failure patients. *Circulation.* 2001;104:3026–3029.

54. Van de Veire NR, Yu CM, et al. Triplane tissue Doppler imaging: a novel three-dimensional imaging modality that predicts reverse left ventricular remodelling after cardiac resynchronisation therapy. *Heart.* 2008;94:e9.

55. Marwick T. Stress Echocardiography – Its Role in the Diagnosis and Evaluation of Coronary Artery Disease. 2nd ed. Boston: Kluwer Academic Publishers; 2003.

56. Pellikka PA, Nagueh SF, Elhendy AA, et al. Stress echocardiography: recommendations for performance, interpretation and application. *J Am Soc Echocardiogr.* 2007;20:1021–1034.

57. Krenning BJ, Vletter WB, Nemes A, et al. Real-time 3-dimensional contrast stress echocardiography: a bridge too far? *J Am Soc Echocardiogr.* 2007;20:1224–1225.

58. Nemes A, Geleijnse ML, Vletter WB, et al. Role of parasternal data acquisition during contrast enhanced real-time three-dimensional echocardiography. *Echocardiography.* 2007;24:1081–1085.

59. Yoshitani H, Takeuchi M, Mor-Avi V, Otsuji Y, Hozumi T, Yoshiyama M. Comparative diagnostic accuracy of multiplane and multislice three-dimensional dobutamine stress echocardiography in the diagnosis of coronary artery disease. *J Am Soc Echocardiogr.* 2009;22:437–442.

60. Jenkins C, Haluska B, Marwick TH. Assessment of temporal heterogeneity and regional motion to identify wall motion abnormalities using treadmill exercise stress three-dimensional echocardiography. *J Am Soc Echocardiogr.* 2009;22:268–275.

61. Walimbe V, Lalude O, Garcia M, et al. Quantitative real-time 3-dimensional stress echocardiography: a preliminary investigation of feasibility and effectiveness. *J Am Soc Echocardiogr.* 2007;20:13–22.

62. Nemes A, Leung KY, van Burken G, et al. Side-by-side viewing of anatomically aligned left ventricular segments in three-dimensional stress echocardiography. *Echocardiography.* 2009;26:189–195.

63. Zwas DR, Takuma S, Mullis-Jansson S, et al. Feasibility of real-time 3-dimensional treadmill stress echocardiography. *J Am Soc Echocardiogr.* 1999;12:285–289.

64. Peteiro J, Pinon P, Perez R, et al. Comparison of 2- and 3-dimensional exercise echocardiography for the detection of coronary artery disease. *J Am Soc Echocardiogr.* 2007;20:959–967.

65. Yang HS, Pellikka PA, McCully RB, et al. Role of biplane and biplane echocardiographically guided 3-dimensional echocardiography during dobutamine stress echocardiography. *J Am Soc Echocardiogr.* 2006;19:1136–1143.

66. Matsumura Y, Hozumi T, Arai K, et al. Noninvasive assessment of myocardial ischaemia using new real-time three-dimensional dobutamine stress echocardiography: comparison with conventional two-dimensional methods. *Eur Heart J.* 2005; 26:1625–1632.

67. Eroglu E, D'hooge J, Herbots L, et al. Comparison of real-time triplane and conventional 2D dobutamine stress echocardiography for the assessment of coronary artery disease. *Eur Heart J.* 2006; 27:1719–1724.

68. Takeuchi M, Otani S, Weinert L, et al. Comparison of contrast-enhanced realtime live 3-dimensional dobutamine stress echocardiography with contrast 2-dimensional echocardiography for detecting stress-induced wall-motion abnormalities. *J Am Soc Echocardiogr.* 2006;19:294–299.

69. Varnero S, Santagata P, Pratali L, et al. Head to head comparison of 2D vs. 3D dipyridamole stress echocardiography. *Cardiovasc Ultrasound.* 2008;6:31.

70. Pulerwitz T, Hirata K, Abe Y, et al. Feasibility of using a real-time 3-dimensional technique for contrast dobutamine stress echocardiography. *J Am Soc Echocardiogr.* 2006;19:540–545.

71. Nemes A, Geleijnse ML, Krenning BJ, et al. Usefulness of ultrasound contrast agent to improve image quality during real-time three-dimensional stress echocardiography. *Am J Cardiol.* 2007; 99:275–278.

72. Krenning BJ, Nemes A, Soliman OI, et al. Contrast-enhanced three-dimensional dobutamine stress echocardiography: between Scylla and Charybdis? *Eur J Echocardiogr.* 2008;9:757–760.

73. Ahmad M, Xie T, McCulloch M, et al. Real-time three-dimensional dobutamine stress echocardiography in assessment of ischemia: comparison with two-dimensional dobutamine stress echocardiography. *J Am Coll Cardiol.* 2001;37:1303–1309.

74. Aggeli C, Giannopoulos G, Misovoulos P, et al. Real-time three-dimensional dobutamine stress echocardiography for coronary artery disease diagnosis: validation with coronary angiography. *Heart.* 2007;93:672–675.

75. Bohs LN, Trahey GE. A novel method for angle independent ultrasonic imaging of blood flow and tissue motion. *IEEE Trans Biomed Eng*. 1991;38:280–286.

76. Amundsen BH, Helle-Valle T, Edvardsen T, et al. Noninvasive myocardial strain measurement by speckle tracking echocardiography: validation against sonomicrometry and tagged magnetic resonance imaging. *J Am Coll Cardiol*. 2006;47:789–793.

77. Notomi Y, Lysyansky P, Setser RM, et al. Measurement of ventricular torsion by two-dimensional ultrasound speckle tracking imaging. *J Am Coll Cardiol*. 2005;45:2034–2041.

78. Nishikage T, Nakai H, Mor-Avi V, et al. Quantitative assessment of left ventricular volume and ejection fraction using two-dimensional speckle tracking echocardiography. *Eur J Echocardiogr*. 2009;10:82–88.

79. Suffoletto MS, Dohi K, Cannesson M, Saba S, Gorcsan J 3rd. Novel speckle-tracking radial strain from routine black-and-white echocardiographic images to quantify dyssynchrony and predict response to cardiac resynchronization therapy. *Circulation*. 2006;113:960–968.

80. Pérez de Isla L, Vivas D, Zamorano J. Three-dimensional speckle tracking. *Echocardiography*. 2008;1:25–29.

81. Nesser HJ, Mor-Avi V, Gorissen W, et al. Quantification of left ventricular volumes using three-dimensional echocardiographic speckle tracking: comparison with MRI. *Eur Heart J*. 2009;30:1565–1573.

82. Pérez de Isla L, Balcones DV, Fernández-Golfín C, et al. Three-dimensional-wall motion tracking: a new and faster tool for myocardial strain assessment: comparison with two-dimensional-wall motion tracking. *J Am Soc Echocardiogr*. 2009;22:325–330.

83. Saito K, Okura H, Watanabe N, et al. Comprehensive evaluation of left ventricular strain using speckle tracking echocardiography in normal adults: comparison of three-dimensional and two-dimensional approaches. *J Am Soc Echocardiogr*. 2009 Jun 23. [Epub ahead of print]

84. Lepper W, Belcik T, Wei K, Lindner JR, Sklenar J, Kaul S. Myocardial contrast echocardiography. *Circulation*. 2004;109:3132–3135.

85. Toledo E, Lang RM, Collins KA, et al. Imaging and quantification of myocardial perfusion using real-time three-dimensional echocardiography. *J Am Coll Cardiol*. 2006;47:146–154.

86. Veronesi F, Caiani EG, Toledo E, et al. Semi-automated analysis of dynamic changes in myocardial contrast from real-time three-dimensional echocardiographic images as a basis for volumetric quantification of myocardial perfusion. *Eur J Echocardiogr*. 2009;10:485–490.

87. Badano LP. Contrast enhanced real-time three-dimensional echocardiography for quantification of myocardial perfusion: a step forward. *Eur J Echocardiogr*. 2009;10:465–466.

88. Bae RY, Belohlavek M, Tanabe K, Greenleaf JF, Seward JB. Rapid three-dimensional myocardial contrast echocardiography: volumetric quantitation of nonperfused myocardium after intravenous contrast administration. *Echocardiography*. 1999;16:357–365.

89. Yao J, De Castro S, Delabays A, Masani N, Udelson JE, Pandian NG. Bulls-eye display and quantitation of myocardial perfusion defects using three-dimensional contrast echocardiography. *Echocardiography*. 2001;18:581–588.

90. Camarano G, Jones M, Freidlin RZ, Panza JA. Quantitative assessment of left ventricular perfusion defects using real-time three-dimensional myocardial contrast echocardiography. *J Am Soc Echocardiogr*. 2002;15:206–213.

91. Chen LX, Wang XF, Nanda NC, et al. Real-time three-dimensional myocardial contrast echocardiography in assessment of myocardial perfusion defects. *Chin Med J (Engl)*. 2004;117:337–341.

92. Pemberton J, Li X, Hickey E, et al. Live real-time three-dimensional echocardiography for the visualization of myocardial perfusion – a pilot study in open-chest pigs. *J Am Soc Echocardiogr*. 2005;18:956–958.

Three-Dimensional Echocardiography of Aortic Valve

Jarosław D. Kasprzak

8.1 Introduction

The most commonly used non-invasive cardiac imaging technique – two-dimensional echocardiography (2DE) – presents cardiac anatomy in multiple cross-sectional views. Due to anatomical limitations, desired cross-sections of the heart may not be available in all patients which is especially true for small, rapidly moving objects such as aortic valve (AV). Therefore, proper assessment of important aspects of cardiac morphology and function including optimal linear and planar measurements (e.g., planimetry of valvular orifices) may not be always possible. Furthermore, reliable understanding of cardiac anatomy requires tedious mental reconstruction based on a limited number of 2D cross-sections. Such mental reconstruction is extremely difficult in cases of complex abnormal cardiac morphology and is facilitated by a novel technique – three-dimensional echocardiography (3DE).

Similarly, volume measurements, mandatory for the evaluation of cardiac function, necessitate the introduction of imprecise assumptions regarding the cavities geometry when based on 2DE. Diagnostic confidence of linear and planar measurements can also be less precise when a unique scan rather than operator-optimized cross-section or spatial perspective based on complete 3D dataset is used. These limitations are valid for the echocardiographic studies of AV.

8.2 Methods

3DE examination can be currently performed in two distinct implementations –as a real-time volumetric sampling or 3D off-line reconstruction of cross-sectional data.[1] The older technique – *off-line reconstruction* – requires ECG and respiratory gated acquisition of two-dimensional cross-sections with simultaneous recording of spatial orientation of registered 2D images. Thereafter, using 2D images acquired from precardial, transesophageal or intracardiac window, stored with corresponding spatial information, 3DE dataset is reconstructed off-line applying intensive interpolation. Off-line reconstruction method cannot be used for the evaluation of rapid, transient phenomena occurring e.g. during stress echocardiography or contrast perfusion imaging and is less effective in irregular rhythm or in case of chaotic motion (vegetations). Other well-known limitations include prolonged acquisition, postprocessing and analysis time, as well as the presence of "stitching" or "malalignment" artifacts. Gated reconstruction is still performed, mainly using rotational, computer-controlled transesophageal acquisition and clinical usefulness of such approach has been convincingly demonstrated.[2] The feasibility of obtaining aortic valve data of excellent quality (59%), or adequate quality (22%) was high and additional clinically relevant information was provided in 31% patients as compared with the two-dimensional echocardiographic findings (Fig. 8.1).[3] Nowadays, transthoracic 3DE is performed using real-time 3D echocardiography,[4] allowing volumetric scanning with matrix transducer containing a large number (up to 3,000) of miniaturized piezoelectric elements. This is currently the basic 3DE acquisition modality for AV studies from transthoracic windows, and intraoperative epicardial acquisitions have recently been reported.[5] An important limitation of real-time technology is scan volume size (especially with color Doppler flow mapping) but it has been recently overcome with new generation scanners. Alternatively, larger grayscale or volumetric color Doppler datasets can be obtained using a brief ECG-gated acquisition with fusion of several spatially neighboring subvolumes can be performed (full-volume mode). Over the last few years, real-time volumetric three-dimensional echocardiographic imaging has become available from transesophageal window (Fig. 8.2) which represents a significant step forward due to new opportunities for improved diagnostic imaging, monitoring of surgical or transvascular procedures[6] and follow-up studies. However, feasibility of transesophageal real-time 3D aortic valve imaging remains lower than that of atrioventricular valves or interatrial septum. Optimal quality

J.D. Kasprzak
II Chair and Department of Cardiology, Bieganski Hospital Medical University of Łódź, Kniaziewicza 1/5, 91-347 Łódź
e-mail: kasprzak@ptkardio.pl

L.P. Badano et al. (eds.), *Textbook of Real-Time Three Dimensional Echocardiography*,
DOI: 10.1007/978-1-84996-495-1_8, © Springer-Verlag London Limited 2011

Fig. 8.1 Three dimensional reconstruction of the normal aortic valve from transesophageal rotational, ECG and respiration gated acquisition. Views from the ascending aorta at end diastole and end-systole

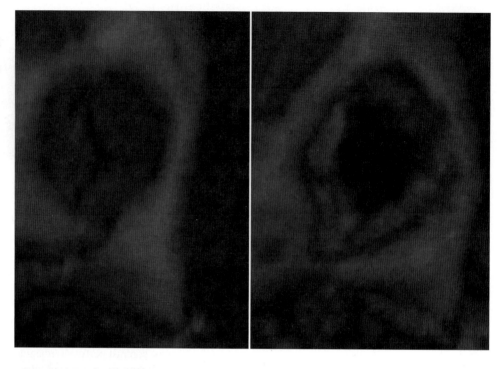

8.3 3D Imaging in Aortic Valve Disease

Real-time scanning of the aortic valve is usually accomplished from parasternal window (Fig. 8.3). When parasternal views of good quality are not available, there is a possibility to visualize the valve in apical views modified from five-chamber position – Fig. 8.4). This approach offers lower resolution for cusp morphology but may be sufficient to identify bicuspid morphology or dynamic motion of vegetations as well as left ventricular outflow tract anatomy. In transesophageal imaging upper esophageal views offer optimal imaging window.

The main problem in aortic valve imaging lies in the fine structure and moderate echogenicity of cusps, although this holds true for healthy valves only. Diseased thickened valves have better definition of cusps although image deterioration is encountered when severe calcifications are present. High quality, volume rendered views of aortic valve are usually obtained in views projected from ascending aorta (looking downwards) although views from left ventricular outflow tract (looking upwards) may be useful for the assessment of vegetations or valve tumors. Long-axis derived views are clinically less contributory.

Handling of volumetric aortic valve data is based on 2D cross-sectional images displayed on standard monitor panel although attempts have been made to apply advanced display modes such as holography, virtual reality or even tangible stereolithographic models.[8]

To analyze an optimized 2D cutplane across the aortic valve, arbitrary cross-sectional image can be selected from

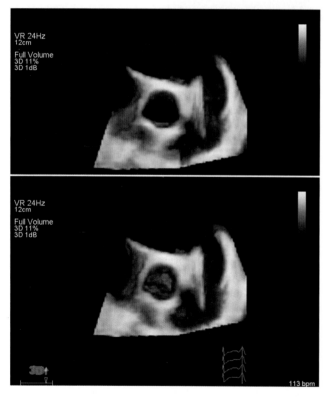

Fig. 8.2 Three dimensional real-time imaging of the normal aortic valve from transesophageal acquisition showing views from the ascending aorta at end diastole and end-systole

acquisitions are reported to occur in 18–22% studies[7] although this rate is expected to rapidly improve with technological progress.

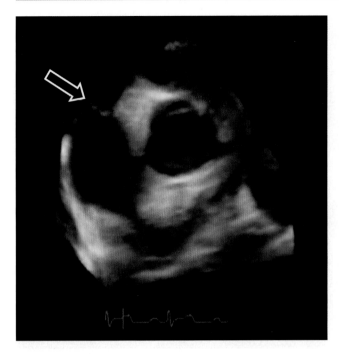

Fig. 8.3 Real-time transthoracic imaging of normal aortic valve seen in opened position from the ascending aorta. Note the anatomical relationships – proximal left coronary artery is seen at 3 o'clock and proximity of the right coronary cusp and septal tricuspid valve leaflet (near 10 o'clock, arrow) is evident

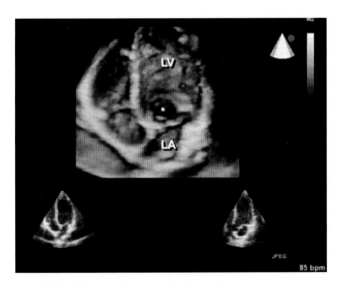

Fig. 8.4 Trileaflet aortic valve anatomy and normal opening area (asterisk) visualized in a non-standard approach – acquisition from apical window, display from left ventricular cavity towards its outflow tract. *LA* left atrium, *LV* left ventricle

the volumetric dataset (in anyplane or "slice" mode) as a specific freehand selection or a series of coaxial (omniplane method) or parallel cross-sections (paraplane/multislice method) (Fig. 8.5). Alternatively, the impression of anatomical perspective for global morphology assessment is digitally

created in volumetric, "three-dimensional" presentations (volume-rendering techniques). 3D images may be freely rotated and sectioned, thus facilitating visualization and detailed analysis of the region of interest. Depending on the image settings (shading, opacity) the structure may appear solid or transparent and thus providing information about structures underneath. Importantly, with these types of display grayscale information is lost and no tissue characterization attempts should be made (e.g., regarding calcifications). 3D color Doppler data can be displayed simultaneously with anatomical information[9] (Fig. 8.6). Future developments will be focused on automatization of workflow by developing algorithms for computer-assisted extraction of aortic valve and neighboring structures followed by automatic orifice and aortic root measurements.

All above mentioned imaging modes can be effectively applied for the assessment of aortic valve. The main benefits of 3DE examination in aortic valve disease include:

- Optimized anatomical display of pathomorphology from any desired viewpoint
- Optimized measurements of dimensions and orifice areas with optimal selection of viewing plane
- Volumetry of the left ventricle offering optimal accuracy for function assessment among the echocardiographic modalities.

8.4 Morphological Assessment

Detailed assessment of aortic valve including anatomy and shape,[8] cusps number[10] (Fig. 8.7), commissural fusion (Fig. 8.8) etc. is usually easy; this advantage can be used for monitoring the outcome of therapeutic interventions.[4,11–15] Better depiction of unusual findings such as perforations or prolapse determines improved accuracy and concordance with intraoperative findings.[5,11] Prosthetic valves are more difficult to image from transthoracic window but transesophageal 3DE reconstruction allows accurate measurements of area[16] or definition of other pathology although aortic position is usually more difficult for imaging.[17] However, successful imaging of postoperative complications such as ring dehiscence has been reported (Fig. 8.9).[18] Initial reports on real-time 3DE transesophageal imaging of prostheses indicate that 3/4of prosthetic rings in aortic position can be evaluated whereas prosthesis leaflets can be rendered in a minority of patients (Fig. 8.10).[19] Similarly, endocarditis-related lesions,[20,21] Lambl excrescences[22] or valve tumors[23] can be reliably shown in any 3DE technique with high feasibility rate. Additional data are provided regarding attachment site, extent and mobility of pathological structures such as vegetations (Figs. 8.11 and 8.12). There is a possibility of exact volumetry of

Fig. 8.5 Paraplane (9 slice mode) imaging for planimetry of a sclerotic aortic valve. Orifice is visualized in optimized cutplane derived from a real-time three-dimensional dataset (central panel) and traced for a reliable area measurement

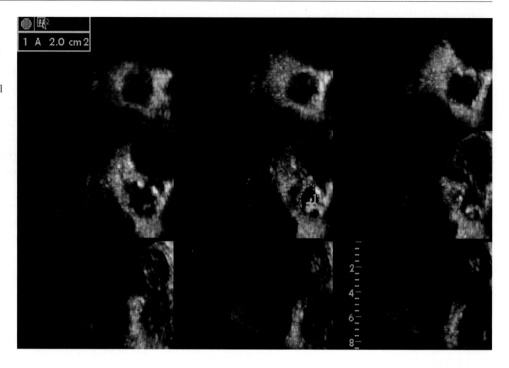

irregularly shaped objects although clinical implications are not established. Straightforward presentation facilitates communication with surgeons and procedure planning. 3DE is also capable of defining and quantification of LVOT narrowing in differential diagnostics of aortic valve disease (Fig. 8.13).[24,25]

8.5 Clinical Applications of 3DE in Aortic Stenosis

The aortic stenosis severity depends on anatomical limitation of aortic orifice which creates pressure gradient. Therefore, additional benefit from 3DE can result from improvements in planimetry or in improved understanding of valve morphology. 3D color Doppler plays a minor role in aortic stenosis except for patients with fixed immobile orifice where it facilitates detection of its contour.

It has been shown that 3DE reconstruction from transesophageal echocardiography allows precise measurements of aortic orifice due to unrestricted optimization of measurement plane positioning exactly a the level of minimal valve orifice (Fig. 8.14).[26,27] Planimetry of aortic orifice was highly reproducible and showed excellent agreement with area estimates in invasive and 2D echocardiographic studies with 88% feasibility. It was demonstrated that minor deviations from the proper measurement plane lead to significant overestimation of valve area, calculated as 0.1 cm²

per every 10 degrees of inappropriate angulation and per each 1.5 mm of plane shift.[5]

This experience in "anyplane" planimetric measurements of aortic valve area was extended onto direct planimetry in reconstructed 3D volumetric datasets (Fig. 8.15) ("surgical views").[28] 3DE derived aortic valve area was consistent with the value obtained by Gorlin formula or Doppler continuity equation as opposed to 2D transesophageal planimetry which significantly overestimated both reference orifice area estimates. However, another study[29] indicated on possible limitations with clear trend towards area underestimation in measurements performed in volume-rendered views with suboptimal image quality. This paper thus suggested that anyplane measurements might be better suited for quantification.

The utility of real-time 3DE has also been tested for aortic orifice planimetry showing significant benefits with significant impact upon correct diagnosis of severe aortic stenosis.[30,31] Direct comparison between real-time 3DE and 3D-guided two-dimensional planimetry (3D/2D), available with matrix probes was recently performed using 2D transesophageal echocardiographic planimetry and Gorlin invasive method as reference. 3D-based methods showed optimal interobserver reproducibility and best correlation (Figs. 8.16 and 8.17) (r = 0.86 for 3DE and 0.81 for 3D/2D). Thus, 3DE is a viable alternative for transesophageal planimetry if acoustic window is sufficient.

A potential issue limiting the accuracy of aortic valve area assessment in 3DE is temporal resolution usually ranging

Fig. 8.6 Paraplane views including color Doppler imaging of diseased aortic valve flow in systole (*top*) showing acceleration of flow in cross-sections of LVOT and turbulent stenotic flow coded in green at the level of stenotic valve and above. Paraplane cuts across LVOT in diastole display concomitant regurgitation coded in green (*bottom panel*)

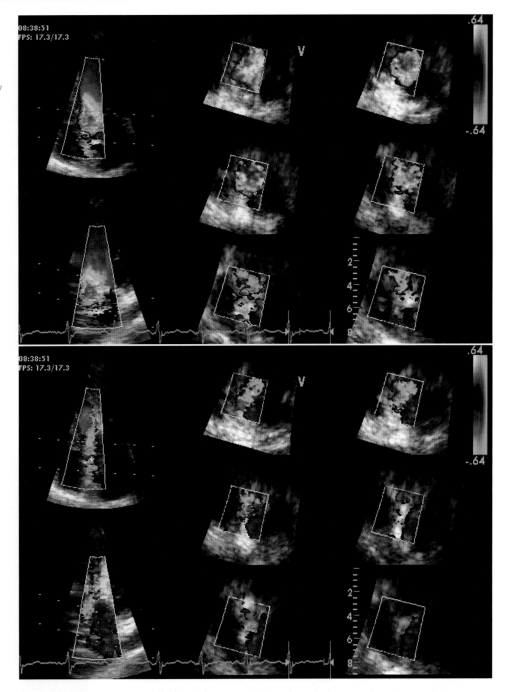

20–25 volumes per second in real-time scanning or reconstruction. This might cause problems with identification of fully opened aortic valve, particularly in patients with low cardiac output). Attempts have been made to increase temporal resolution and latest generation systems offer volume rates twice as high as those previously available. Prototype high volume-rate systems demonstrated three-dimensional aortic cusps motion with unprecedented quality with temporal resolution up to 168Hz.[32] This allows studying novel aspects of valve physiology such as area change rate (opening/closing velocity) in specific heart cycle periods.[33]

Applications of 3DE in aortic stenosis reach beyond improved planimetry, including improved quantification of myocardial mass regression after valve replacement.[34] 3D analysis improved understanding of aortic annulus blood flow velocity profiles[35] and importance of stenotic aortic valve shape proximal to the orifice for the determination of flow physiology. Indeed, there was evidence of significantly smaller effective areas and higher pressure gradients for flat-shaped rather than dome-shaped valves[8] which extends our understanding of valve disease beyond the orifice area in determining the physiological consequences of valvular aortic stenosis.

Fig. 8.7 Detailed visualization of partially fused aortic commissure (between the right and non-coronary cusp) in transthoracic real-time 3DE study

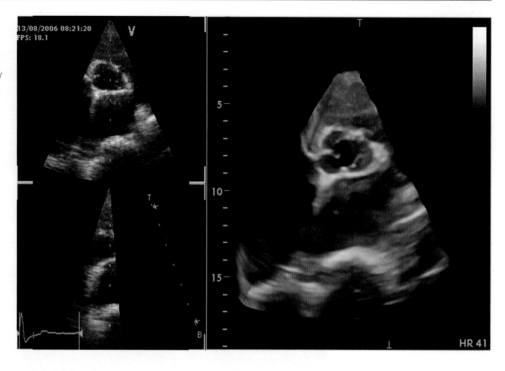

Fig. 8.8 Real-time transesophageal (left) and transthoracic (right) 3DE study showing a bicuspid morphology of the aortic valves with visible raphe but without marked calcifications on a anatomically right sided (left-sided on the figure) cusp

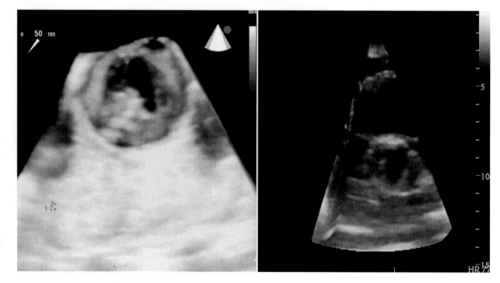

Importantly, 3DE measurements can be used to facilitate precise calculation of functional aortic valve orifice from continuity equation. The main obstacle for classic approach are geometric assumptions related to left ventricular outflow tract cross-sectional area and derived stroke volume value. 3DE allows for direct measurement of left ventricular outflow tract area which is not circular.[36,37] Indeed, orthogonal diameters of elliptical left ventricular outflow tract cross-section below the aortic valve vary in 50% of humans by more than 20% (especially in end-systole) and standard geometrical method underestimates left ventricular outflow tract area by 15% or absolute value of 0.55 cm^2 (3.18 = −0.73 cm^2 vs. 3.73 + −0.95 cm^2 in 3DE).[38] Incorporation of true, 3DE planimetered left ventricular outflow tract area improved the concordance of 3DE-enhanced continuity equation results with alternative methods.[39]

Alternatively, aortic stroke volume may be obtained by accurate volumetry of left ventricular volumes (in the absence of mitral regurgitation). This practical approach allowed the improvement in aortic valve area reproducibility as compared to standard continuity equation and optimization of stenosis flow cross-section and this concept has been experimentally validated for aortic stenosis.[42]

8.6 Aortic Regurgitation

Direct visualization of regurgitant aortic orifice is infrequently possible both in two and three-dimensional echocardiography (Fig. 8.18). However, 3D imaging of the aortic regurgitant jets may be easily obtained, especially in real-time technique. The use of 3D color Doppler flow mapping combined with 3D morphologic data provides clinically relevant supplementary information, enabling exact definition of number of jets, their origin and relationship to adjacent structures.[4] 3D color coded jets can be displayed separately from morphologic data with potential for volume quantification of regurgitation.[43] There is experimental evidence that 3D, but not 2D measurements of aortic regurgitation correlate with true regurgitant flow.[44] Another approach is to compare accurate, 3D derived left ventricular and right ventricular stroke volume values when aortic regurgitation is a sole valvular problem.[45] Furthermore, the shape of the flow convergence region – significantly different from commonly assumed hemisphere – can also be appreciated. This leads to direct measurement of the proximal isovelocity surface area[46] and volume, which proved to minimize aortic regurgitant jet underestimation in experimental study.[47] A simpler application is to improve the measurements of vena contracta width from 3D datasets.[48] Additionally, 3D with color Doppler allowed new insights in pathophysiology of eccentric regurgitation jets correlating them with abnormal leaflet function.[49]

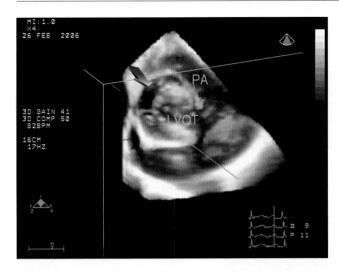

Fig. 8.9 Large dehiscence (*arrow*) of mechanical aortic valve ring causing severe regurgitation seen from left ventricular outflow tract. *LVOT* left ventricular outflow tract, *PA* pulmonary artery (Courtesy of Dr. YFM Nosir, Dr. H Chamsi-Pasha, KFAFH Jeddah)

severity grading vs. Gorlin method. Stroke-volume based 3DE method slightly underestimated aortic area (difference 0.13 cm²) and optimal cutoff for severe aortic stenosis according to Gorlin was established at 1.06 cm².[40]

Thus, 3DE derived, more accurate left ventricular outflow tract stroke volume values may improve the clinical applicability of modified continuity equation to calculate true aortic valve area. 3DE allows also the integration of true velocity profile and cross-sectional flow area to optimize stroke volume calculation.[41] Thus, expected developments include automatic integration of 3D flow data and corresponding

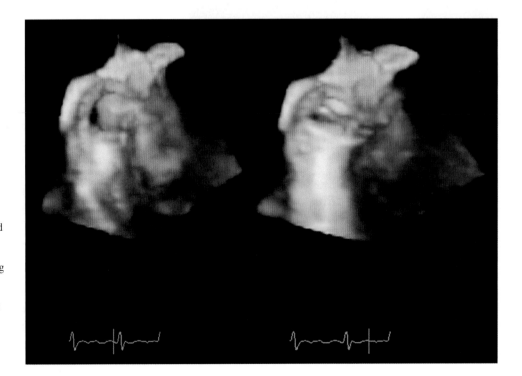

Fig. 8.10 Three dimensional transesophageal real-time imaging of mechanical bicuspid prosthesis showing open disks with shadow artifact from anterior disk from the ascending aorta. There is a signal dropout due to acoustic shadowing in systole and the image of closed leaflets could not be obtained (Courtesy of Dr. YFM Nosir, Dr H Chamsi-Pasha, KFAFH Jeddah)

Fig. 8.11 Aortic valve vegetation originating from the non-coronary aortic cusp (*arrow*) seen in the left ventricular outflow tract in diastole from two different angles. Diastolic prolapse of the vegetation into the left ventricular cavity is demonstrated. Transthoracic real-time study

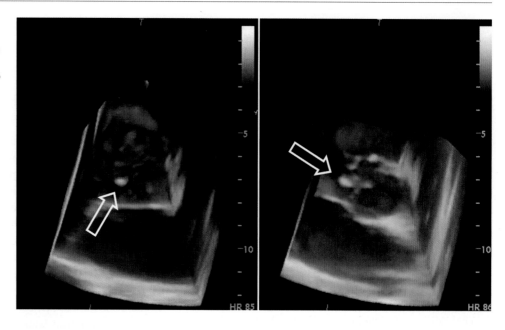

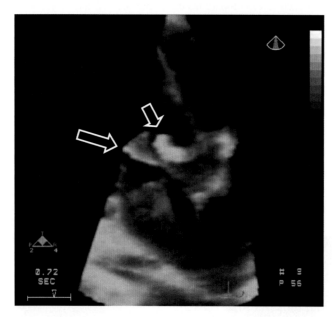

Fig. 8.12 Aortic valve vegetation seen prolapsing to left ventricular outflow tract in diastole. Note the proximity of the anterior mitral leaflet (*arrow*) and a long vegetation (*short arrow*) originating from the right coronary aortic cusp. Transthoracic real-time study

8.7 Intraprocedural Studies of Aortic Valve

Three-dimensional echocardiography can be readily applied for intraoperative or interventional procedure monitoring, communication and feedback. This has been shown for transesophageal reconstruction approach.[11] In a prospective study the feasibility of intraoperative application was 93% with 3D reconstruction and analysis time below 15 minutes. In 84% all major pathologies were readily confirmed whereas in 25% patients, 3DE provided new additional information absent in 2DE, including a case of surgical strategy change. This proves that even more cumbersome 3D transesophageal reconstruction is feasible in routine clinical intraoperative setting. This is even more valid for real-time imaging.[4,11,50] Recent reports indicate on the benefits of real-time 3DE online monitoring of transvascular aortic valve implantation procedures due to fast and complete information about the underlying pathomorphology, spatial orientation, and complications.[12–15] These benefits may accelerate the learning curve and translate into increased safety and efficacy of interventional therapy.

8.8 Summary and Perspectives

In twenty-first century, 3DE has already become a part of routine diagnostic pathway with a high feasibility rate, including patients with aortic valve disease, and providing additional qualitative or quantitative information in up to 47% of cases.[51] The main benefits of the method in aortic valve disease includes unrestricted plane imaging and improved quantification, especially for aortic orifice as well as for left ventricular volume and function measurements for decision making. This is particularly important with the advent and expected wide dissemination of less invasive, transvascular aortic valve interventions and growing interest in demanding valve repair surgery. Surgical perspective facilitates the objective assessment of the aortic valve and aortic root pathomorphology and explanation of unexpected anatomy such as vegetations or complicated postoperative conditions. Expected developments include improved software for structure extraction, computer-assisted cropping and view positioning and standardized, computer assisted or fully automated quantification, possibly with integration of flow and structural data (Figs. 8.19–8.21).

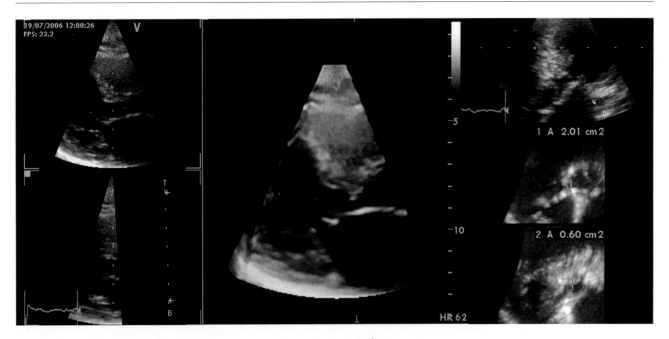

Fig. 8.13 Transthoracic 3D echocardiographic evaluation of subaortic stenosis – there is a subaortic discrete narrowing below the sclerotis aortic valve. Optimized anyplane planimetry is shown in the right panel, proving mild valvular lesion with area of 2 cm² and severe subaortic obstruction –0.6 cm²

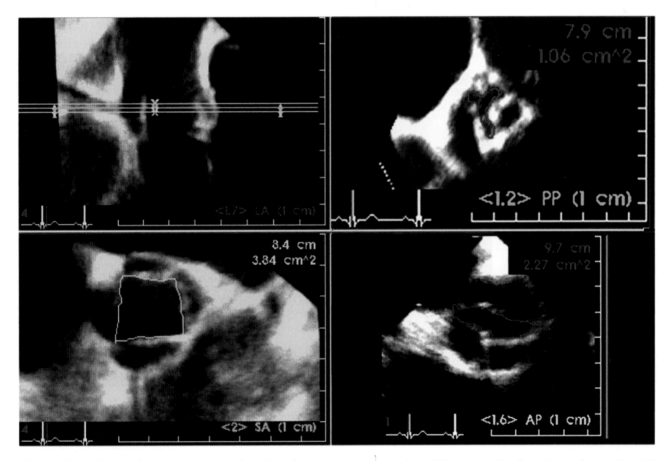

Fig. 8.14 Quantification of aortic valve area in optimized anyplace views from transesophageal 3D reconstruction from datasets showing bicuspid, tricuspid and quadricuspid aortic valve

Fig. 8.15 Heavily calcified aortic
stenosis with 0.7 cm² slit-like
orifice seen from aortic root with
0.7 cm² slit-like orifice (*arrow*).
Transthoracic real time 3DE
study. PA – pulmonary artery
bifurcation, RV – right ventricle

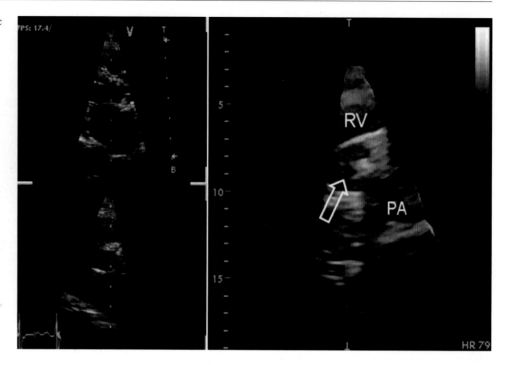

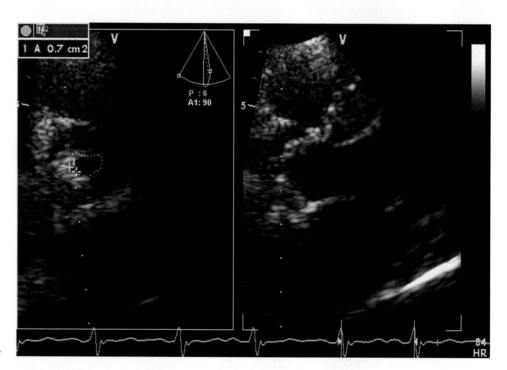

Fig. 8.16 Stenotic aortic
valve – optimized 3D-guided
(biplane mode obtained using a
matrix transducer) 2D planimetry

Fig. 8.17 Moderately stenotic aortic valve – standard 2D planimetry corresponding with precise volume-rendered view of the valve orifice from the aorta

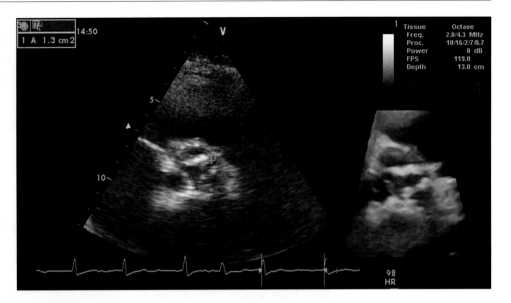

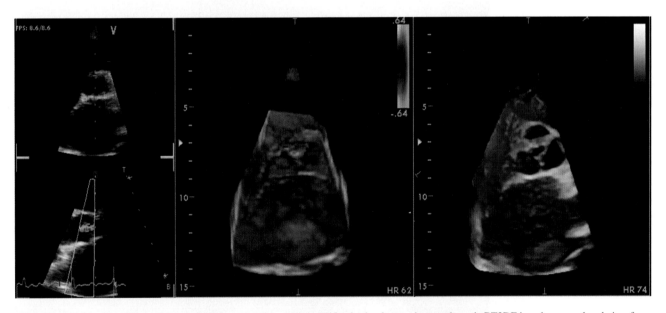

Fig. 8.18 Aortic valve with severe regurgitation – central regurgitant orifice is clearly seen in transthoracic RT3DE in volume-rendered view from the left ventricular outflow tract (*right panel*) and in real-time color Doppler 3DE study in diastole

Fig. 8.19 Computer-assisted
extraction and quantification of
aortic annulus, root and valve
area (Courtesy of Tomtec
Imaging Systems)

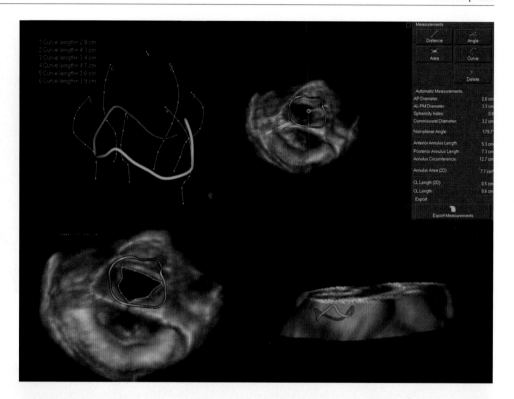

Fig. 8.20 Fully automatic aortic
valve and root mesh rendering
and tissue rendering (Courtesy of
Siemens Healthcare – Ultrasound
Division)

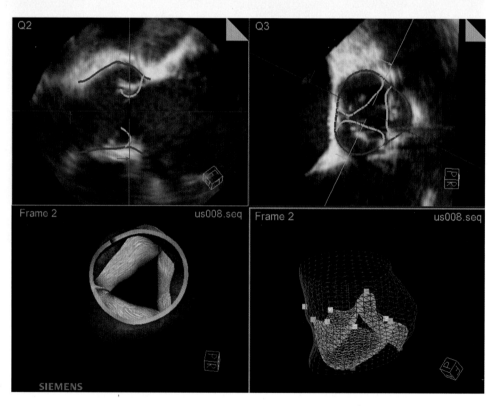

Fig. 8.21 Fully automatic aortic valve surface rendering and area quantification (Courtesy of Siemens Healthcare – Ultrasound Division)

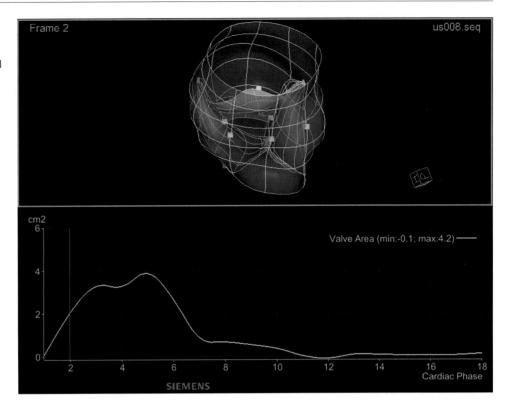

References

1. Roelandt JRTC, Yao J, Kasprzak JD. Three-dimensional echocardiography. *Curr Opin Cardiol*. 1998;13:386–396.
2. Ciesielczyk M, Drozdz J, Krzeminska-Pakula M et al. Clinical application of 3-dimensional echocardiography-a 3-year single center experience. *Przegl Lek*. 2002;59:658–662.
3. Kasprzak JD, Salustri A, Roelandt JR, Ten Cate FJ. Three-dimensional echocardiography of the aortic valve: feasibility, clinical potential, and limitations. *Echocardiography*. 1998;15:127–138.
4. Wang XF, Deng YB, Nanda NC, et al. Live three-dimensional echocardiography: imaging principles and clinical application. *Echocardiography*. 2003;20:593–604.
5. Vida VL, Hoehn R, Larrazabal LA, Gauvreau K, Marx GR, del Nido PJ. Usefulness of intra-operative epicardial three-dimensional echocardiography to guide aortic valve repair in children. *Am J Cardiol*. 2009;103:852–856.
6. Balzer J, Kühl H, Rassaf T, Hoffmann R, Schauerte P, Kelm M, Franke A. Real-time transesophageal three-dimensional echocardiography for guidance of percutaneous cardiac interventions: first experience. *Clin Res Cardiol*. 2008;97:565–574.
7. Sugeng L, Shernan SK, Salgo IS, Weinert L, Shook D, Raman J, Jeevanandam V, Dupont F, Settlemier S, Savord B, Fox J, Mor-Avi V, Lang RM. Live 3-dimensional transesophageal echocardiography initial experience using the fully-sampled matrix array probe. *J Am Coll Cardiol*. 2008;52:446–449.
8. Gilon D, Cape EG, Handschumacher MD, Song JK, Solheim J, VanAuker M, King ME, Levine RA. Effect of three-dimensional valve shape on the hemodynamics of aortic stenosis: three-dimensional echocardiographic stereolithography and patient studies. *J Am Coll Cardiol*. 2002;40:1479–1486.
9. De Simone R, Glombitza G, Vahl CF, et al. Three-dimensional color Doppler: a clinical study in patients with mitral regurgitation. *J Am Coll Cardiol*. 1999;33:1646–1654.
10. Espinola-Zavaleta N, Munoz-Castellanos L, Attie F, Hernandez-Morales G, Zamora-Gonzalez C, Duenas-Carbajal R, Granados N, Keirns C, Vargas-Barron J. Anatomic three-dimensional echocardiographic correlation of bicuspid aortic valve. *J Am Soc Echocardiogr*. 2003;16:46–53.
11. Abraham TP, Warner JG Jr, Kon ND, Lantz PE, Fowle KM, Brooker RF, Ge S, Nomeir AM, Kitzman DW. Feasibility, accuracy, and incremental value of intraoperative three-dimensional transesophageal echocardiography in valve surgery. *Am J Cardiol*. 1997;80:1577–1582.
12. Scohy TV, Soliman OI, Lecomte PV, McGhie J, Kappetein AP, Hofland J, Ten Cate FJ. Intraoperative real time three-dimensional transesophageal echocardiographic measurement of hemodynamic, anatomic and functional changes after aortic valve replacement. *Echocardiography*. 2009;26:96–99.
13. Balzer J, Kelm M, Kühl HP. Real-time three-dimensional transesophageal echocardiography for guidance of non-coronary interventions in the catheter laboratory. *Eur J Echocardiogr*. 2009;10:341–349.
14. Janosi RA, Kahlert P, Plicht B, Bose D, Wendt D, Thielmann M, Jakob H, Eggebrecht H, Erbel R, Buck T. Guidance of percutaneous transcatheter aortic valve implantation by real-time three-dimensional transesophageal echocardiography – A single-center experience. *Minim Invasive Ther Allied Technol*. 2009;1:142–148.
15. Perk G, Lang RM, Garcia-Fernandez MA, Lodato J, Sugeng L, Lopez J, Knight BP, Messika-Zeitoun D, Shah S, Slater J, Brochet E, Varkey M, Hijazi Z, Marino N, Ruiz C, Kronzon I. Use of real time three-dimensional transesophageal echocardiography in intracardiac catheter based interventions. *J Am Soc Echocardiogr*. 2009;22:865–882.
16. Mannaerts H, Li Y, Kamp O, Valocik G, Krudova J, Ripa S, Visser C. Quantitative assessment of prosthetic mechanical valve area by 3-dimensional echocardiography. *J Am Soc Echocardiogr*. 2001;14:723–731.
17. Sezai A, Shiono M, Orime Y, Hata H, Yagi S, Tsukamoto S, Nakata K, Hasegawa M, Sezai Y, Tanigawa N. Three-dimensional

transesophageal echocardiographic assessment for prosthetic valves. *Nippon Kyobu Geka Gakkai Zasshi.* 1997;45:1084–1089.

18. Mukhtari O, Horton CJ Jr, Nanda NC, Aaluri SR, Pacifico A. Transesophageal color Doppler three-dimensional echocardiographic detection of prosthetic aortic valve dehiscence: correlation with surgical findings. *Echocardiography.* 2001;18:393–397.

19. Sugeng L, Shernan SK, Weinert L, Shook D, Raman J, Jeevanandam V, DuPont F, Fox J, Mor-Avi V, Lang RM. Real-time three-dimensional transesophageal echocardiography in valve disease: comparison with surgical findings and evaluation of prosthetic valves. *J Am Soc Echocardiogr.* 2008;21:1347–1354.

20. Kasprzak JD, Salustri A, Roelandt JR, Cornel JH. Comprehensive analysis of aortic valve vegetation with anyplane, paraplane, and three-dimensional echocardiography. *Eur Heart J.* 1996; 17: 318–320.

21. Nemes A, Lagrand WK, McGhie JS, ten Cate FJ. Three-dimensional transesophageal echocardiography in the evaluation of aortic valve destruction by endocarditis. *J Am Soc Echocardiogr.* 2006; 19:355.

22. Samal AK, Nanda N, Thakur AC, Narayan VK, Ocak O, Lee TY, Voros S, Jindal A, Winokar TS. Three-dimensional echocardiographic assessment of Lambl's excrescences on the aortic valve. *Echocardiography.* 1999;16:437–441.

23. Dichtl W, Muller LC, Pachinger O, Schwarzacher SP, Muller S. Improved preoperative assessment of papillary fibroelastoma by dynamic three-dimensional echocardiography. *Circulation.* 2002; 106:1300.

24. Ge S, Warner JG Jr, Fowle KM, Kon ND, Brooker RF, Nomeir AM, Kitzman DW. Morphology and dynamic change of discrete subaortic stenosis can be imaged and quantified with three-dimensional transesophageal echocardiography. *J Am Soc Echocardiogr.* 1997; 10:713–716.

25. Dall'Agata A, Cromme-Dijkhuis AH, Meijboom FJ, Spitaels SE, McGhie JS, Roelandt JR, Bogers AJ. Use of three-dimensional echocardiography for analysis of outflow obstruction in congenital heart disease. *Am J Cardiol.* 1999;83:921–925.

26. Nanda NC, Roychoudhury D, Chung SM, Kim KS, Ostlund V, Klas B. Quantitative assessment of normal and stenotic aortic valve using transesophageal three-dimensional echocardiography. *Echocardiography.* 1994;11:617–625.

27. Kasprzak JD, Nosir YF, Dall'Agata A, Elhendy A, Taams M, Ten Cate FJ, Roelandt JR. Quantification of the aortic valve area in three-dimensional echocardiographic data sets: analysis of orifice overestimation resulting from suboptimal cut-plane selection. *Am Heart J.* 1998;135:995–1003.

28. Ge S, Warner JG Jr, Abraham TP, Kon ND, Brooker RF, Nomeir AM, Fowle KM, Burgess P, Kitzman DW. Three-dimensional surface area of the aortic valve orifice by three-dimensional echocardiography: clinical validation of a novel index for assessment of aortic stenosis. *Am Heart J.* 1998;136:1042–1050.

29. Handke M, Schafer DM, Heinrichs G, Magosaki E, Geibel A. Quantitative assessment of aortic stenosis by three-dimensional anyplane and three-dimensional volume-rendered echocardiography. *Echocardiography.* 2002;19:45–53.

30. Vengala S, Nanda NC, Dod HS, Singh V, Agrawal G, Sinha A, Khanna D, Upendram SK, Chockalingam A, McGiffin DC, Kirklin JK, Pacifico AD. Usefulness of three-dimensional echocardiography in aortic valve stenosis evaluation. *Am J Geriatr Cardiol.* 2004; 13:279–284.

31. Goland S, Trento A, Iida K, Czer LS, De Robertis M, Naqvi TZ, Tolstrup K, Akima T, Luo H, Siegel RJ. Assessment of aortic stenosis by three-dimensional echocardiography: an accurate and novel approach. *Heart.* 2007;93:801–807.

32. Handke M, Jahnke C, Heinrichs G, Schlegel J, Vos C, Schmitt D, Bode C, Geibel A. New three-dimensional echocardiographic system using digital radiofrequency data – visualization and quantitative

analysis of aortic valve dynamics with high resolution: methods, feasibility, and initial clinical experience. *Circulation.* 2003;107: 2876–2879.

33. Handke M, Heinrichs G, Beyersdorf F, Olschewski M, Bode C, Geibel A. In vivo analysis of aortic valve dynamics by transesophageal 3-dimensional echocardiography with high temporal resolution. *J Thorac Cardiovasc Surg.* 2003;125:1412–1419.

34. Kuhl HP, Franke A, Puschmann D, Schondube FA, Hoffmann R, Hanrath P. Regression of left ventricular mass one year after aortic valve replacement for pure severe aortic stenosis. *Am J Cardiol.* 2002;89:408–413.

35. Haugen BO, Berg S, Brecke KM, Torp H, Slordahl SA, Skaerpe T, Samstad SO. Blood flow velocity profiles in the aortic annulus: a 3-dimensional freehand color flow Doppler imaging study. *J Am Soc Echocardiogr.* 2002;15:328–333.

36. Menzel T, Mohr-Kahaly S, Wagner S, Fischer T, Bruckner A, Meyer J. Calculation of left ventricular outflow tract area using three-dimensional echocardiography. Influence on quantification of aortic valve stenosis. *Int J Card Imaging.* 1998;14:373–379.

37. Pérez de Isla L, Zamorano J, Pérez de la Yglesia R, Cioccarelli S, Almeria C, Rodrigo JL, Aubele AL, Herrera D, Mataix L, Serra V, Macaya C. Quantification of aortic valve area using three-dimensional echocardiography. *Rev Esp Cardiol.* 2008;61:494–500.

38. Doddamani S, Bello R, Friedman MA, Banerjee A, Bowers JH Jr, Kim B, Vennalaganti PR, Ostfeld RJ, Gordon GM, Malhotra D, Spevack DM. Demonstration of left ventricular outflow tract eccentricity by real time 3D echocardiography: implications for the determination of aortic valve area. *Echocardiography.* 2007;24: 860–866.

39. Khaw AV, von Bardeleben RS, Strasser C, Mohr-Kahaly S, Blankenberg S, Espinola-Klein C, Münzel TF, Schnabel R. Direct measurement of left ventricular outflow tract by transthoracic real-time 3D-echocardiography increases accuracy in assessment of aortic valve stenosis. *Int J Cardiol.* 2009;136:64–71.

40. Gutiérrez-Chico JL, Zamorano JL, Prieto-Moriche E, Hernandez-Antolin RA, Bravo-Amaro M, Pérez de Isla L, Sanmartin-Fernandez M, Baz-Alonso JA, Iniguez-Romo A. Real-time three-dimensional echocardiography in aortic stenosis: a novel, simple, and reliable method to improve accuracy in area calculation. *Eur Heart J.* 2008;29:1296–1306.

41. Haugen BO, Berg S, Brecke KM, Samstad SO, Skjaerpe T, Slørdahl SA, Torp H. Measurement of volumetric mitral and aortic blood flow based on a new freehand three-dimensional colour flow imaging method. An in vivo validation. *Eur J Echocardiogr.* 2000;1: 204–212.

42. Poh KK, Levine RA, Solis J, Shen L, Flaherty M, Kang YJ, Guerrero JL, Hung J. Assessing aortic valve area in aortic stenosis by continuity equation: a novel approach using real-time three-dimensional echocardiography. *Eur Heart J.* 2008;29:2526–2535.

43. Acar P, Jones M, Shiota T, Masani N, Delabays A, Yamada I, Sahn DJ, Pandian NG. Quantitative assessment of chronic aortic regurgitation with 3-dimensional echocardiographic reconstruction: comparison with electromagnetic flowmeter measurements. *J Am Soc Echocardiogr.* 1999;12:138–148.

44. Shiota T, Jones M, Tsujino H, Qin JX, Zetts AD, Greenberg NL, Cardon LA, Panza JA, Thomas JD. Quantitative analysis of aortic regurgitation: real-time 3-dimensional and 2-dimensional color Doppler echocardiographic method-a clinical and a chronic animal study. *J Am Soc Echocardiogr.* 2002;15:966–971.

45. Irvine T, Stetten GD, Sachdev V, Zetts AD, Jones M, Mori Y, Ramsperger C, Castellucci JB, Kenny A, Panza JA, von Ramm OT, Sahn DJ. Quantification of aortic regurgitation by real-time 3-dimensional echocardiography in a chronic animal model: computation of aortic regurgitant volume as the difference between left and right ventricular stroke volumes. *J Am Soc Echocardiogr.* 2001;14:1112–1118.

46. Li X, Shiota T, Delabays A, et al. Flow convergence flow rates from 3-dimensional reconstruction of color Doppler flow maps for computing transvalvular regurgitant flows without geometric assumptions: An in vitro quantitative flow study. *J Am Soc Echocardiogr.* 1999;12:1035–1044.

47. Pirat B, Little SH, Igo SR, McCulloch M, Nosé Y, Hartley CJ, Zoghbi WA. Direct measurement of proximal isovelocity surface area by real-time three-dimensional color Doppler for quantitation of aortic regurgitant volume: an in vitro validation. *J Am Soc Echocardiogr.* 2009;22:306–313.

48. Fang L, Hsiung MC, Miller AP, Nanda NC, Yin WH, Young MS, Velayudhan DE, Rajdev S, Patel V. Assessment of aortic regurgitation by live three-dimensional transthoracic echocardiographic measurements of vena contracta area: usefulness and validation. *Echocardiography.* 2005;22:775–781.

49. Sato Y, Kamata J, Izumoto H, Nasu M, Kawazoe K. Morphological analysis of aortic root in eccentric aortic regurgitation using anyplane two-dimensional images produced by transesophageal three-dimensional echocardiography. *J Heart Valve Dis.* 2003;12: 186–196.

50. Usui A, Araki Y, Sakurai K, Murayama H, Yoshikawa M, Akita T, Ueda Y. Real time 3-D echocardiography in cardiac surgery. *Jpn J Thorac Cardiovasc Surg.* 2004;52:509–514.

51. Kasprzak JD, Lipiec P, Drozdz J, Krzeminska-Pakula M. Real-time three-dimensional echocardiography: still a research tool or an imaging technique ready for daily routine practice? A pilot feasibility study in a tertiary cardiology centre. *Kardiol Pol.* 2004; 61:303–308.

Three-Dimensional Echocardiographic Evaluation of the Right Ventricle

9

Gloria Tamborini and Mauro Pepi

9.1 The Right Ventricle

The right ventricle is a structurally and functionally complex chamber whose importance has been partially neglected previously. Right ventricular dimensions and function are known to be of diagnostic as well of prognostic importance in patients with cardiac disease.[1-6] Unfortunately an accurate and rapid non-invasive assessment of right ventricular performance is challenging due to the complex structure and anatomy of the ventricle and its unfavourable position in the thorax behind the sternum. The right ventricle is in fact composed by several anatomic and functional subunits extending from the tricuspid valve annulus to the proximal os infundibulum, then extending from the right ventricular outflow tract to the pulmonary valve as well as the right ventricular body extending to the apex. Understanding of right ventricular morphology in general is greatly aided by considering the ventricle in three parts: inlet, trabecular (apex) and outlet. The right ventricle is highly trabeculated, with several trabeculations including the septoparietal trabeculations and the moderator band. From a functional point of view, due to the orientation of right ventricular fibres, global assessment of the right ventricle is difficult with the two main portions of the right ventricle contracting perpendicular to each other: the proximal (inflow) longitudinally and the distal (outflow) circumferentially.

Echocardiographic measurements of fractional shortening area in the four chamber view and fractional shortening diameter of the right ventricular outflow tract distinctly analyse free wall movements of the inflow and outflow right ventricular portions. M-mode tricuspid annular plane systolic excursion (TAPSE) and the corresponding tissue Doppler peak systolic velocity evaluate base-apical movements of the right ventricle. These relatively simple 2D, M-mode and tissue Doppler imaging methods have been demonstrated to be feasible during a routine complete echocardiographic exam and correlate to the systolic function of the right ventricle (a sort of surrogate of the right ventricle ejection fraction).[7-9] However, these methods have several limitations: they do not allow an accurate volumetric measurement of right ventricular dimensions nor a complete estimation of global right ventricular function.

3DE overcome geometric limitations of 2DE methods with volumes assessment obtained through a true volume dataset without any geometrical assumption. Transthoracic (or transesophageal) 3DE using matrix array probe is becoming a robust, accurate and reproducible modality for right ventricular volumes and function in children and adults with different pathologies. Recent papers have clearly demonstrated the feasibility of the method and validated the accuracy vs. multiplanar magnetic resonance.[10-14]

Several methods and softwares have been proposed. 3D data are acquired in a full volume set from the apical approach adapted to encompass the entire right ventricle. Full-volume analysis may result in the acquisition of a wider pyramidal volume (full-volume mode gated to ECG which acquires four or seven wedges of volumes over four or seven beats). New ultrasound units allow also a one beat acquisition of the 3D data set. Figure 9.1 shows examples of acquisition of RV 3D data sets with different technical modalities.

Depending of the companies and different softwares, generally 3D dataset are digitally stored and then off-line post-processing and 3D reconstruction are performed through a dedicated system. On-board dedicated 3D right ventricular analysis softwares will be available soon, similarly to those for 3D left ventricular analysis (this will further facilitate the use of these measurements). 3D-right ventricular analysis software program allows the display of the sagittal, four chamber and coronal views obtained from the 3D dataset.

A variety of options for off-line 3D reconstruction of the right ventricular exists. Several studies demonstrated the feasibility of the method of discs. After the acquisition and automatic display of the right ventricle (end-diastolic and end-systolic frames) with different cut planes (generally orthogonal views of the right ventricle) a contour of the right ventricle is traced manually by the operator in the axial plane. The traced contour generated bricks or discs of fixed height (generally 10 mm) but varying lengths and widths as

M. Pepi (✉)
Cardiovascular Imaging Department,
Centro Cardiologico Monzino, IRCCS, Milan, Italy
e-mail: mpepi@ccfm.it

L.P. Badano et al. (eds.), *Textbook of Real-Time Three Dimensional Echocardiography*,
DOI: 10.1007/978-1-84996-495-1_9, © Springer-Verlag London Limited 2011

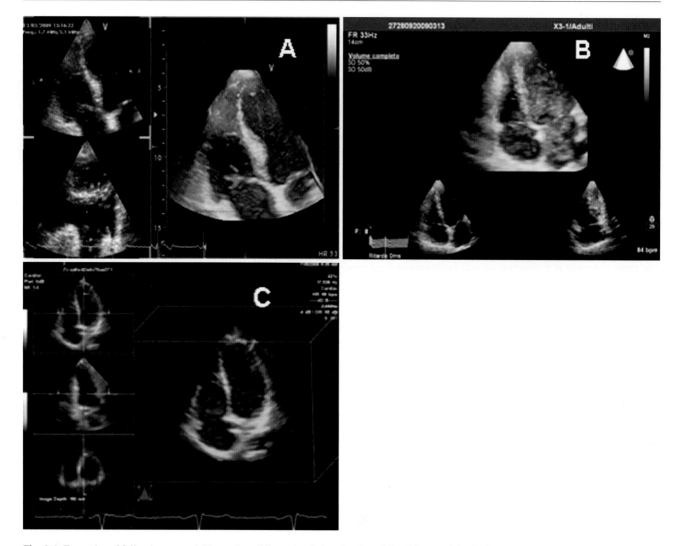

Fig. 9.1 Examples of full volume acquisitions adapted for optimal visualization of the right ventricle obtained through three different modalities: four beat method (*panel A*), seven subsequent beat method (*panel B*) or (*panel C*) one beat acquisition method

visualized in the other right ventricular cut planes. The volume of the right ventricular cavity was computed by summating the known areas of the axial traces obtained 10-mm apart and the fixed height of 10 mm, i.e., disc summation. The number of discs required to cover the right ventricle from the base to apex varies (seven or eight slices depending on heart size).

Another dedicated commercial method analyses the acquired data through the tracings of the endocardial borders at end-diastolic and end-systolic frames on sagittal (to outline the tricuspid valve in the best possible view), four-chamber (to outline the apex) and coronal (to outline the right ventricular outflow tract) cross-sections. The operator can manually adjust the traced contours in each frame prior to quantification. Trabeculations are generally included in the endocardial rim, but the apical component of the moderator band is excluded from the cavity. The right ventricular volumes are calculated by summating the areas for each slice through the complete data set. Each volume data set is imported into the application and manipulated by rotating, angulating and slicing in any of the 3 displayed orthogonal planes. The software analysis uses a semiautomated border detection algorithm with manual correction options on in vivo normal as well as pathologic right ventricular modelling that was performed to design this program. Through this method, volumes of the right ventricle are reconstructed (Fig. 9.2). The computer analysis for 3DE uses a semiautomated border detection algorithm over complete heart cycle with manual correction option and right ventricular end diastolic and end systolic volume automatically calculated as well as ejection fraction. Moreover segmental analysis of the RV of the 3 main portions of the chamber (inlet, apex and outflow segments) may also be performed allowing measurements of RV segmental function. Curves of global and regional right ventricular function may be therefore generated and analysed (Fig. 9.3).

Fig. 9.2 Manual tracing of end-systolic frames in sagittal (**a**), four chamber (**b**) and coronal views (**c**). *Panel D* shows the 3D reconstruction of right ventricle (end-systolic frame)

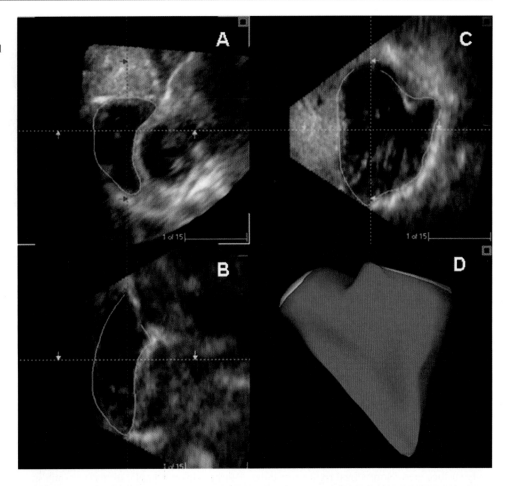

Fig. 9.3 Example of segmental analysis of the RV main portions: inlet (*green*), outlet (*yellow*) and apex (*pink*). Segmental time-volume curves are calculated and plotted, frame by frame, throughout the cardiac cycle

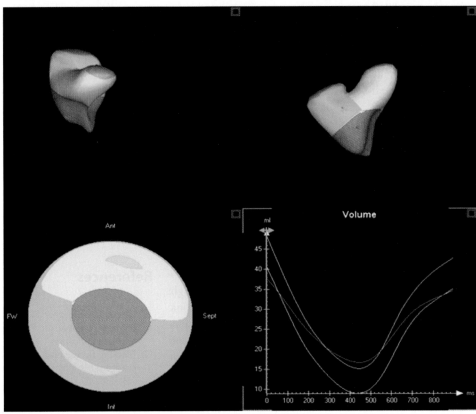

Fig. 9.4 Examples of 3D real time morphologic evaluation of the RV cavity. *Left panel*: normal RV (*arrow*). *Right panel*: hypertrabeculated and enlarged RV (*arrow*) in a case of RV arrhythmogenic dysplasia. *RV* right ventricle

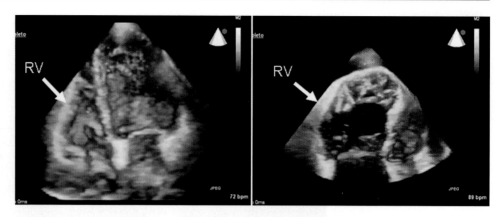

Differences between men (129 ± 25 ml) and women (102 ± 33 ml) have been demonstrated, however adjusting to lean body mass (but not to body surface area or height) eliminated this difference.[15] Very recently a study provides normal reference values for right ventricular volumes and function that may be useful for identification of clinical abnormalities.[16] A total of 245 cases, including 15–20 subjects for each gender and age decile, were studied. Dedicated 3D acquisitions for RV were obtained in all subjects. Mean right ventricular end-diastolic and end-systolic volumes resulted in 49 ± 10 ml/m^2 and 16 ± 6 ml/m^2 respectively while right ventricular ejection fraction was 67% ± 8%. Significant correlations were observed between right ventricular parameters and body surface area. Normalized right ventricular volumes significantly correlated with age and gender. Right ventricular ejection fraction was smaller in males, but differences across age deciles were not evident.

Niemann et al.[11] studied 14 normal subjects and 16 patients with major congenital heart disease with both 3DE and MRI analysing right ventricular size and function. Although there was a slightly higher variability measuring right ventricular ejection fraction and volumes by echo compared with MRI, both imaging methods showed closely correlated results. Recently the feasibility of the method in large (200) series of cases[17] has been evaluated. This new quantitative 3D method to assess right ventricular volumes and function was feasible, relatively simple and not time consuming. Three-dimensional evaluation of the right ventricle was well correlated with standard echo and Doppler methods and could differentiate normal vs. pathologic subjects.

All these data suggest that this new method may be introduced in the clinical practise in selected cases in whom right ventricular dysfunction is relevant such as acute and chronic heart failure and lung disease, primary and secondary pulmonary vascular disease, congenital heart disease. In patients with secundum atrial septal defect (3D TEE acquisition), Tetralogy of Fallot repair, Ebstein's anomaly and right ventricular cardiomyopathy the use of transthoracic 3DE has been validated.[18–20] It has also been reported the feasibility

and utility of real-time 3DTTE to guide right ventricular endomyocardial biopsies in children.[21]

Moreover it has been demonstrated that 3DE may overcome limitations of the standard 2DE and Doppler methods (TAPSE and tissue Doppler imaging of the tricuspid annulus) in patients with a previous cardiac surgery.[22] In 40 patients undergoing surgical mitral valve repair without complications TAPSE and tissue Doppler imaging of the tricuspid annulus were markedly reduced after surgery (at 3, 6 and 12 months) while 3D right ventricular ejection fraction did not change. The reduction of the longitudinal echo parameters after cardiac surgery is a well known phenomenon which is not coherent to the clinical conditions of patients without complications (not only in valve disease but also in coronary artery disease). Therefore this study not only support the hypothesis that geometric rather then functional changes of the right ventricular chamber occur after surgery, but clearly support this new 3D methodology as an ideal technique for the evaluation of right ventricular function in these cases.

As concerns morphology of the right ventricular chamber and evaluation of the right ventricular cavity there are few data. Potentially 3D real time or full volume images of the right ventricle allows a very complete definition of chamber morphology, valves and intracavitary pathologies. Figure 9.4 shows an example of an hypertrabeculated right ventricle in a case of RV dysplasia (in comparison with a normal RV). Selected cases of right ventricular tumors or thrombi are also reported.

References

1. Lualdi J, Goldhaber S. Right ventricular dysfunction after acute pulmonary embolism. Pathophysiologic factors, detection and therapeutic implications. *Am Heart J*. 1995;130:1276–1282.
2. Madsen B, Egeblad H, Melchior T, et al. Prognostic value of echocardiography compared to other clinical findings. *Cardiology*. 1995;86:157–162.
3. Sun J, James K, Yang X, et al. Comparison of mortality rates and progression of left ventricular dysfunction in patients with idiopathic

dilated cardiomyopathy and dilated versus nondilated ventricular cavities. *Am J Cardiol.* 1997;80:1583–1587.

4. Patel A, Dubrey S, Mendes L, et al. Right ventricular dilation in primary amyloidosis: an independent predictor of survival. *Am J Cardiol.* 1997;80:486–492.

5. De Groote P, Millaire A, Foucher-Hossein C, et al. Right ventricular ejection fraction is an independent predictor of survival in patients with moderate heart failure. *J Am Coll Cardiol.* 1998;32:948–954.

6. Ghio S, Gavazzi A, Campana C, et al. Independent and additive prognostic value of right ventricular systolic function and pulmonary artery pressure in patients with chronic heart failure. *J Am Coll Cardiol.* 2001;37:183–188.

7. Ueti OM, Camargo EE, Ueti Ade A, de Lima-Filho EC, Nogueira EA. Assessment of right ventricular function with Doppler echocardiographic indices derived from tricuspid annular motion: comparison with radionuclide angiography. *Heart.* 2002; 88:244–248.

8. Meluzin J, Spiranova L, Bakala J, et al. Pulsed Doppler tissue imaging of the velocity of tricuspidal annular systolic motion; a new, rapid, and non-invasive method of evaluating right ventricular systolic function. *Eur Heart J.* 2001;22:340–348.

9. Tamborini G, Pepi M, Galli CA, Maltagliati A, Celeste F, Muratori M, Salehi R, Veglia F. Feasibility and accuracy of a routine echocardiographic assessment of right ventricular function. *Int J Cardiol.* 2007;115:86–89.

10. Shiota T, Jones M, Chikada M, Fleishman CE, Castellucci JB, Cotter B. Real time three- dimensional right ventricular stroke volume in an animal model of chronic right ventricular volume overload. *Circulation.* 1998;97:1897–1900.

11. Niemann PS, Pinho L, Balbach T, Galuschky C, Blankenhagen M, Silberbach M, Broberg C, Jerosch-Herold M, Sahn DJ. Anatomically oriented right ventricular volume measurements with dynamic three-dimensional echocardiography validated by 3-Tesla magnetic resonance imaging. *J Am Coll Cardiol.* 2007;50:1668–1676.

12. Kjaergaard J, Petersen CL, Kjaer A, Schaadt BK, Oh JK, Hassager C. Evaluation of right ventricular volume and function by 2D and 3D echocardiography compared to MRI. *Eur J Echocardiogr.* 2006;7(6):430–438.

13. Gopal AS, Chukwu EO, Iwuchukwu CJ, Katz AS, Toole RS, Shapiro W, Reichek N. Normal values of right ventricular size and function by real time 3-dimensional echocardiography: comparison with cardiac resonance imaging. *J Am Soc Echocardiogr.* 2007; 20:445–455.

14. Shiota T. 3D echocardiography: evaluation of the right ventricle. *Curr Poin Cardiol.* 2009;24:410–414.

15. Kjaaergaard J, Sogaard P, Hassager C. Quantitative echocardiographic analysis of the right ventricle in healthy individuals. *J Am Soc Echocardiogr.* 2006;19:1365–1372.

16. Tamborini G, Ajmone Marsan N, Gripari P, Maffessanti F, Brusoni D, Muratori M, Caiani E, Fiorentini C, Pepi M. Reference values for right ventricular volumes and ejection fraction with real time three-dimensional echocardiography: evaluation in a large series of normal subjects. *J Am Soc Echocardiogr.* 2010;23: 109–115.

17. Tamborini G, Brusoni D, Torres Molina J, Galli C, Maltagliati A, Muratori M, Susini F, Colombo C, Maffessanti F, Pepi M. Feasibility of a new generation three-dimensional echocardiography for right ventricular volumetric and functional measurements. *Am J Cardiol.* 2008;102:499–505.

18. Liang X, Cheung E, Wong S, Cheung Y. Impact of right ventricular volume overload on three-dimensional global left ventricular mechanical dyssynchrony after surgical repair of tetralogy of Fallot. *Am J Cardiol.* 2008;102:1731–1736.

19. Acar P, Abadir S, Roux D, et al. Ebstein's anomaly assessed by real-time 3D echocardiography. *AnnThorac Surg.* 2006;82:731–733.

20. Kjaergaard J, Hastrup Svendsen J, Sogaard P et al: Advanced quantitative echocardiography in arrhythmogenic right ventricular cardiomyopathy. *J Am Soc Echocardiogr.* 2007;20:27–35.

21. Scheurer M, Bandisode V, Ruff P et al: Early experience with real-time three-dimensional echocardiographic guidance of right ventricular biopsy in children. *Echocardiography.* 2006;23:45–49.

22. Tamborini G, Muratori M, Brusono D, Celesate F, Maffessanti F, Caiani E, Alamanni F, Pepi M. Is right ventricular systoli function reduced after cardiac surgery? A two- and three-dimensional echocardiographic study. *Eur J Echocardiogr.* 2009;10:630–634.

Three-Dimensional Echocardiography in Congenital Heart Disease

10

Girish S. Shirali, Anthony M. Hlavacek, and G. Hamilton Baker

10.1 Introduction

Complex intracardiac anatomy and spatial relationships are inherent to congenital heart defects. Beginning over 30 years ago and until recently, the clinician's ability to image the heart non-invasively was limited to 2DE.[1] However, 2D imaging has fundamental limitations. The very nature of a 2DE slice, which has no thickness, necessitates the use of multiple orthogonal "sweeps." The imager then mentally reconstructs the anatomy, and uses the structure of the report to express this mentally reconstructed vision. This means that the only 3D image of the heart is the "virtual image" that exists in the mind of the imager, who then translates this vision into words. It is not easy for an untrained observer to understand the images obtained in the course of a sweep; expert interpretation is required. Importantly, since myocardial motion occurs in 3D, 2D techniques inherently do not lend themselves to accurate quantitation. Recognition of these limitations of 2DE has led to burgeoning research and clinical interest in 3D imaging.

10.2 Clinical Applications

3DE currently has three broad areas of clinical application among patients with congenital heart disease: (1) visualization of morphology, (2) quantitation of chamber sizes and ventricular function, and (3) image-guided interventions.

10.3 Visualization of Morphology

From early in development of 3DE, the structural complexity inherent to congenital heart disease has been identified as

G.S. Shirali (✉)
Department of Pediatrics, Pediatric Cardiology, Medical University of South Carolina, 165 Ashley Avenue, MSC 915, Charleston, South Carolina, SC 29125, USA
e-mail: shiralig@musc.edu

fertile substrate for exploration. The utility of this technology has been established in a wide spectrum of defects.

10.3.1 The Atrioventricular Valves

3DE is valuable in delineating the morphology of the atrioventricular valves. Espinola-Zavaleta et al. described the role of 3DE in delineating congenital abnormalities of the mitral valve.[2] Rawlins et al. demonstrated the additive value of 3DE and improved image quality using intraoperative epicardial 3DE to delineate the anatomy of atrioventricular valves.[3] Seliem et al. studied 41 patients with atrioventricular valve abnormalities and found that 3DE imaging was helpful in delineating the morphology of the valve leaflets and their chordal attachments, the subchordal apparatus, the mechanism and origin of regurgitation, and the geometry of the regurgitant volume.[4] Vettukatil et al. examined the role of 3DE in patients with Ebstein's anomaly of the tricuspid valve. They demonstrated that 3DE provided clear visualisation of the morphology of the valve leaflets, including the extent of their formation, the level of their attachment, and their degree of coaptation. They were also able to visualize the mechanism of regurgitation or stenosis.[5] We have found that 3DE provides unparalleled surgeon's views of the tricuspid valve *en face*.

10.3.2 Atrioventricular Septal Defect

Hlavacek et al. studied 52 datasets on 51 patients with atrioventricular septal defects and showed that gated 3DE views could be cropped to obtain *en face* views of the atrial and ventricular septa.[6] These views provide a clear understanding of the relationships of the bridging leaflets to the septal structures. These views have been useful to determine the precise location of the interventricular communication relative to the bridging leaflets, and to demonstrate how these relationships determine the level of shunting (atrial, ventricular or both atrial and ventricular). They found that 3DE on unrepaired

L.P. Badano et al. (eds.), *Textbook of Real-Time Three Dimensional Echocardiography*,
DOI: 10.1007/978-1-84996-495-1_10, © Springer-Verlag London Limited 2011

balanced atrioventricular septal defects and repaired atrioventricular septal defects with residual lesions was more often additive/useful (33/36; 92%) than on repaired atrioventricular septal defects without residual lesions or unbalanced atrioventricular septal defects (9/16 (56%), P=0.009). 3DE was additive or useful in all 3 patients with unbalanced atrioventricular septal defects being considered for biventricular repair. Useful information obtained by 3DE included: precise characterization of mitral regurgitation and leaflet anatomy, unique images such as views of a cleft mitral valve (Figs. 10.1

and 10.2), substrate for subaortic stenosis, valve anatomy, and presence and location of additional septal defects.

10.3.3 The Atrial and Ventricular Septa

Tantengco et al. showed that 3DE reconstructions provided unique *en face* views of atrial and ventricular septal defects.[7] Cheng et al. studied 38 patients with atrial and/or ventricular septal defects using 3DE, and compared their results to 2DE and surgical findings. They demonstrated novel 3DE views of both atrial and ventricular septal defects and improved accuracy of quantification of the size of the defect by 3DE compared to 2DE (r = 0.92 vs. r = 0.69).[8] This approach has also been used to demonstrate the morphology of muscular ventricular septal defects.[9] We have found 3DE to be of great value in evaluating the ventricular septum *en face* (Fig. 10.3) and to assess malformations that involve malalignment of the outlet septum (Fig. 10.4).

10.3.4 The Aortic Arch, Pulmonary Arteries and Aortopulmonary Shunts

3DE color flow Doppler has been used to provide echocardiographic 'angiograms' of flow patterns in the aortic arch

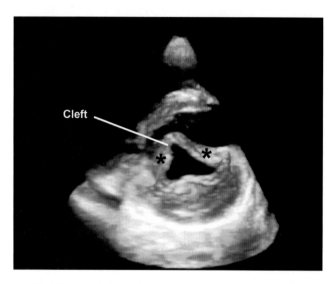

Fig. 10.1 Parasternal short axis live 3D image demonstrates a cleft in the anterior leaflet of the mitral valve. Asterisks mark the free edges of the cleft

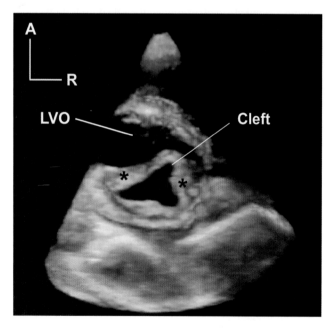

Fig. 10.2 The same image that was demonstrated in Fig. 10.1 has been rotated 180 degrees to view the mitral valve from the left atrium, looking down. This shows the trifoliate nature of the mitral valve. *A* anterior, *R* right, *LVO* left ventricular outflow tract

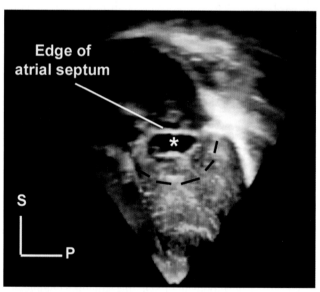

Fig. 10.3 *En face* view of the ventricular septum in a patient with the partial form of atrioventricular septal defect, looking from left to right. The free walls of the left atrium and left ventricle have been cut away. Note the primum atrial septal defect (*asterisk*) between the crescentic inferior margin of the atrial septum and the atrioventricular valves, and the scooped-out edge of the interventricular septum (*dashed lines*). The image can be rotated to view the right ventricular aspect of these structures as well. *P* posterior, *S* superior

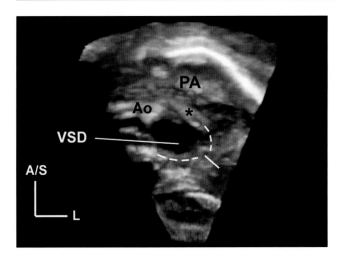

Fig. 10.4 Subcostal long axis view in tetralogy of Fallot demonstrates several of the classic features of this defect. The anterior surface of the right ventricle has been cropped away, and the viewing perspective is from below upwards. Note the septal band (*solid line*) that divides into anterosuperior and posteroinferior limbs (*dashed lines*). An asterisk marks the outlet septum, which is malaligned anteriorly, and has fused with the anterosuperior limb of the septal band. This malalignment leads to narrowing of the subpulmonary outflow tract (PA), an overriding aorta (aAo) and a large ventricular septal defect (VSD). The image can be rotated to view the VSD from the left ventricular aspect. *A/S* anterosuperior, *L* left

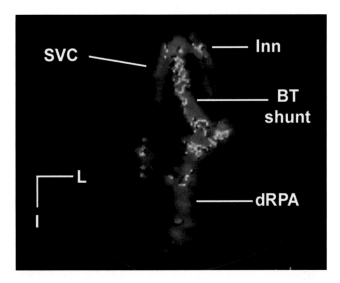

Fig. 10.5 Suprasternal notch view of a Blalock-Taussig shunt (BT shunt). The grayscale image has been suppressed, yielding an "echocardiographic angiogram." The shunt is seen throughout its length, originating from the innominate artery (Inn). Note the proximity of the shunt to the superior vena cava (SVC). Flow is visualized well into the distal right pulmonary artery (dRPA). This image can be rotated and tilted to evaluate the shunt in an unlimited number of viewing perspectives

(coarctation of the aorta), the branch pulmonary arteries (the Lecompte maneuver) and across Blalock-Taussig shunts.[10] These authors examined echocardiographic "angiograms" in 26 patients (Fig. 10.5). 3DE provided additional diagnostic information in 10 of 26 patients (38%). In 17 of 26 patients

(65%), validation of the 3DE diagnosis was available at surgery, cardiac catheterization, MRI or computerized tomography angiography.

10.3.5 The Aortic Valve and Outflow Tract

Sadagopan et al. examined the role of 3DE in 8 children who subsequently underwent surgery for congenital aortic valve stenosis. They showed that 3DE was accurate in providing measurements of aortic valve annulus, number of valve leaflets, in identifying sites of fusion of the leaflets as well as nodules and excrescences that characterized dysplastic valves.[11] Bharucha et al. studied 16 patients with subaortic stenosis. Using a form of 3DE reconstruction known as multiplanar reconstruction, which provides access to an unlimited number of 2DE planes, they demonstrated abnormalities of mitral valve leaflet or chordal apparatus attachments (14 patients), abnormal ventricular muscle band (11 patients) and abnormal increased aorto-mitral separation (2 patients).[12]

10.3.6 Characterization of Left Ventricular Noncompaction

Baker et al. evaluated four patients with left ventricular noncompaction using 3DE.[13] They found that 3DE enabled diagnosis and provided detailed characterization of the affected myocardium, including easy visualization of entire trabecular projections, intertrabecular recesses, endocardial borders and wall motion abnormalities of the affected myocardium. 3DE enabled easy differentiation between compact and noncompact portions of the myocardium.

10.4 Quantitation of Chamber Dimensions, Valve Apparatus, Function and Flows

In congenital heart defects ranging from tetralogy of Fallot to congenitally corrected transposition to hypoplastic left heart syndrome, the pulmonary and/or systemic ventricles are characterized by abnormal shapes, sizes and loading conditions that may well persist after surgery. As the results of surgery continue to improve and patients survive into adulthood, it is clear that the functional outcomes in such patients will be related to ventricular remodeling as a function of time and somatic growth, with the attendant alterations in ventricular loading conditions. With its potential ability to capture the entire ventricular volume, 3DE has the potential to steer away from older formula-dependent techniques of ventricular volumetrics, and to provide geometry-independent ability to quantify ventricular size and function.

10.5 Left Ventricular Volumetrics in Children

Bu et al. compared 3DE measurements of left ventricular volumetrics to those obtained using MRI.[14] They demonstrated that 3DE measurements of left ventricular end-systolic volume, end-diastolic volume, mass, stroke volume and ejection fraction in children using a rapid full volume acquisition strategy are feasible, reproducible and comparable with MRI measurements. They found good correlations between the two methods, but a tendency towards mild underestimation of volumes by 3DE. Interestingly, estimates of ejection fraction were in closer agreement. Baker et al. evaluated the feasibility of 3DE left ventricular volumetrics, as well as the resource utilization, learning curve, inter- and intra-observer reproducibility of this technique. The study design involved 15 datasets and four observers who had varying degrees of (self-rated) experience with 3DE quantitation.[15] They found that in 59 of 60 instances, observers were able to obtain 3D left ventricular ejection fraction in less than 3 min (median time 1 min and 27 s). They demonstrated a learning curve for the observer with the lowest level of self-rated experience. Their study also showed excellent inter- and intra-observer reproducibility for 3DE left ventricular volumetrics.

10.6 Left Ventricular Mass

Studies in adults have validated 3DE as an accurate method for measuring left ventricular mass.[16,17] While studies in children have been limited in number and scope, Riehle et al. recently demonstrated excellent correlations between left ventricular mass measured by 3DE and MRI.[18]

10.7 Left Ventricular Dyssynchrony

The 3DE approach to measuring intra-ventricular dyssynchrony utilizes the American Society of Echocardiography's 16-segment model of the left ventricle.[19] It measures the time of each subvolume from maximal (end-diastolic) volume to minimal volume, and the standard deviation of these time intervals. The higher is the value of the standard deviation, the higher the implied degree of intra-ventricular dyssynchrony. Baker et al. examined the association between left ventricular dysfunction and intra-ventricular

dyssynchrony in children using 3DE.[20] They studied 9 children with dilated cardiomyopathy and an equal number of age- and body size-matched normals. They found that normal patients had 3DE dyssynchrony indices that were below 3%. Among children with dilated cardiomyopathy, there was a clear threshold value of left ventricular ejection fraction: at a left ventricular ejection fraction below 35–40%, intra-ventricular dyssynchrony was the rule. In contrast, patients whose left ventricular ejection fraction was higher than 40% exhibited no significant dyssynchrony. This method of evaluation of dyssynchrony has correlated well with tissue-Doppler based indices of dyssynchrony.[21] 3DE has demonstrated left ventricular dyssynchrony in patients who had undergone repair of right heart lesions including tetralogy of Fallot.[22]

10.8 Right Ventricular Volumetrics

Advances in the area of right ventricular volumetrics have been relatively recent; this is unsurprising given the complex architecture of the right ventricle, and the technical difficulty of imaging it adequately. Niemann et al. studied right ventricular volumes by 3DE using a new and robust protocol that utilizes multiplanar reconstruction and tracing with semi-automated border detection in 16 children with congenital heart disease.[23] They found excellent correlations between MRI and 3DE for measurement of right ventricular volumes and ejection fraction. Soriano et al. quantified right ventricular volumes in children with functionally univentricular hearts with systemic right ventricles.[24] Calculations of diastolic volumes by three dimensional echocardiography proved to be smaller than those made by MRI, but systolic volumes and mass showed good agreement. Ejection fraction correlated less well, with an intraclass correlation coefficient of 0.64; measurements by 3DE were lower than those obtained using MRI by 6%. Inter- and intra-observer reproducibility was excellent. In a reflection of the speed with which technology is advancing, this study, which was published in March 2008, used a transducer that is already outdated in terms of quality of microelectronics, which translates directly into image quality and frame rates. In addition, the frequencies emitted by the transducer ranged from 2 to 4 megahertz. This is probably too low for optimal imaging in most of the children who were studied (weight 3–31 kg, median 7 kg). It is likely that the improved spatial and temporal resolution, and higher frequency of state-of-the-art transducers and machines that is available today, will lead to further improvements in accuracy.

As these tools become more widely available, user-friendly and accurate, we may well see the emergence of a new paradigm in the use of echocardiographic parameters as surrogate outcome measures in clinical trials of medications and pacing strategies.

10.9 Visualization and Quantitation of 3DE Color Flow

Multiplanar reconstruction tools provide the ability to not only visualize but also to trace and measure the area of valve regurgitant orifices at the level of the *vena contracta*. While this technique is new and has not been validated, it has been shown to be feasible, and has already yielded new insights into the shape of regurgitant jets, and holds promise as a tool to enhance the echocardiographer's ability to serially quantify valve regurgitation.[25]

Pemberton et al. developed and validated a technique for quantifying non-aliased 3DE color flow jets on open-chest pigs. When compared to measurements obtained from flow probes positioned on the ascending aorta, they obtained excellent correlations between the two methods.[26] They compared 143 individual measurements of cardiac output and found excellent correlation between the two techniques (r^2 = 0.93). 3DE quantification of color flow has recently been validated in adults by comparison to cardiac outputs obtained by thermodilution.[27] Application of this technique to pathologic states could lead to potentially more accurate measurements of regurgitant volumes and fractions.

10.10 Pressure:Volume Loops

Research using ventricular pressure:volume loop analysis has played a fundamental role in developing current concepts of cardiac pathophysiology and performance.[28,29] It provides vital information regarding systolic and diastolic cardiac performance, myocardial energetics, and ventriculovascular interactions.[30] However, pressure:volume loop analysis has failed to make the transition from a research application to widespread clinical use. One of the major reasons for this failure is the difficulty of acquiring data under varying conditions of ventricular loading. While accurate and effective, these methods are cumbersome and expensive. Recently, innovative techniques have been developed to derive pressure:volume indices without load alteration using a single cardiac cycle.[31] Our laboratory is currently working on methodology that utilizes 3DE to capture left ventricular volume and mass, paired with simultaneously collected pressure data, to yield pressure:volume loops that can be easily obtained during a diagnostic catheterization (Fig. 10.6). If the application is successful, it would transform this highly robust measurement of ventricular function into a clinically-practical modality.

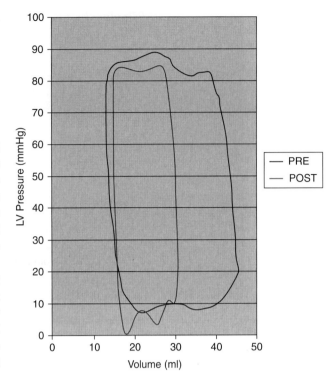

Fig. 10.6 Example of a 3DE pressure:volume loop of the left ventricle in a patient before and after device closure of a patent ductus arteriosus. *LV* left ventricular; *mmHg* millimeters of mercury, *ml* milliliters

10.11 Image-Guided Intervention: Trans-thoracic 3DE

Scheurer et al. demonstrated the use of live 3DE to guide the performance of endomyocardial biopsy in children.[32] In their experience, the use of live 3DE guidance was associated with no complications, including no new tricuspid valve leaflet flail or pericardial effusion. 3DE proved to be a reliable noninvasive modality to accurately direct the bioptome to the desired site of biopsy within the right ventricle. As familiarity with this technique increased, the need for fluoroscopic guidance of bioptome manipulation in the right ventricle was minimized. Del Nido et al. have extended the concept of image-guided intervention to the very novel approach of epicardial live 3DE-guided, open-chest, closed-heart, off-bypass cardiac surgery.[33–35] They began with in vitro validation of the ability of live 3DE to guide the performance of common surgical tasks. More recently, they have undertaken closure of small atrial septal defects in the porcine model using live 3DE guidance.

10.12 Image-Guided Intervention: Trans-esophageal 3DE

Transesophageal 3DE is a new application with great potential in the care of patients with congenital heart disease.[36] We found this modality to be useful in routine diagnostic studies

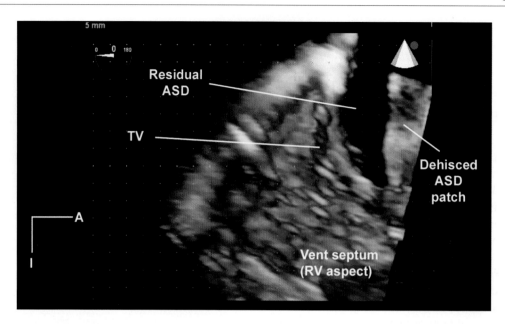

Fig. 10.7 Transesophageal (TEE) 3DE in a patient who had undergone surgical partitioning of common atrium. At follow-up, transthoracic echocardiograms revealed that the atrial septal defect patch was more mobile than is typical. TEE was performed to delineate the anatomy. In this view, the viewing perspective is from right to left. We are examining the right side of the septal structures, after having cropped off the free walls of the right heart chambers. This demonstrates a large, crescent-shaped residual atrial septal defect that is located posteriorly. The free edge of the dehisced atrial septal defect patch is seen. The grid marks are 5 mm apart in the horizontal and vertical planes, providing a clear indication of the large size of the residual defect. The image can be rotated 180 degrees to view the leftward aspect of the defect. *A* anterior, *I* inferior

(Figs. 10.7 and 10.8) as well as the perioperative setting and to guide trans-catheter interventions, particularly for guiding percutaneous interventions involving the atrial septum. We have been able to use this probe in patients who weigh over 22 kg. The development of a miniaturized probe should increase the practicality of this modality in patients with congenital heart disease.

10.13 Learning Curve

The learning curve with 3DE is steep but negotiable. Our experience would suggest that the success of 3DE in a program requires advocacy and an investment of time by both echocardiographers and sonographers. The acceptance of 3DE is increasing on a global level, albeit at an early stage of the technology cycle. We have developed and implemented an interactive teaching course that utilizes simulations using 3DE datasets with rehearsal and direct mentoring; this has been shown to be useful in overcoming the steep part of the learning curve.[37]

10.14 Future Directions

Over the next decade, advances in the 3DE arena will involve technical enhancements such as miniaturization, holographic displays, a wide range of validated software tools for quantification, and enhancements to work flow. New, multimodality applications will increasingly bring 3DE into the mainstream. Refinements in transducer technology will make high-resolution 3DE available across the spectrum of patient sizes. We anticipate a 3DE TEE probe miniaturized for pediatric usage. With the growing interest in multi-modality imaging, 3DE volumetric data will eventually be integrated with the pressure data that is available during cardiac

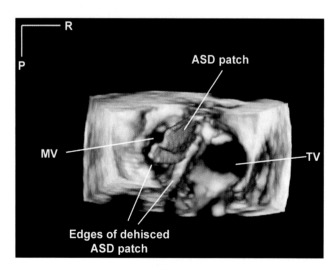

Fig. 10.8 This image is from the same patient and study as Fig. 10.7. The viewing perspective is from above downwards. This provides a unqiue perspective of how the patch remains attached anteriorly, but has dehisced posteriorly

catheterization, yielding pressure-volume loops that can be obtained as a matter of routine clinical practice.

10.15 Conclusion

Recent innovations in the field of 3DE has allowed this modality to offer unique and clinically useful information in the evaluation of patients with congenital heart disease. 3DE offers excellent anatomical imaging and functional analysis in a manner that is easily obtained and clinically practical. Sustained progress in the development of this modality will continue to improve our diagnostic and management capabilities in patients with congenital heart disease.

References

1. Tajik AJ, Seward JB, Hagler DJ, Mair DD, Lie JT. Two-dimensional real-time ultrasonic imaging of the heart and great vessels. Technique, image orientation, structure identification, and validation. *Mayo Clin Proc.* 1978;53:271–303.
2. Espinola-Zavaleta N, Vargas-Barron J, Keirns C, et al. Three-dimensional echocardiography in congenital malformations of the mitral valve. *J Am Soc Echocardiogr.* 2002;15(5):468–472.
3. Rawlins DB, Austin C, Simpson JM. Live three-dimensional paediatric intraoperative epicardial echocardiography as a guide to surgical repair of atrioventricular valves. *Cardiol Young.* 2006;16(1): 34–39.
4. Seliem MA, Fedec A, Szwast A, et al. Atrioventricular valve morphology and dynamics in congenital heart disease as imaged with real-time 3-dimensional matrix-array echocardiography: comparison with 2-dimensional imaging and surgical findings. *J Am Soc Echocardiogr.* 2007;20(7):869–876.
5. Vettukattil JJ, Bharucha T, Anderson RH. Defining Ebstein's malformation using three-dimensional echocardiography. *Interact Cardiovasc Thorac Surg.* 2007;6(6):685–690.
6. Hlavacek AM, Crawford FA, Jr., Chessa KS, Shirali GS. Real-time three-dimensional echocardiography is useful in the evaluation of patients with atrioventricular septal defects. *Echocardiography.* 2006;23:225–231.
7. Tantengco MV, Bates JR, Ryan T, et al. Dynamic three-dimensional echocardiographic reconstruction of congenital cardiac septation defects. *Pediatr Cardiol.* 1997;18(3):184–190.
8. Cheng TO, Xie MX, Wang XF, et al. Real-time 3-dimensional echocardiography in assessing atrial and ventricular septal defects: an echocardiographic-surgical correlative study. *Am Heart J.* 2004;148(6):1091–1095.
9. Mercer-Rosa L, Seliem MA, Fedec A, et al. Illustration of the additional value of real-time 3-dimensional echocardiography to conventional transthoracic and transesophageal 2-dimensional echocardiography in imaging muscular ventricular septal defects: does this have any impact on individual patient treatment? *J Am Soc Echocardiogr.* 2006;19(12):1511–1519.
10. Hlavacek A, Lucas J, Baker H, et al. Feasibility and utility of three-dimensional color flow echocardiography of the aortic arch: the "echocardiographic angiogram". *Echocardiography.* 2006;23(10): 860–864.
11. Sadagopan SN, Veldtman GR, Sivaprakasam MC, et al. Correlations with operative anatomy of real time three-dimensional echocardiographic imaging of congenital aortic valvar stenosis. *Cardiol Young.* 2006;16(5):490–494.
12. Bharucha T, Ho SY, Vettukattil JJ. Multiplanar review analysis of three-dimensional echocardiographic datasets gives new insights into the morphology of subaortic stenosis. *Eur J Echocardiogr.* 2008; 9(5):614–620.
13. Baker GH, Pereira NL, Hlavacek AM, et al. Transthoracic real-time three-dimensional echocardiography in the diagnosis and description of noncompaction of ventricular myocardium. *Echocardiography.* 2006;23(6):490–494.
14. Bu L, Munns S, Zhang H, et al. Rapid full volume data acquisition by real-time 3-dimensional echocardiography for assessment of left ventricular indexes in children: a validation study compared with magnetic resonance imaging. *J Am Soc Echocardiogr.* 2005;18(4): 299–305.
15. Baker G, Flack E, Hlavacek A, et al. Variability and resource utilization of bedside three-dimensional echocardiographic quantitative measurements of left ventricular volume in congenital heart disease. *Congenital Heart Dis.* 2006;1(6):309–314.
16. Mor-Avi V, Sugeng L, Weinert L, et al. Fast measurement of left ventricular mass with real-time three-dimensional echocardiography: comparison with magnetic resonance imaging. *Circulation.* 2004;110(13):1814–1818.
17. Caiani EG, Corsi C, Zamorano J, et al. Improved semiautomated quantification of left ventricular volumes and ejection fraction using 3-dimensional echocardiography with a full matrix-array transducer: comparison with magnetic resonance imaging. *J Am Soc Echocardiogr.* 2005;18(8):779–788.
18. Riehle TJ, Mahle WT, Parks WJ, et al. Real-time three-dimensional echocardiographic acquisition and quantification of left ventricular indices in children and young adults with congenital heart disease: comparison with magnetic resonance imaging. *J Am Soc Echocardiogr.* 2008;21(1):78–83.
19. Kapetanakis S, Kearney MT, Siva A, et al. Real-time three-dimensional echocardiography: a novel technique to quantify global left ventricular mechanical dyssynchrony. *Circulation.* 2005;112(7):992–1000.
20. Baker GH, Hlavacek AM, Chessa KS, et al. Left ventricular dysfunction is associated with intraventricular dyssynchrony by 3-dimensional echocardiography in children. *J Am Soc Echocardiogr.* 2008;21(3):230–233.
21. Vieira ML, Cury AF, Naccarato G, et al. Analysis of left ventricular regional dyssynchrony: comparison between real time 3D echocardiography and tissue Doppler imaging. *Echocardiography.* 2009; 26(6):675–683.
22. Raedle-Hurst TM, Mueller M, Rentzsch A, Schaefers HJ, Herrmann E, Abdul-Khaliq H. Assessment of left ventricular dyssynchrony and function using real-time 3-dimensional echocardiography in patients with congenital right heart disease. *Am Heart J.* 2009;157:791–798.
23. Niemann PS, Pinho L, Balbach T et al. Anatomically oriented right ventricular volume measurements with dynamic three-dimensional echocardiography validated by 3-Tesla magnetic resonance imaging. *J Am Coll Cardiol.* 2007;50:1668–1676.
24. Soriano BD, Hoch M, Ithuralde A, et al. Matrix-array 3-dimensional echocardiographic assessment of volumes, mass, and ejection fraction in young paediatric patients with a functional single ventricle. A comparison study with cardiac magnetic resonance. *Circulation.* 2008;117:1842–1848.
25. Sugeng L, Weinert L, Lang RM. Real-time 3-dimensional color Doppler flow of mitral and tricuspid regurgitation: feasibility and initial quantitative comparison with 2-dimensional methods. *J Am Soc Echocardiogr.* 2007;20(9):1050–1057.
26. Pemberton J, Li X, Karamlou T, et al. The use of live three-dimensional Doppler echocardiography in the measurement of cardiac output: an in vivo animal study. *J Am Coll Cardiol.* 2005;45(3): 433–438.
27. Lodato JA, Weinert L, Baumann R, et al. Use of 3-dimensional color Doppler echocardiography to measure stroke volume in

human beings: comparison with thermodilution. *J Am Soc Echocardiogr*. 2007;20(2):103–112.

28. Burkhoff D, Mirsky I, Suga H. Assessment of systolic and diastolic ventricular properties via pressure-volume analysis: a guide for clinical, translational, and basic researchers. *Am J Physiol Heart Circ Physiol*. 2005;289:H501–512.

29. Grossman W, Braunwald E, Mann T, McLaurin LP, Green LH. Contractile state of the left ventricle in man as evaluated from end-systolic pressure-volume relations. *Circulation*. 1977;56:845–852.

30. Sugawa K. *Cardiac Contraction and the Pressure-Volume Relationship*. New York: Oxford University Press; 1988.

31. Karunanithi MK, Feneley MP. Single-beat determination of preload recruitable stroke work relationship: derivation and evaluation in conscious dogs. *J Am Coll Cardiol*. 2000;35:502–513.

32. Scheurer M, Bandisode V, Ruff P, et al. Early experience with real-time three-dimensional echocardiographic guidance of right ventricular biopsy in children. *Echocardiography*. 2006;23(1):45–49.

33. Suematsu Y, Martinez JF, Wolf BK, et al. Three-dimensional echo-guided beating heart surgery without cardiopulmonary bypass: atrial septal defect closure in a swine model. *J Thorac Cardiovasc Surg*. 2005;130(5):1348–1357.

34. Suematsu Y, Marx GR, Triedman JK, et al. Three-dimensional echocardiography-guided atrial septectomy: an experimental study. *J Thorac Cardiovasc Surg*. 2004;128(1):53–59.

35. Vasilyev NV, Martinez JF, Freudenthal FP, et al. Three-dimensional echo and videocardioscopy-guided atrial septal defect closure. *Ann Thorac Surg*. 2006;82(4):1322–1326; discussion 1326.

36. Baker GH, Shirali G, Ringewald JM, Hsia TY, Bandisode V. Usefulness of live three-dimensional transesophageal echocardiography in a congenital heart disease center. *Am J Cardiol*. 2009;103:1025–1028.

37. Jenkins C, Monaghan M, Shirali G, et al. An intensive interactive course for 3D echocardiography: Is "Crop Till You Drop" an effective learning strategy? *Eur J Echocardiogr*. 2008;9(3):373–380.

11.1 Introduction

Echocardiography is the most frequently used imaging modality in the assessment of intra-cardiac masses. Historically, this evaluation had been based on the analysis of two-dimensional (2D) slices of the heart. The information obtained from orthogonal tomographic planes from several acoustic windows, was used in an attempt to mentally reconstruct a model, of how the mass would actually appear in three dimensions, and how it would relate to the adjacent structures.

New technology using matrix-array transducers, has made possible the development of real-time 3D echocardiography (3DE), bringing cardiac imaging to a new dimension.

This new imaging modality provides valuable clinical information, that empowers echocardiographers with new levels of confidence in the diagnosis of heart disease.[1]

This chapter discusses the added value of this new technology in the echocardiographic assessment of intra-cardiac masses.

11.2 Echocardiographic Assessment of Intra-cardiac Masses

The complete echocardiographic evaluation of a cardiac mass is summarized in Table 11.1. It starts with a thorough description of its location, and relationship to adjacent structures. Masses can be either intra or extra-cardiac. The description should include the location and mechanism of implantation of the mass (i.e., pedunculated mass attached to the apical segment of the inferior wall through a long stalk), or the route of access of the mass to the heart (superior, inferior vena cava or pulmonary veins), if the mass is not primarily attached to the heart (Fig. 11.1).

The characterization of the shape, longest dimensions, and ideally volume of the mass, is essential. Additionally, a description of the hemodynamic consequences of the mass, should also be reported. The echocardiographer should then integrate all the information to generate a differential diagnosis. Finally, an essential part of the assessment, is the accurate calculation of volumes, ejection fraction and definition of regional wall function. Once all this information is obtained, a decision can be made as to the most appropriate treatment for the patient (anticoagulation, chemotherapy or surgery).

11.3 The 3D Examination

Three acquisition modes are used with 3DE in the evaluation of intra-cardiac masses: Full volume, live 3D, and 3D zoom (smaller, magnified pyramidal data at a higher resolution).[2]

Imaging with narrow angles (live 3D) is recommended if high-resolution images of the cardiac mass are desired.

11.4 Real Time 3D Evaluation of Cardiac Masses

In our Institution, the evaluation of a cardiac mass using transthoracic 3DE, includes at the minimum the performance of a full-volume acquisition in the parasternal long axis, and in the apical-four-chamber views. If the mass in question is located in the right atrium, a full volume acquisition and live 3D images are obtained from the right modified inflow, and sub-costal windows as well.

Live 3D images of the right parasternal and supraclavicular windows, have been used in the echocardiographic assessment of thrombus in the innominate vein, and the superior vena cava.[3] If the clinical questions are not successfully answered by the transthoracic 3DE, a trans-esophageal 3DE is performed. In addition to the images obtained following our lab protocol, a full volume acquisition of the left ventricle is obtained. Depending upon the location of the mass in

J.C. Plana
Department of Cardiology, The University of Texas
M.D. Anderson Cancer Center, 1515 Holcombe Boulevard,
Houston, Texas 77030, USA
e-mail: jcplana@mdanderson.org

L.P. Badano et al. (eds.), *Textbook of Real-Time Three Dimensional Echocardiography*,
DOI: 10.1007/978-1-84996-495-1_11, © Springer-Verlag London Limited 2011

Table 11.1 Echocardiographic evaluation of cardiac masses

1. Characterization of the mass
   a. Location. Intra or extra-cardiac
   b. Relationship with adjacent structures
   c. Site and mechanism of implantation
   d. Route of access to the heart
   c. Shape, size and volume
   e. Hemodynamic consequences
2. Differential diagnosis
   a. Benign
      1. Embryonic remnants
      2. Normal variants (false chords, heavy trabeculation, accessory papillary muscles)
      3. Thrombi (mural or associated with catheter or devices)
      4. Benign cardiac tumors
      5. Cardiomyopathy (apical HCM, non-compaction cardiomyopathy)
      6. Vegetations
   b. Malignant
      1. Primary
      2. Metastatic
      3. Accurate estimation of LV volumes and ejection fraction
      4. Therapeutic decision making

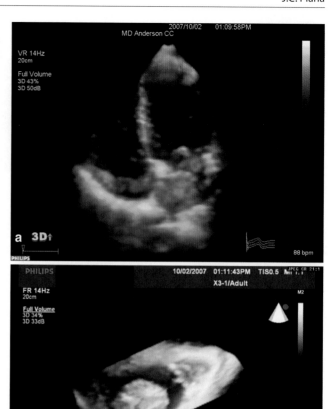

Fig. 11.1 Full volume acquisition (**a**) and cropped image (**b**) obtained from the apical 4-chamber view of a 22-year-old male with a recurrent metastatic osteosarcoma. The images show the tumor accessing the heart through the right upper pulmonary vein

question, 3D-zoom captures are obtained from the mitral valve, the tricuspid valve, the left atrial appendage, the left upper pulmonary vein, and the interatrial septum. A full volume acquisition and live 3D imaging in the bi-caval view are useful in the characterization of masses in the superior vena cava, inferior vena cava, and right atrium.

11.5 Differential Diagnosis

The differential diagnosis of intra-cardiac masses, includes tumors (benign, malignant or metastatic), normal structures or their variants, embryonic remnants, thrombi, cardiomyopathy (apical hypertrophic cardiomyopathy, non-compaction cardiomyopathy, and hypereosinophilic syndrome) and masses, or complications associated with device implantation (Table 11.1).

Primary tumors, are far less common than metastatic tumors in the heart, occurring in at least 7/10.000 people (Fig. 11.2).[4] Benign primary cardiac tumors occur more frequently than malignant ones. The most common cardiac tumor is the myxoma. In a large single-institution series of primary cardiac tumors at the University of Minnesota, 42% were cardiac myxomas, and 16% were malignant tumors (sarcomas).[5]

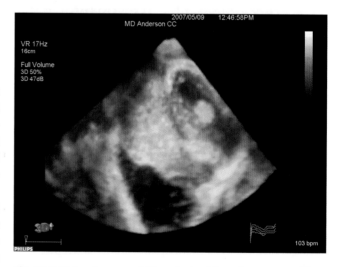

Fig. 11.2 Full volume acquisition obtained from the parasternal long axis view of a 35-year-old female with a primary cardiac sarcoma. There is evidence of a large exophytic mass originating from the base and mid segments of the inferolateral wall. An intracavitary mass is also visualized, originating from the mid-segment of the inferior wall

11.6 Added Value of 3D Echocardiography in the Assessment of Intra-cardiac Benign, Malignant, and Metastatic Cardiac Tumors

11.6.1 Unlimited Slicing and Cropping

Once a 3D data set is acquired, it can be sliced and cropped in many different manners. It also allows the manipulation of images in the space, obtaining views, and planes, and aligning structures in ways that were impossible to get before, with 2D imaging.

This feature is particularly useful in the way in which echocardiography is practiced in the United States, where the images captured by an echo technician, are interpreted later on by the physician, at times when the patient is no longer available, if additional images are needed. The availability of the full volume acquisition allows the echocardiographer to slice and crop the heart, the way that he or she had done if he/she had been the one directly imaging the patient (Fig. 11.3). The full volume allows for a detailed description of the location, shape, attaching interface and relationship to adjacent structures of the cardiac masses (Fig. 11.4). In addition, it is well known that 2D echocardiography, is very operator dependant. 3DE on the other hand, permits the acquisition of the images of the cardiac mass, from any ultrasound window, with less dependence on the skill of the technician. It is also important to realize that the availability of all of the information in just one capture, can significantly reduce the time that would otherwise be needed to fully characterize the mass.

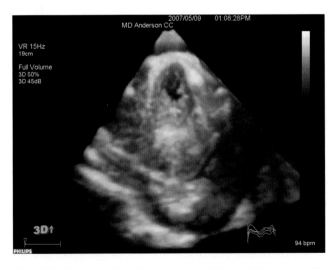

Fig. 11.3 Cropping of a full volume acquisition obtained from the apical 4 chamber view of the patient with primary cardiac sarcoma mentioned in Fig. 10.2. The tumor originates from the inferior, inferolateral and anterolateral walls of the left ventricle. A large pleural effusion is seen with large amounts of echodense material visualized floating in the space

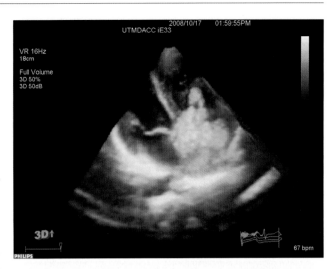

Fig. 11.4 Full volume acquisition obtained from a modified right ventricular inflow view of a 31-year-old patient with hepatocellular carcinoma. The mass access the heart through the inferior vena cava. The mass prolapses into the right ventricle through the tricuspid valve

11.6.2 Evaluation of the Composition of the Mass

Emphasis should also be put on the evaluation of the composition of the cardiac mass (Fig. 11.5). Mehmood et al. demonstrated in a preliminary study the superiority of live 3D over transthoracic 2DE in the assessment of left atrial tumors in patients with myxomas and hemangiomas. Because of the unique ability of live 3DE to systematically section and view the contents of an intra-cardiac mass, left atrial myxomas in the patients studied could be more confidently diagnosed by noting isolated echoluscent areas consistent with hemorrhage/necrosis in the tumor mass. In patients with hemangiomas, live 3DE showed much more extensive and closely packed echolucencies with little solid tissue as compared to a myxoma consistent with a highly vascularized tumor.[6] Overall, 3DE provides a more comprehensive assessment of the inner structure of the mass, which correlates better with pathologic findings (necrosis, hemorrhage, cystic areas or fibrotic bands).[7,8]

11.6.3 Unparalleled Level of Anatomic Detail

Sugeng et al. recently published the initial experience of her group using transesophageal 3DE. They tested the feasibility and clinical utility of this new technology in the imaging of different cardiac structures including mitral, aortic, and tricuspid valves; interatrial septum; left atrial appendage and pulmonic veins. The percentage of patients in whom each cardiac structure was assigned an optimal score of 2 was 85–91% of all scallops for both mitral valve leaflets, 84% of

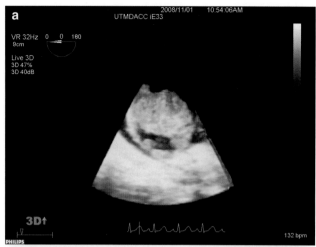

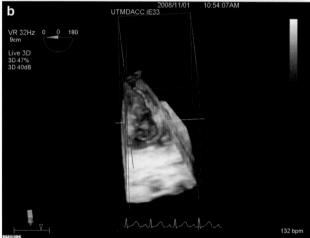

Fig. 11.5 Orthogonal views from live 3DMTEE obtained at 0 degrees from a 61-year old male with a metastatic thymoma. The mass appears homogenously echodense in panel A. When the mass is cropped from the orthogonal plane, it appears to have a cystic component as well

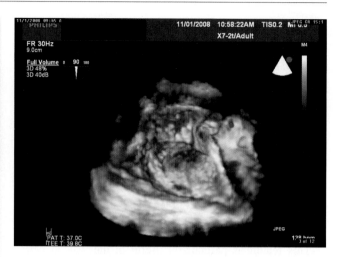

Fig. 11.6 Cropped full volume acquisition obtained from a 3D-MTEE at 90 degrees from the patient with metastatic thymoma mentioned in Fig. 10.5. The tumor completely obliterates the superior vena cava (SVC), and extends through the right atrium into the tricuspid valve annulus. Please note the mass is heterogeneous. The mass appears uniformly echodense in the SVC and at the cavo-atrial junction, while appears cystic as it gets close to the tricuspid valve annulus

11.6.4 Evaluation of the Size of the Cardiac Mass

Echocardiography is the method of choice for diagnosis and prognosis of cardiac masses, whether they are thrombi, vegetations, or tumors.[10] Maximum diameter measurements from 2DE are routinely used to determine mass size. The size of an intracardiac mass has important clinical relevance as a predictor for embolic events, congestive heart failure and death, and as an efficacy assessment after treatment (anticoagulation, antibiotics and chemotherapy).[10]

However, most masses are irregularly shaped, making it difficult to accurately image or select the largest diameter. Nanda et al. reported that 2D measurements from a transthoracic or a transesophageal study underestimates the true maximum diameter of irregularly shaped structures.[11] In the case of cardiac masses, this can lead to a misrepresentation of the patient's prognosis. 3DE images the entire volume of a mass allowing for accurate measurements in multiple planes. Asch et al. conducted a study testing the hypothesis that measurements of the maximum diameter of a mass by 3DE, are larger than those obtained by 2D.

He reported that 2D transthoracic, and 2D transesophageal consistently underestimated the maximum diameter by 24.6% (p<0.001), and 19.8% (P=0.01), as compared to 3DE. The measurements were fast and with excellent intra and inter observer variability (better then 2DE).

The authors suggested that 3DE may be the technique of choice for the noninvasive evaluation of intracardiac mass size.[10]

the interatrial septum, 86% of the left atrial appendage, and 77% of the left ventricular endocardium.[9]

One of the biggest limitations of 2DE in the assessment of cardiac masses is the possibility of "missing" the mass during the evaluation. As mentioned above, orthogonal planes are used to evaluate them, and if the mass happens to be located in an area between the imaging planes, the mass would not become apparent during the examination.

Transesophageal 3DE has allowed us the possibility to visualize the full volume of 3D structures with an unparalleled level of anatomic detail (Fig. 11.6). We are now able to really understand the 3D nature of the left atrial appendage, and its unique anatomic relationship with the ridge, and the left upper pulmonary vein. With this new technology, we are also able to visualize the foramen ovale of the inter-atrial septum from the left or the right atrium taking advantage of its posterior location.

11.7 Visualization of the True Apex, and Calculation of Left Ventricular Volumes and Ejection Fraction

A variety of methods are available for calculation of ejection fraction using 2DE. Unfortunately, they all have two big limitations. They are based on geometrical models that didn't take in consideration the architecture of the sick heart, and they are strongly affected by foreshortening.

3DE has emerged as a solution to these problems. The ability to capture a full volume acquisition of the left ventricle, allows for accurate identification of the true apex of the heart. An algorithm based on the detection of the endocardial border, then allows for direct quantification of left ventricular volumes, without multiplane tracing or geometric modeling.

Jacobs et al. compared 2D and 3DE against cardiac magnetic resonance imaging, in their ability to accurately calculate the end diastolic volume, end systolic volume, and ejection fraction. 3DE measurements of left ventricular volumes correlated highly with the cardiac MRI values (r = 0.96, 0.97 and 0.93 for end-diastolic and end-systolic volumes, and ejection fraction respectively).[12]

Left ventricular volume assessment and calculation of ejection fraction by 3DE is a rapid, accurate and reproducible method, superior to the conventional 2D methods. The small negative biases of the calculation of volumes and ejection fraction, as compared to the MRI, would hopefully be reduced as we gain experience with this new technique, and as we learn to trace the endocardium, underneath the trabeculations, and not on top of them.[1]

More recently, contrast has been used to enhance 3DE images. Contrast enhancement was found not only to improve the accuracy and reproducibility of left ventricular volume measurements in patients with poor image quality, but also to enhance the assessment of regional wall motion from 3DE datasets. The authors found that with the use of selective dual triggering to minimize bubble destruction by ultrasound energy, contrast enhancement increased the accuracy of 3DE-based analysis of regional left ventricular function against MRI reference, and its reproducibility to levels similar to those noted in patients with optimal imaging quality.[13]

The improved accuracy and reproducibility of 3DE-based left ventricular volumes and ejection fraction measurements are of vital importance in the patient with cardiac tumors, since clinical decision making relies heavily in this measurement. The mainstay in the treatment of cardiac sarcomas is anthracyclines, well known to cause cardiac toxicity in the form of systolic dysfunction. Hence, the accurate calculation of volumes and ejection fraction is essential in the initial and follow-up evaluations of these patients, as they are treated with this cardio-toxic regimens. In the study mentioned above by Jacobs, there was evidence of a wider limit of agreement for volumes and ejection fraction for 2DE (29%,

24% and 9.5%) as compared to 3DE (17%, 16%, 6.4%).[12] This means that when using 2DE, the ejection fraction can be potentially miscalculated by 9.5 points.

In our institution, anthracyclines are discontinued if patients drop their ejection fraction below 50%, or if they have a drop of 10 points of ejection fraction as compared to baseline. The mis-calculation of the ejection fraction by 2DE, can lead to the decision by the oncologist to stop the anthracycline based regimen due to concern for toxicity, in a patient that actually doesn't have it, where the mistake in the calculation is solely the result of the inherent limitations of the technology used.

11.8 Evaluation of Associated Abnormalities

3DE can also enhance the ability of the echocardiographer to detect associated abnormalities and conditions that predispose to the development of a mass (aneurisms or rheumatic mitral valve disease.)[14–17]

11.9 Surgical Planning

Muller at al conducted a study evaluating the value of transesophageal 3DE as an adjunct to conventional 2D imaging in preoperative evaluation of cardiac masses. In 37% of the patients, transesophageal 3DE revealed one or more items of additional information regarding type and site of attachment, surface features, and spatial relationship to surrounding structures. It is estimated by them that in at least 18% of all intra-cardiac masses, transesophageal 3DE can be expected to deliver supplementary information. In six of their patients the additional findings led to decisions deviating from those made on the basis of transesophageal 2DE. The authors concluded that the information revealed by 3D imaging facilitates therapeutic decision making and especially the choice of an optimal surgical access prior to the removal of the intracardiac mass (Fig. 11.7).[18]

Sugeng et al. demonstrated that transesophageal 3DE consistently provided excellent quality volume-rendered images of mitral valve components, including anterior and posterior leaflets, as well as the annulus and subvalvular structures. This finding suggests that transesophageal 3DE may become one of the modalities of choice to assess this valve during preoperative planning of mitral valve surgery, including the resection of tumors from the valve.[9,19] Le Tourneau et al. reported on the use of live transesophageal 3DE in the assessment of tumors of the aortic valve (papillary fibroelastomas). In their opinion, the use of this technology improved their operative planning.[20] The visualization of the aortic valve by

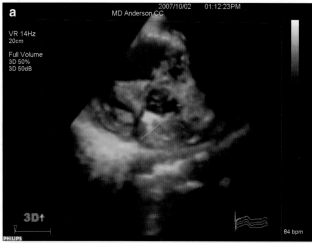

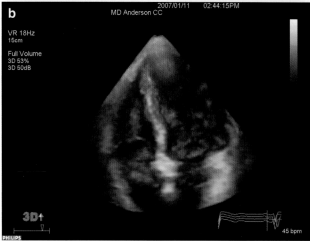

Fig. 11.7 (**a**) Full-volume acquisition obtained from the short axis view of the patient with osteosarcoma shown in Figs. 10.2 and 10.3. The mass was not amenable for surgical resection as it involved the aortic root. (**b**) Full volume acquisition obtained from the apical 4 chamber view of a 60-year-old male with metastatic squamous cell carcinoma of the penis. The mass was not thought to involve the tricuspid valve by 2DTTE. RT3DE revealed involvement of the tricuspid valve

transesophageal 3DE appears to be more challenging (optimal visualization of the aorta was possible only in 18–22% of the patients, from both the aorta and the left ventricular perspectives) as it is an anteriorly located cardiac structure.[9] Transesophageal 3DE has also been used, in the assessment of neoplasms of the pulmonic valve.[21]

11.10 Added Value in the Evaluation of Embryonic Remnants and Normal Variants

Normal cardiac structures (moderator band or false chords), or their variants (accessory papillary muscles), can be confused with cardiac masses in a 2DE.

In addressing these questions, we find very useful to obtain a full volume acquisition, and to crop the structure understanding its 3D relations.

We also have frequent referrals to our echo lab for the characterization of masses in the right atrium, where the differential diagnosis includes a normal structure (prominent inferior vena cava ridge or a crista terminalis), embryonic remnants (prominent Eustachian valve or a Chiari network), a thrombus, a tumor, or a tumor-thrombus arising from the inferior vena cava.[22–24] The ability to use the live-3D mode to see these 3D structures in motion, has allowed us in many instances to answer the questions without the need of a more invasive testing like a transesophageal 3DE.

11.11 Added Value in the Evaluation of Thrombi

Cardiac thrombi are most frequently seen in the apex, in the left atrial appendage, and in the right atrium/superior vena cava.

11.11.1 Apical Thrombi

The evaluation of cardiac masses at the apex can be extremely challenging using orthogonal planes, as it is customary with 2DE.

As mentioned above, it is the ability of 3DE to show the structure and function of the true apex of the heart what differentiates this technology from 2D. This feature has also opened a window of opportunity for a more refined assessment of the left and right ventricular apex (Fig. 11.8).

We find useful the administration of ultrasound contrast while obtaining a full volume acquisition of the left ventricle. This allows us the opportunity to carefully crop the ventricle from apex to base, fully confirming or ruling out the presence of an apical thrombus.

Sinha reported on the usefulness of live 3D in the morphological assessment of a left ventricular thrombus. Using live 3DE, the thrombus could be easily viewed end-on and from the sides. In addition, by cropping the 3D images sequentially in transverse (horizontal and short axis), longitudinal (vertical or long axis), frontal, and oblique planes, the degree and extent of lysis within the thrombus, which represents an integral part of the clot-resolution process, could be comprehensively assessed. The site of attachment of the thrombus in the left ventricular apex and its morphology can be fully evaluated in three dimensions by live 3DE.[25]

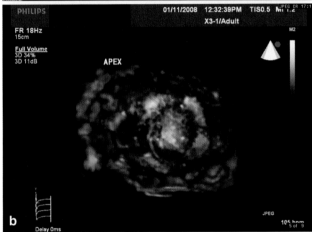

Fig. 11.8 Full volume (**a**) and cropped images (**b**) obtained from the apical-4-chamber view of a 41-year-old female with dilated cardiomyopathy. An apical thrombus is visualized

11.11.2 Thrombi and the Left Atrial Appendage

The left atrium is the most important location for the formation of thrombi in many cardiovascular conditions. Most of these clots occur in the left atrial appendage, which is a finger-like outpouching of the left atrium. The shape and location of the left atrial appendage allow for stasis of blood in atrial fibrillation, mitral stenosis, and other conditions with low cardiac output, particularly states with poor left ventricular function, or enlargement of the left atrium. The left atrial appendage is generally a 1.2–4.5 cm long structure, formed during the third week of gestation from the left wall of the primary atrium. Its multilobulated structure has been described by Venoit et al. at the Mayo clinic based on autopsy studies of about 500 specimens. The left atrial appendage may have anywhere between 1 and 4 lobes in 80% of the general population, with about 54% having 2 lobes. It is internally lined by pectinate muscles which are arranged in a parallel fashion, giving a web-like appearance. Most pectinate muscles are

greater than 1 mm in size.[26] Traditionally, it has been difficult to visualize by 2DE, and in most cases transesophageal 2DE has been used as the tool to evaluate its morphology and its pathology. It has been believed that the left atrial appendage is not well visualized by 2DE. Hence, the accepted gold standard for the assessment of the left atrial appendage has been transesophageal 2DE. Karakus et al. compared combined transthoracic 2DE and 3DE with transesophageal 2DE in evaluating the left atrium and the left atrial appendage for thrombus. Their preliminary study suggested that combined transthoracic 2DE and 3DE has a comparable accuracy to transesophageal 2DE in evaluating the left atrium and left atrial appendage for thrombus. In some patients the transesophageal 2DE, but not transthoracic 3DE, may misdiagnose pectinate musculature as thrombus.[27]

More recently, we have used transesophageal 3DE in the evaluation of patients with pathology suspected in the left atrial appendage and left upper pulmonary vein. A 3D zoom of the left atrial appendage, shows this finger-like outpouching in its three dimensions, with full display of its multi-lobular architecture, allowing us to conclusive differentiate thrombi from pectinate muscles, or bilobar left atrial appendages. We also take advantage of this technology in the characterization of masses accessing the heart through the left upper pulmonary vein.

In our institution, we frequently have patients with atrial fibrillation at risk for stroke, who have absolute contraindications to taking warfarin. The left atrial appendage occlusion devices may provide a novel treatment option for these patients, and randomized clinical trials for left atrial appendage occlusion devices are ongoing. Shah et al. recently performed a study evaluating the feasibility and accuracy of transesophageal 3DE for the determination of the left atrial appendage geometry. They concluded that transesophageal 3DE for the visualization and quantitative assessment of left atrial appendage orifice is feasible and correlates well with 64-slice cardiac computerized tomography.[28]

11.12 Added Value in the Evaluation of Masses Associated with Cardiomyopathy

Non-compaction cardiomyopathy is a congenital cardiomyopathy that affects children and adults. It results from the failure of myocardial development during embryogenesis.

It is characterized by a two-layered structure with a compacted thin epicardial layer, and a thicker non-compacted layer of trabecular meshwork with deep endomyocardial spaces. A maximal end-systolic ratio of noncompacted to compacted >2 is diagnostic.[29] We find useful the cropping of a full volume acquisition of the apical four chamber view, from apex to base at end-systole, to easily demonstrate the presence of the above mentioned ratio (Fig. 11.9a). 3DE also supplements 2DE in making a definitive diagnosis of clots coexisting with trabeculations in the left ventricle. Mobility of clots and the presence of central echolucencies consistent with clot lysis were best demonstrated with 3DE and served to confidently differentiate clots from adjacent trabeculations.

In the hypereosinophilic syndrome, cardiac involvement is often bi-ventricular, with mural endocardial thickening of the inflow portions and apex of the ventricles. The echocardiogram commonly demonstrates localized thickening of the posterobasal left ventricular wall, with absent or markedly limited motion of the posterior leaflet of the mitral valve. There may be obliteration of the apex by thrombus.

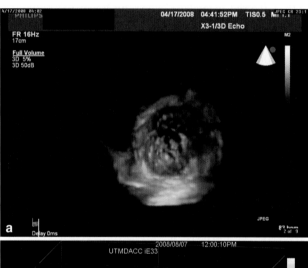

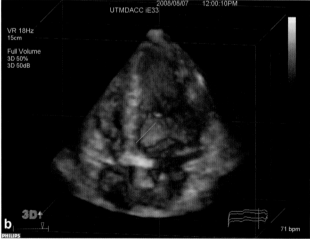

Fig. 11.9 (**a**) Cropped images obtained from a full volume acquisition of a 22-year-old –female with diagnosis of non-compaction cardiomyopathy. The image shows the spongiform appearance of the LV apex, with numerous trabeculation and recesses. (**b**) Full volume acquisition obtained from the apical-4-chamber view of a 72-year-old male with hypereosinophilic syndrome. The apex appears obliterated with thrombus

3DE is very useful in the evaluation of these patients, as the obliteration of the apex (Fig. 11.9b), the thickening of the posterobasal, and the limited motion of the left ventricular wall can be easily demonstrated with the cropping of the full volume acquisition images.

Contrast can further assist in the definition of the trabeculations and the recesses in the non-compaction cardiomyopathy, as well as in the definition of the obliteration of the apex in the patients with the hypereosinophilic syndrome.

11.13 Added Value in the Evaluation of Masses and Complications Associated with Devices

Thrombi or vegetations can occur as a complication of the implantation of catheters or pacemakers. The most common situation for the formation of a thrombus in the right atrium, is the presence of a catheter with its tip far beyond the junction of the superior vena cava and the right atrium. The jet of fluid then hits on the wall of the right atrium, denuding the endothelium, and provoking the formation of a thrombus in that location. We find useful the use of live 3DE, and 3D zoom, in the evaluation of these cardiac masses. Anticoagulation as well as correction of the position of the catheter (pulling the tip to the junction of the superior vena cava and right atrium) are essential.

3DE can also be used in the diagnosis of complications associated with placement of pacemakers. Daher et al. reported on the use of a full volume acquisition to demonstrate a pacemaker lead perforation of the interventricular septum with location of the pacer tip in the left ventricle.[30]

11.14 Conclusions

3D transthoracic and transesophageal echocardiography have revolutionized the assessment of cardiac structure and function.

The use of 3D echocardiography adds value in the assessment of a cardiac mass. A detailed characterization of the mass size, composition, location, and relationship to adjacent structures; in conjunction with an accurate assessment of left ventricular volumes and ejection fraction, empowers the echocardiographer with a new level of confidence in the diagnosis, follow up, and surgical planning of the patient with a cardiac mass.

11.15 Disclosure

Our laboratory has received equipment grants from Philips and General Electric. Dr. Plana is on the speakers' bureau for Philips and General Electric.

References

1. Mor-Avi V, Sugeng L, Lang RM. Real-time 3-dimensional echocardiography: an integral component of the routine echocardiographic examination in adult patients? *Circulation*, 2009;119(2):314–329.
2. Hung J, et al. 3D echocardiography: a review of the current status and future directions. *J Am Soc Echocardiogr*. 2007;20(3): 213–233.
3. Upendram S, et al. Live three-dimensional transthoracic echocardiographic assessment of thrombus in the innominate veins and superior vena cava utilizing right parasternal and supraclavicular approaches. *Echocardiography*. 2005;22(5):445–449.
4. Reynen K. Cardiac myxomas. *N Engl J Med*. 1995;333(24): 1610–1617.
5. Molina JE, Ward HB. Primary cardiac tumors: experience at the University of Minnesota. *Thorac Cardiovasc Surg*. 1990;38: 183–191.
6. Mehmood F, et al. Live three-dimensional transthoracic echocardiographic assessment of left atrial tumors. *Echocardiography*. 2005;22(2):137–143.
7. Pothineni KR, et al. Live/real time three-dimensional transthoracic echocardiographic description of chordoma metastatic to the heart. *Echocardiography*. 2008;25(4):440–442.
8. Suwanjutah T, et al. Live/real time three-dimensional transthoracic echocardiographic findings in primary left atrial leiomyosarcoma. *Echocardiography*. 2008;25(3):337–339.
9. Sugeng L, et al. Live 3-dimensional transesophageal echocardiography initial experience using the fully-sampled matrix array probe. *J Am Coll Cardiol*. 2008;52(6):446–449.
10. Asch FM, et al. Real-time 3-dimensional echocardiography evaluation of intracardiac masses. *Echocardiography*. 2006;23(3): 218–224.
11. Nanda NC, A.-E.R.S., Khatry G, et al. Incremental value of three-dimensional echocardiography over transesophageal multiplane two-dimensional echocardiography in qualitative and quantitative assessment of cardiac masses and defects. *Echocardiography*. 1995;12:619–628.
12. Jacobs LD, et al. Rapid online quantification of left ventricular volume from real-time three-dimensional echocardiographic data. *Eur Heart J*. 2006;27(4):460–468.
13. Corsi C, et al. Quantification of regional left ventricular wall motion from real-time 3-dimensional echocardiography in patients with poor acoustic windows: effects of contrast enhancement tested against cardiac magnetic resonance. *J Am Soc Echocardiogr*. 2006;19(7):886–893.
14. Stewart JA, et al, Echocardiographic documentation of vegetative lesions in infective endocarditis: clinical implications. *Circulation*. 1980;61(2):374–380.
15. Zamorano J, et al. Real-time three-dimensional echocardiography for rheumatic mitral valve stenosis evaluation: an accurate and novel approach. *J Am Coll Cardiol*. 2004;43(11):2091–2096.
16. Zamorano J, et al. Non-invasive assessment of mitral valve area during percutaneous balloon mitral valvuloplasty: role of real-time 3D echocardiography. *Eur Heart J*. 2004;25(23):2086–2091.
17. Monaghan MJ, Role of real time 3D echocardiography in evaluating the left ventricle. *Heart*. 2006;92(1):131–136.
18. Muller S, et al. Value of transesophageal 3D echocardiography as an adjunct to conventional 2D imaging in preoperative evaluation of cardiac masses. *Echocardiography*. 2008;25(6):624–631.
19. Handke M, et al. Myxoma of the mitral valve: diagnosis by 2-dimensional and 3-dimensional echocardiography. *J Am Soc Echocardiogr*. 1999;12(9):773–776.
20. Le Tourneau T, et al. Assessment of papillary fibroelastomas with live three-dimensional transthoracic echocardiography. *Echocardiography*. 2008;25(5):489–495.
21. Singh A, et al. Papillary fibroelastoma of the pulmonary valve: assessment by live/real time three-dimensional transthoracic echocardiography. *Echocardiography*. 2006;23(10):880–883.
22. Pothineni KR, et al. Live/real time three-dimensional transthoracic echocardiographic visualization of Chiari network. *Echocardiography*. 2007;24(9):995–997.
23. McKay T, Thomas L. Prominent crista terminalis and Eustachian ridge in the right atrium: Two dimensional (2D) and three dimensional (3D) imaging. *Eur J Echocardiogr*. 2007;8(4):288–291.
24. Roldan FJ, et al. Three-dimensional transesophageal echocardiography of the atrial septal defects. *Cardiovasc Ultrasound*. 2008; 6:38.
25. Sinha A, et al. Morphological assessment of left ventricular thrombus by live three-dimensional transthoracic echocardiography. *Echocardiography*. 2004;21(7):649–655.
26. Veinot JP, et al. Anatomy of the normal left atrial appendage: a quantitative study of age-related changes in 500 autopsy hearts: implications for echocardiographic examination. *Circulation*. 1997;96(9):3112–3115.
27. Karakus G, et al. Comparative assessment of left atrial appendage by transesophageal and combined two- and three-dimensional transthoracic echocardiography. *Echocardiography*. 2008;25(8): 918–924.
28. Shah SJ, et al. Real-time three-dimensional transesophageal echocardiography of the left atrial appendage: initial experience in the clinical setting. *J Am Soc Echocardiogr*. 2008;21(12): 1362–1368.
29. Jenni R, et al. Echocardiographic and pathoanatomical characteristics of isolated left ventricular non-compaction: a step towards classification as a distinct cardiomyopathy. *Heart*. 2001;86(6): 666–671.
30. Daher IN, et al. Live three-dimensional echocardiography in diagnosis of interventricular septal perforation by pacemaker lead. *Echocardiography*. 2006;23(5):428–429.

Real Time Three Dimensional Transesophageal Echocardiography for Guidance of Catheter Based Interventions

12

Miguel Angel Garcia Fernandez, Gila Perk, Muhamed Saric, and Itzhak Kronzon

12.1 Introduction

Over the recent years, percutaneous catheter-based intracardiac procedures have gained growing acceptance into the cardiac procedural armamentarium allowing treatment of increasingly complex cardiac pathologies via a non surgical, catheter based approach.[1–6] Guidance of these procedures is usually by fluoroscopy. However, this technique has limited resolution for soft tissue differentiation, and involves radiation exposure as well as occasional iodinated contrast injection. Other guiding techniques include intracardiac echocardiography or transesophageal 2DE.[7–14] Intracardiac echocardiography is a useful, yet invasive and expensive technique. The disposable ultrasound catheter is inserted via a central venous approach and is for single-use only. Additionally, intracardiac echocardiography transducers are limited monoplane transducers and allow only several imaging planes. Transesophageal 2DE is commonly used for guiding purposes, however it has several limitations. The main limitation of transesophageal 2DE is related to the tomographic nature of this imaging technique. Since only a "slice" of the heart is imaged at any given view, intra-cardiac catheters cannot be fully visualized without acquisition from multiple imaging planes, which may be time consuming and distracting during a procedure. The relative location of an intra-cardiac catheter and the surrounding anatomical structures can be challenging with a two-dimensional tomographic view, especially for the interventionalist who may be less familiar with the various transesophageal echocardiographic planes.

Transesophageal 3DE is a new imaging modality that may become the technique of choice for guiding catheter-based interventions. The main advantages of this technique include real time visualization of the entire length of all intracardiac catheters and devices, as well as multiple views, including en-face view, of cardiac structures (e.g. atrial septum, mitral valve) which permit clear delineation of the relative location of the catheters and the surrounding anatomy.

12.2 General Considerations

Transesophageal 3DE guided procedures are generally performed under general anesthesia, or if a short, uncomplicated procedure is anticipated, conscious sedation under close supervision and monitoring by an anesthesiologist can be used. The echocardiography unit is connected to a screen which is placed alongside the hemodynamic and fluoroscopy monitors, such that images are available to the interventional cardiologist.

Often the procedure is performed by two operators; one manipulates the probe while the other operates the machine, to optimize image quality. Sonographers trained in 3DE imaging can serve as the second operators during such procedures. Of note, during a catheter-based intervention, when the patient is under general anesthesia, the imaging can also be easily performed by one operator.

Most protocols include a pre-procedure, comprehensive transesophageal 2D and 3DE. This is done for obtaining clear anatomic definition of the cardiac pathology being intervened on, as well ruling out any possible contraindications for percutaneous corrective procedure (e.g., ruling out intra-cardiac thrombus prior to mitral balloon valvuloplasty for mitral stenosis).

During the procedure, imaging is done continuously, with switching between 2D and 3D modes. Most probe adjustments are done based on the 2D imaging, although as the operator experience grows, increasingly more adjustments and image optimizations can be performed based on the 3D image alone, with less need to switch back and forth between the two imaging modalities. Most procedure-related decisions are done based on the real-time imaging modes (3D zoom mode and narrow angle acquisitions) although periodically, full volume loops are acquired which can be further processed

I. Kronzon (✉)
NYU School of Medicine, 550 First Ave, TH-2, HW-228,
New York, 10016 NY
e-mail: itzhak.kronzon@nyumc.org

L.P. Badano et al. (eds.), *Textbook of Real-Time Three Dimensional Echocardiography*,
DOI: 10.1007/978-1-84996-495-1_12, © Springer-Verlag London Limited 2011

off line. This can be done post procedure, however can also be quickly performed during the procedure, with the advantage of a higher frame rate of the images acquired in this mode.

12.3 Specific Procedures

12.3.1 Atrial Septal Defect and Patent Foramen Ovale Closure

Over the recent years, percutaneous closure of ostium secundum atrial septal defects and patent foramen ovale has become the standard of care in appropriately selected patients.[3–5,15,16] Pre-procedure transesophageal 3DE with en-face view of the atrial septum, allows clear anatomic delineation of the septal defect, including definition of its shape (which is often not perfectly round), size, presence of adequate tissue rim around the defect (which is crucial for successful device closure) and existence of any ridges or tissue membranes across the defect (Fig. 12.1 panels A and B).

The procedure is performed via a central venous access. A guiding catheter is advanced through the atrial septal defect (or the patent foramen ovale) (Fig. 12.1 panel C). In atrial septal defect closure procedures, a sizing balloon is used to measure the size of the defect and choose the correct size occlusion device. Verification of complete occlusion of the defect by the balloon is done using both direct visualization (using the 3D zoom mode), as well as color Doppler imaging to demonstrate cessation of flow across the septum.

Once the device size has been chosen, the collapsed device is advanced through the guiding catheter into position across the inter-atrial septum. 3DE allows continuous visualization of the entire length of the intra-cardiac catheter, including its tip, thus minimizing the complication potential. Once the device has been deployed, proper positioning, complete occlusion of the defect and shunt termination are verified using both direct inspection of the septum (using the 3D zoom mode) and color Doppler imaging. If malpositioning has occurred (Fig. 12.1 panel D), it can be easily identified with 3DE and repositioning of the device should be attempted, until optimal occlusion has been achieved.

In a small percentage of patients with ostium secundum atrial septal defect, the defect anatomy can be more complex than what might be seen on 2DE imaging. Some atrial septal defects can be fenestrated or can have a tissue strip across the defect. This may create a wrong estimation of the defect's size in 2DE, as the entire septum cannot be visualized in one view. 3DE imaging, with the 3D zoom mode, allows for the en-face view of the entire inter-atrial septum, thus eliminating the need to "mentally

Fig. 12.1 Atrial septal defect (ASD) closure. **Panel A**: ASD as seen from the left atrial perspective. Using commercially available software, the defect margins can be traced for a precise measurement of its size and shape. **Panel B**: En face view of the ASD allowing assessment of the presence of adequate tissue rim around the defect, to determine suitability for percutaneous closure. **Panel C**: Guiding catheter passed through the septal defect, as seen from the left atrial perspective. **Panel D**: En face view of the closure device in place as seen from the left atrial perspective

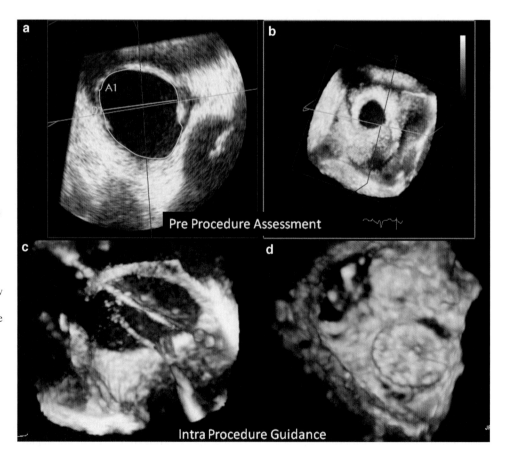

reconstruct" the anatomy. This translates into proper sizing and selection of closure device, minimizing potential complications (e.g. distal device embolization if a small size device is introduced through a larger atrial septal defect). Rarely, two closure devices need to be placed in order to achieve optimal occlusion of a dual-orifice atrial septal defect. Transesophageal 3DE is crucial in these cases as it allows verification of passing the two guiding catheters through the two different orifices (which is not discernable by a 2D imaging modality).

12.3.2   Percutaneous Closure of Ventricular Septal Defect

Catheter based closure of ventricular septal defect has been recently described.[17–19] Ventricular septal defects, congenital or acquired, have been traditionally treated by open heart surgery. Catheter based closure allows avoiding open heart surgery, and in the case of post-infarction ventricular septal defect eliminates the need to suture into a friable, necrotic, recently infracted area. This has the potential to improve outcome of patients suffering from this highly risky complication.

3D imaging is an essential component of attempted percutaneous closure of ventricular septal defects. Pre-procedure imaging allows en-face view of the interventricular septum, thus allowing accurate assessment of the size and shape of the defect. Post infarction ventricular septal defects commonly have complex anatomy with tracks through the septum and

bizarre geometrical shapes. This cannot be ascertained by 2D imaging; however the en-face view of the ventricular septal defect allows better understanding of this complex morphology (Fig. 12.2 panels A and B). Device size can be chosen based on the 3D assessment of the defect.

The procedure is done via an arterial and a central venous approach. One guiding catheter is placed in the left ventricle via a retrograde approach, and another in the right ventricle via a central venous approach (Fig. 12.2 panel C). The closure device is introduced through the arterial guide, while the right ventricular catheter is used to snare the device across the septum (Fig. 12.2 panel D).

Transesophageal 3DE during the procedure allows continuous visualization of all the catheters, guides and devices that are used. This uninterrupted monitoring of every tip of every intra-cardiac catheter allows safer manipulation, thus minimizing the risk of complications. Once the device has been deployed, correct positioning is verified by direct visualization (using the 3D zoom mode) as well as color Doppler imaging.

12.3.3   Mitral Valve Clipping

Mitral clipping procedure is a newly developed technique for the percutaneous treatment of mitral regurgitation. In this procedure, a clip is placed between the mitral valve leaflet tips, grasping together the central part of the anterior and posterior leaflets, essentially creating an "Alfieri Stitch" repair. It offers an alternative to open heart surgery for high risk patients, or

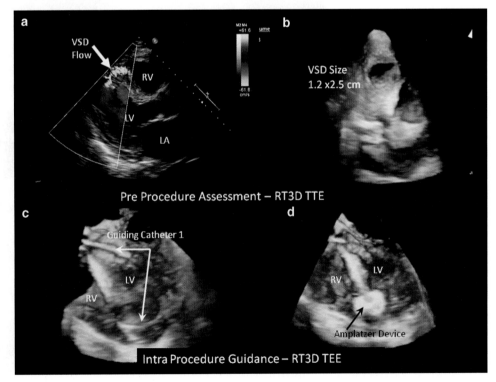

Fig. 12.2 Ventricular septal defect (VSD) closure. **Panel A**: Transthoracic 2-dimensional echocardiography (TTE) with color Doppler demonstrating the presence of a VSD in the apical portion of the interventricular septum. **Panel B**: En face view of the VSD as seen from the right ventricular perspective, allowing clear visualization of the shape and extent of the defect, as well as accurate measurement of its size, which enables proper device selection. **Panel C**: Image taken during percutaneous closure procedure. The left ventricular catheter enters the ventricle via the aortic valve (retrograde arterial approach). The entire length of catheter can be seen throughout its course in the heart. **Panel D**: Closure device deployed in the VSD, achieving complete occlusion of the defect

those who wish to avoid open heart surgery. The procedure is still experimental, yet with so far promising results.[20,21]

The procedure is performed via a central venous access and a transseptal puncture. Performing the transseptal puncture at an appropriate place in the interatrial septum is a critical part of this procedure. Since all further catheters and devices will be advanced via the passage created, correct location of the puncture will facilitate easy accessibility to the mitral valve and perfect positioning of the clip. Transesophageal 3DE imaging, with 3D zoom mode, allows for the en-face visualization of the interatrial septum, thus facilitating precise localization of the transseptal puncture (Fig. 12.3 panel A).

The clip is then passed through the guiding catheter towards the mitral valve leaflets (Fig. 12.3 panels B and C). The clip arms are opened and positioned such that they are perpendicular to the mitral valve closure line. Correct positioning is essential for optimal grasping of the leaflets and subsequent reduction in the mitral regurgitation. This step is also greatly facilitated by the use of transesophageal 3DE imaging. Viewing the mitral valve en-face allows identification of the closure line and accurate alignment of the clip arms (Fig. 12.3 panel D). Without the use of 3D imaging, this stage generally requires either a transgastric view (which is occasionally hard to obtain) or a transthoracic, parasternal short axis view (which is extremely hard

to obtain during a procedure where the patient lies supine, sedated, draped and underneath a fluoroscopy tube).

Once a clip is deployed, immediate assessment of the severity of the remaining mitral regurgitation can be obtained (using both 2D, 3D[22] and color Doppler imaging). If a second clip is deemed necessary, transesophageal 3DE imaging is key to the success of the deployment of the second clip. Using the 3D zoom mode and the en-face view, verification of passing the guiding catheter through the larger remaining orifice of the valve can be accomplished, thus allowing placement of the second clip at the correct spot. Discerning the two orifices created by the first clip and the catheter location relative the clip on 2D imaging is challenging and sometimes impossible.

12.3.4 Mitral Balloon Valvulotomy for Mitral Stenosis

Since it was first described in 1989 by Inoue, percutaneous mitral valve balloon valvulotomy has become a standard treatment option for patients with mitral stenosis and suitable valve anatomy; it is currently considered to be the first-line treatment for symptomatic, suitable patients.[23,24]

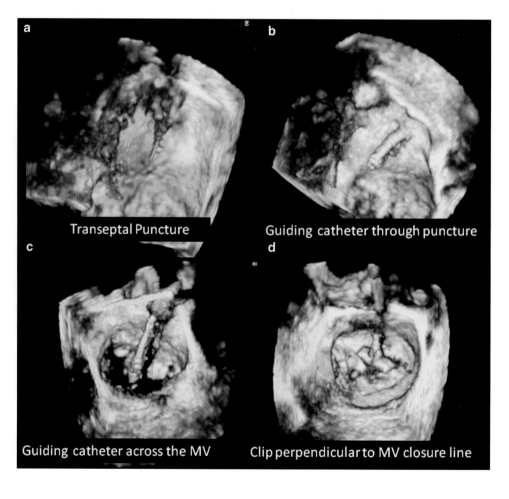

Fig. 12.3 Mitral valve clipping procedure. **Panel A**: Trans-septal needle across the atrial septum and seen from the left atrial perspective. **Panel B**: Guiding catheter across the inter-atrial septum. The entire length of the catheter is easily seen, as well as its relative relation to other left atrial structures. **Panel C**: Guiding catheter across the mitral valve, seen from the left atrial perspective. **Panel D**: Mitral clip advanced towards the valve, seen from the left atrial perspective. The clip arms are still open and can be easily adjusted such that they are perpendicular to the mitral valve closure line (optimal positioning for proper grasping)

Transeptal Puncture

Guiding catheter through puncture

Guiding catheter across the MV

Clip perpendicular to MV closure line

Traditionally, transesophageal 2DE has been employed as the guiding technique during percutaneous intervention to assist in the positioning of the balloon, and to immediately assess the valvulotomy results.

Recent studies have confirmed that the degree of commissural opening, before and after the procedure, is an important prognostic determinant, and thus should be systematically evaluated during and after mitral balloon valvulotomy.[25,26]

Transesophageal 3DE allows accurate anatomical assessment of the mitral valve, including the degree of commissural fusion. During the procedure, transesophageal 3DE facilitates the accurate positioning of the Inoue balloon through the mitral valve (Fig. 12.4). It also allows immediate assessment of results of the valvulotomy, with real-time anatomical analysis of the commissural opening as well as assessment for the presence of complications (e.g., leaflet tear). This analysis overcomes the difficulties and limitations involved in making immediate post-intervention measurements of valvular area, thus giving immediate feedback to the operator and guiding decisions regarding need for further balloon inflations.[27]

12.3.5 Percutaneous Closure of Prosthetic Valve Dehiscence

Paravalvular dehiscence is a complication that may occasionally occur in patients with prosthetic valves, especially mechanical prosthetic valves. The reported incidence is approximately 2%–17% of patients post valve surgery, and up to 10% of re-operated patients.[28,29] Factors associated with valve dehiscence include faulty surgical technique, endocarditis operation, advanced patient's age, and presence of calcifications of the valvular ring.[30] The resulting valve regurgitation may produce clinical symptoms of congestive heart failure and/or haemolytic anemia.[31] Traditionally, treatment is surgical with restitution of the valve with re-suture or patch implant. Some authors even propose aggressive surgery in minimally symptomatic patients if the defect is of a significant size.[30,32] However, since by definition these are all re-operation procedures, each intervention carries a significant risk to the patient, with a reported mortality rate of 6%–22%, and recurrence of valve dehiscence in 15%, 22% and 35% of cases in first, second and third re-operations, respectively.[33]

Over the past few years, various percutaneous treatment procedures for paravalvular dehiscence have been described; these allow correction of the defect and the resulting clinical syndrome for those patients who are poor surgical candidates.[31,34–36]

Recently published studies have proven the usefulness of transesophageal 2DE in the evaluation and follow-up of patients with paravalvular mitral dehiscence who were treated by a percutaneous closure technique.[36] The main limitation of transesophageal 2DE is the inability to define the exact anatomical characteristics of the dehisced segment (size, shape and area); such data are of critical importance for the proper

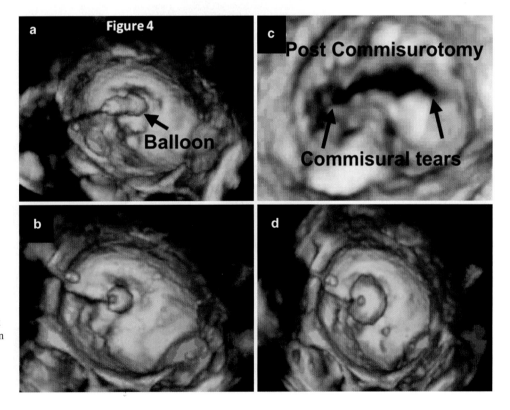

Fig. 12.4 Mitral balloon valvulotomy. Panel A: Guiding catheter with balloon as seen from the left atrial perspective. Panel B: Balloon insertion into the mitral valve. Panel C: Post procedure en face view of the mitral valve as seen from the left atrial perspective. Clear depiction of the resultant commissural tears is demonstrated. Panel D: Balloon inflation at the mitral valve commissure

selection of patients for a percutaneous closure procedure, monitoring and guiding of the actual procedure, and evaluating short-term and long-term results of the intervention. Transesophageal 3DE allows for the accurate anatomical and functional assessment of the dehiscence; number of dehisced segments, location, size and extent of the dehiscence can be ascertained, as well as the presence and severity of para-valvular or trans-valvular regurgitation.[37,38] In a cohort of 52 patients with para-valvular mitral dehiscence treated by a percutaneous closure procedure, only 51.5% had significant reduction in the mitral regurgitation severity. Transesophageal 3DE analysis of those patients in whom the severity of the mitral regurgitation remained unchanged, revealed that this was due to the dehisced segment being large and only partially occluded by the implanted device (Fig. 12.5). These findings were not surprising; patients with very extensive dehiscence or more than one areas of dehiscence are more likely to have significant persistent para-valvular regurgitation following percutaneous closure of the dehiscence. While accurate data regarding para-valvular dehiscence is easily obtainable using transesophageal 3DE imaging, it is essentially impossible to obtain with transesophageal 2DE given the tomographic nature of this technique. Transesophageal 3DE is thus crucial for the pre-procedure screening, to determine suitability for percutaneous closure procedure based on the location, size, shape and extent of the dehisced segment.

In addition, transesophageal 3DE can assist the operator during the procedure itself; confirmation of passing the guide wire through the dehisced segment rather than through the valve itself can be obtained with 3D imaging. Transesophageal 3DE allows also for the continuous visualization of all the intra-cardiac catheters throughout their entire length, including their tips, and their spatial location relative to the dehisced segment and other cardiac structures (Figs. 12.6–12.8).

The assessment of percutaneous closure of aortic prosthetic valve dehiscence with transesophageal 3DE is somewhat limited: The transesophageal 3DE study allows real-time visualization of all intracardiac catheters and their relation to cardiac structures, as well as aids the operator in guiding across the dehiscence and providing an anatomical and functional assessment of the intervention's success (Fig. 12.9). However the size and shape of aortic paravalvular dehiscence is occasionally not well visualized.

12.4 Catheter-Based Aortic Valve Implantation

The incidence of aortic stenosis in patients older than age 65 is estimated at 2%–9%.[39] Generally, the rate of progression of the disease is relatively predictable with gradient increase

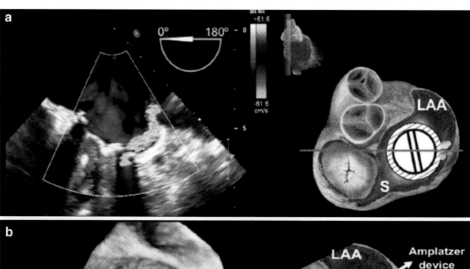
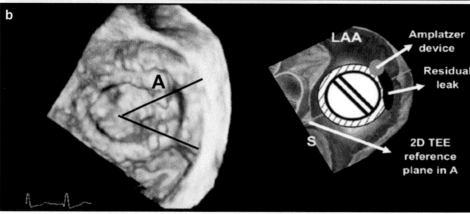

Fig. 12.5 Mitral prosthesis dehiscence. **Panel A**: Pre-intervention study of a paravalvular dehiscence on the outer lateral surface of a mitral tissue prosthesis ring. The patient underwent percutaneous closure performed, however he continued to do poorly three months post-procedure. **Panel B**: Repeat transesophageal echocardiogram, this time with RT3D imaging, demonstrates that the previously placed device (A) does not completely occlude the dehisced segment with a residual dehiscence

Fig. 12.6 Mitral prosthesis dehiscence II. **Panel A**: 2D-TEE view of a corrected extensive dehiscence of mitral tissue prosthesis. **Panel B**: Corresponding RT3D TEE image, seen from the left atrial perspective, showing a clear depiction of the two closure devices that were used to occlude the defects. Note the clear delineation of the spatial relationship of the two closure devices, which is not obtainable by the 2D imaging technique

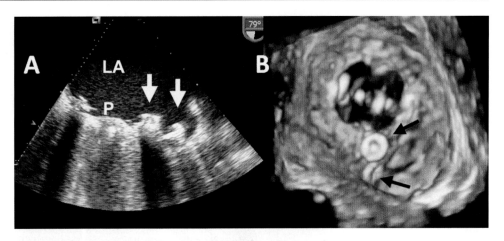

Fig. 12.7 Mitral prosthesis dehiscence III. **Panel A**: Dehisced mitral mechanical prosthesis (*black arrow*) as seen from the left atrial perspective. **Panel B**: 3D color imaging showing minimal transvalvular mitral regurgitation (normal for mechanical prosthesis) as well and significant jet of paravalvular mitral regurgitation. **Panel C**: During a percutaneous closure procedure, the catheters can be seen throughout their entire course in the heart. In this image, the extreme distal portion of the catheter can be observed as it is passed through the dehiscence. **Panel D**: Corresponding 2D TEE image showing the same catheter as in panel C, however demonstrating the difficulties in perceiving the spatial relation between the catheter and the various cardiac structures (*RA* right atrium, *LA* left atrium, *P* mitral prosthesis)

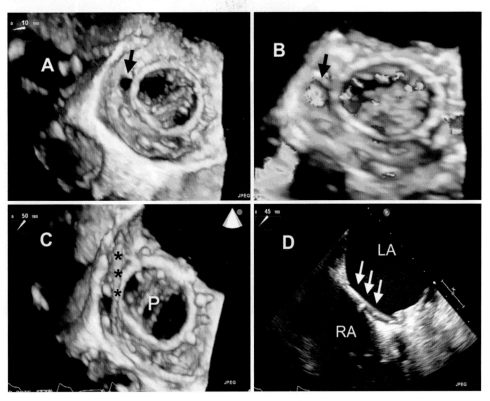

of a mean of 7 mm Hg per year and aortic valve area decrease of 0.1 cm² per year.[40] In patients with symptoms, the prognosis is poor with conservative treatment.[41] Surgical treatment is the procedure of choice and provides excellent results. However, many patients present a very high risk due to co-morbidities: advanced age, ventricular dysfunction, lung disease, and prior surgery. Percutaneous transcatheter aortic valve implantation is an evolving interventional therapy for high-risk patients with severe symptomatic aortic valve stenosis.[42] Two valve models, the Edwards SAPIEN valve (EdwardsLifescience, Irvine, California) and the CoreValve ReValving system (CoreValve Inc., Irvine, California), have thus far been used in over 4,000 cases worldwide for the percutaneous treatment of symptomatic aortic stenosis. Mid-

term follow-up shows no evidence of restenosis or prosthetic valve dysfunction. Transfemoral and transapical delivery routes can be selected depending on ease of vascular access and type of prosthesis used. Randomized trials that are currently underway will confirm procedural safety and guide the applicability of this technology.[43]

Transesophageal echocardiography can play a major role in the selection of candidates and guidance of the procedure for possible reduction in complications. Accurate measurement of the aortic annular size is central to acquiring proper positioning of the prosthesis. The transcatheter heart valve should be slightly larger than the aortic annulus in order to reduce paravalvular aortic regurgitation. However, marked over-sizing of the prosthesis may cause aortic annular rupture in patients with

Fig. 12.8 Mitral prosthesis dehiscence IV. **Panel A**: Mitral prosthesis dehiscence on the external lateral surface of the ring, and in the region joining the ring with the left atrial appendage (LAA). Only a small segment of the catheter can be seen in this view, making it hard to manipulate the catheter safely. **Panel B**: RT3D TEE imaging permits localization of the entire guiding catheter and its tip across the dehisced segment of the mitral prosthesis

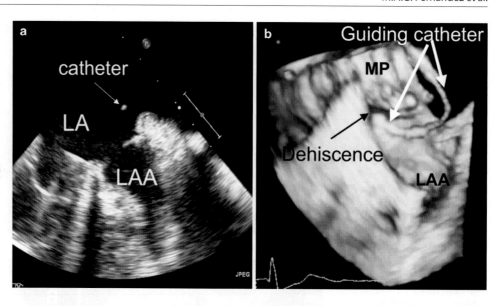

Fig. 12.9 Aortic prosthesis dehiscence. **Panel A**: 2D TEE image of an occluded dehisced aortic prosthesis. Only a section of the device at the aortic level can be seen. **Panel B**: Corresponding RT3D TEE imaging allows proper assessment of the occlusion device in the left ventricular outflow tract (LVOT) and its relation to the different cardiac structures (*MV* mitral valve, *AP* aortic prosthesis, *LA* left atrium)

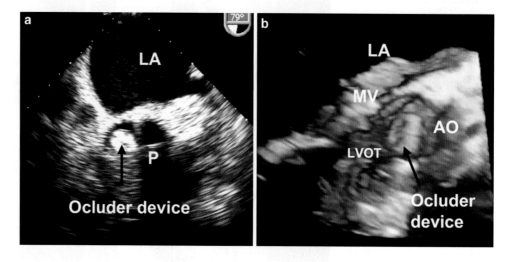

a calcified aortic root. A large aortic annulus may provide inappropriate support for the stent frame and may be associated with valve embolization. While transesophageal 2DE allows measuring of the aortic ring, transesophageal 3DE provides improved evaluation of the native aortic valve and annulus dimension due to unlimited scan plane orientation.

The 3D spatial assessment of the anatomy of both the ring and the aortic valve is vital for successful procedure. For example, patients with bicuspid aortic valves are not optimal candidates for transcatheter heart valve implantation. This is because the valvular orifice is elliptical and may predispose to para-valvular regurgitation.[44]

Transesophageal 3DE is also important during the procedure itself (Fig. 12.10). It allows for the continuous visualization of all intra-cardiac catheters and devices, as well as their relation to cardiac structures (e.g., assessment of the patency of the ostium of the left and right coronary artery [Fig. 12.11]). Transesophageal 3DE also allows an immediate assessment of the results of the procedure; analysis of

correct stent placement along the entire circumference of the aortic ring as well as presence and extent of resultant aortic regurgitation.

12.5 Left Atrial Appendage Obliteration

The left atrial appendage is the most common site for clot formation in patients with atrial fibrillation. For patients who are unable to take anticoagulant therapy, left atrial appendage obliteration has been suggested as a possible procedure to reduce the stroke risk.[6,45–51] Left atrial appendage obliteration can be achieved surgically (e.g., over sewing the left atrial appendage mouth) or percutaneously (using one of several occlusion devices e.g. the Watchman device, PLATO device). So far, this is still considered an experimental procedure, but results are encouraging. The catheter-based procedures are done under transesophageal guidance. Imaging

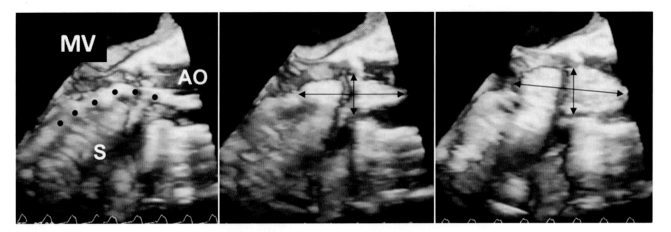

Fig. 12.10 Catheter-based aortic valve implantation. Various balloon dilation phases at the aortic ring tract level can be observed (*S* septum, *Ao* aorta, *MV* mitral valve)

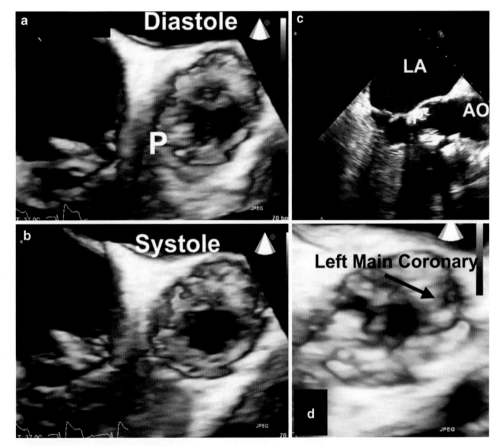

Fig. 12.11 Percutaneous aortic valve replacement. **Panel A**: Systolic frame of a percutaneously implanted aortic valve seen from the left ventricular perspective. **Panel B**: Diastolic frame of a percutaneously implanted aortic valve seen from the left ventricular perspective. **Panel C**: Corresponding 2D TEE image, showing the implanted prosthetic aortic valve. **Panel D**: Patency of the ostium of the left main coronary artery is confirmed with RT3D imaging after valve implantation

guidance is necessary in order to rule out the presence of left atrial appendage clot immediately before starting the procedure, as well as for assessing the position and orientation of the deployed device in the left atrial appendage and confirming total obliteration of the left atrial appendage.

Transesophageal 3DE imaging, with en-face view of the left atrial appendage mouth, allows measurement of the size of the opening of the left atrial appendage, thus aid in choosing the appropriate size device for the procedure. It also allows direct visualization of the deployed occlusion device in the left atrial appendage mouth. Mal-aligned device is easily recognizable in this view, and the device can then be repositioned until correct placement has been achieved (Fig. 12.12). Color Doppler imaging is then used to confirm lack of communication between the main left atrial body and the left atrial appendage.

Fig. 12.12 Left atrial appendage (LAA) obliteration. **Panel A:** LAA occlusion device at the mouth of the LAA. The device was clearly positioned at an off-angle, leaving open communication between the main left atrium and the left atrial appendage. **Panel B:** Proper positioning of an LAA occlusion device. Complete closure of the LAA opening has been achieved with no residual communication between the mail left atrium and the LAA

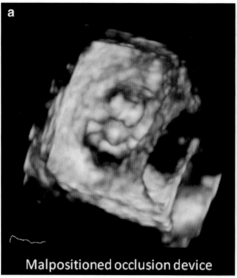
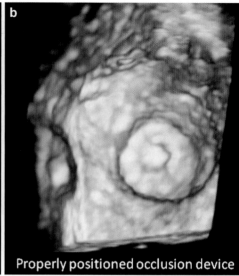

Malpositioned occlusion device

Properly positioned occlusion device

12.6 Pulmonary Vein Ablation for Atrial Fibrillation

Atrial fibrillation is a very common arrhythmia associated with significant morbidity.[52,53] Medical therapy is suboptimal with significant side effects and high recurrence rate. A number of different ablation strategies have been used, including pulmonary vein isolation, targeting of fractionated electrograms, compartmentalizing the atria with linear lesions and various combinations and modifications of these lesion sets. Catheter ablation, particularly targeting the pulmonary veins, is increasingly being performed in recent years; there is some randomized evidence to suggest that radio frequency catheter ablation is superior to long-term antiarrhythmic drugs in keeping patients with drug refractory paroxysmal atrial fibrillation arrhythmia free at 12 months.[54–56]

Pulmonary vein ablation is usually performed under fluoroscopic guidance. For anatomic assessment of the left atrium and pulmonary veins, a 3D reconstruction map of the left atrium superimposed on a previously obtained computed tomographic scan or magnetic resonance of the left atrium is utilized. Traditionally, the real-time imaging methods that have been used during the procedure included intracardiac-echocardiography and X-ray fluoroscopy. More recently transesophageal 3DE has been introduced into usage. Transesophageal 3DE imaging permits easy tracking of the catheters in the left atrium, as well as clear visualization of structures neighboring the left atrial appendage. It also allows verification of the proper catheter placement in the ridge between the left atrial appendage and the left-sided pulmonary veins, which is considered a central area for successful ablation (Fig. 12.13).[37,57,58] Transesophageal 3DE can be useful in the identification of pulmonary vein stenosis, a known complication of the procedure, and in the guidance of its appropriate treatment (Fig. 12.14).

12.7 Current Status and Future Directions

Transesophageal 3DE is a new, powerful imaging tool that has been recently added to clinical practice.[37,59] The key advantages of this technique, over transesophageal 2D imaging are:

1. Ability to visualize intracardiac catheters and devices along their entire length, including their tips and relationship to nearby cardiac structures. This may minimize the

Fig. 12.13 Pulmonary vein ablation. **Panel A:** En face view from left atrium perspective, showing the opening of left atrial appendage, left upper pulmonary vein and the Marshall ligament. **Panel B:** Mapping catheter positioned in the pulmonary vein area. RT3D TEE imaging allows clearer definition of the spatial relation of the catheter and all surrounding cardiac structures (*LAA* left atrial appendage, *LSPV* left superior pulmonary vein)

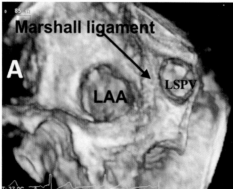
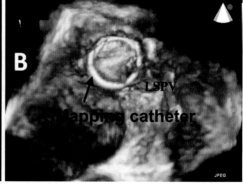

Fig. 12.14 Pulmonary vein ablation – complication. Images taken from a patient with a prior history of two pulmonary vein ablation procedures. The patient developed total occlusion of the left inferior pulmonary vein and severe obstruction of the left superior pulmonary vein (LSPV). **Panels A** and **B**: Color and continuous wave Doppler at the left superior pulmonary vein demonstrating increased flow velocities characteristic of pulmonary vein obstruction. **Panels C** and **D**: RT3D TEE imaging showing a stent implanted in the LSPV with en face view of the left atrial appendage (LAA) and the ridge between the LAA and pulmonary vein

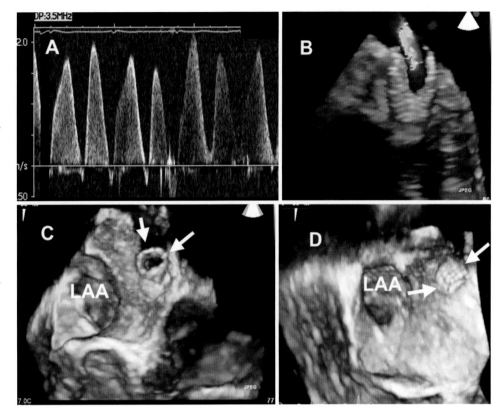

potential for complications, and can facilitate improved results of percutaneous procedures.

2. Ability to view certain intracardiac structures from multiple angles, otherwise not available with any other real-time technique; mainly, visualization of certain structures (interatrial septum, mitral valve, left atrial appendage mouth) "enface". This allows better appreciation of the cardiac anatomy and pathology, which can translate into better patient selection for percutaneous catheter-based interventions.

Future research will be directed towards proving that the new technique affects performance and outcome of percutaneous, catheter-based intervention; both in minimizing complication (both structural as well minimizing fluoroscopy time and iodinated contrast use) rate and optimizing results. Most likely, transesophageal 3DE will become the technique of choice and the standard of care for guidance of percutaneous, catheter-based procedures.

References

1. Hung JS, Chern MS, Wu JJ, Fu M, Yeh KH, Wu YC, et al. Short- and long-term results of catheter balloon percutaneous transvenous mitral commissurotomy. *Am J Cardiol*. 1991;67:854–862.
2. Arora R, Kalra GS, Singh S, Mukhopadhyay S, Kumar A, Mohan JC, et al. Percutaneous transvenous mitral commissurotomy: immediate and long-term follow-up results. *Catheter Cardiovasc Interv*. 2002;55:450–456.
3. Masura J, Gavora P, Pondar T. Long term outcome of transcatheter secundum-type atrial septal defect closure using Amplatzer septal occluders. *J Am Coll Cardiol*. 2005;45:505–507.
4. Balbi M, Casalino L, Gnecco G, Bezante GP, Pongiglione G, Marasini M, et al. Percutaneous closure of patent foramen ovale in patients with presumed paradoxical embolism: periprocedural results and midterm risk of recurrent neurologic events. *Am Heart J*. 2008;56:356–360.
5. Luermans JG, Post MC, Schräder R, Sluysmans T, Vydt T, Vermeersch P, et al. Outcome after percutaneous closure of a patent foramen ovale using the Intrasept device: a multi-centre study. *Catheter Cardiovasc Interv*. 2008;71:822–828.
6. Sievert H, Lesh MD, Trepels T, Omran H, Bartorelli A, Della Bella P, et al. Percutaneous left atrial appendage transcatheter occlusion to prevent stroke in high-risk patients with atrial fibrillation: early clinical experience. *Circulation*. 2002;105:1887–1889.
7. Hung JS, Fu M, Yeh KH, Wu CJ, Wong P. Usefulness of intracardiac echocardiography in complex transseptal catheterization during percutaneous transvenous mitral commissurotomy. *Mayo Clin Proc*. 1996;71:134–140.
8. Zanchetta M. On-line intracardiac echocardiography alone for Amplatzer Septal Occluder selection and device deployment in adult patients with atrial septal defect. *Int J Cardiol*. 2004;95:61–68.
9. Kronzon I, Tunick PA, Schwinger ME, Slater J, Glassman E. Transesophageal echocardiography during percutaneous mitral valvuloplasty. *J Am Soc Echocardiogr*. 1989;2:380–385.
10. Kronzon I, Tunick PA, Glassman E, Slater J, Schwinger M, Freedberg RS. Transesophageal echocardiography to detect atrial clots in candidates for percutaneous transseptal mitral balloon valvuloplasty. *J Am Coll Cardiol*. 1990;16:1320–1322.
11. Vilacosta I, Iturralde E, San Román JA, Gómez-Recio M, Romero C, Jiménez J, et al. Transesophageal echocardiographic monitoring of percutaneous mitral balloon valvulotomy. *Am J Cardiol*. 1992; 70:1040–1044.

12. Goldstein SA, Campbell A, Mintz GS, Pichard A, Leon M, Lindsay J Jr. Feasibility of on-line transesophageal echocardiography during balloon mitral valvulotomy: experience with 93 patients. *J Heart Valve Dis*. 1994;3:136–148.

13. Applebaum RM, Kasliwal RR, Kanojia A, Seth A, Bhandari S, Trehan N, et al. Utility of three-dimensional echocardiography during balloon mitral valvuloplasty. *J Am Coll Cardiol*. 1998; 32:1405–1409.

14. Mazic U, Gavora P, Masura J. The role of transesophageal echocardiography in transcatheter closure of secundum atrial septal defects by the Amplatzer septal occluder. *Am Heart J*. 2001;142:482–488.

15. Podnar T, Martanovic P, Gavora P, Masura J. Morphological variations of secundum-type atrial septal defects: feasibility for percutaneous closure using Amplatzer septal occluders. *Catheter Cardiovasc Interv*. 2001;53:386–391.

16. Acar P, Saliba Z, Bonhoeffer P, Aggoun Y, Bonnet D, Sidi D, et al. Influence of atrial septal defect anatomy in patient selection and assessment of closure with the Cardioseal device; a three-dimensional transesophageal echocardiographic reconstruction. *Eur Heart J*. 2000;21:573–581.

17. Halpern DG, Perk G, Ruiz C, Marino N, Kronzon I. Percutaneous closure of a post-myocardial infarction ventricular septal defect guided by real-time three-dimensional echocardiography. *Eur J Echocardiogr*. 2009; doi: 10.1093/ejechocard/jep021.

18. Mullasari AS, Umesan CV, Krishnan U, Srinivasan S, Rvikumar M, Raghuraman H. Transcatheter closure of post-myocardial infarction ventricular septal defect with Amplatzer septal occluder. *Catheter Cardiovasc Interv*. 2001;54:484–487.

19. Holzer R, Balzer D, Amin Z, Ruiz C, Feinstein J, Bass J, et al. Transcatheter closure of postinfarction ventricular septal defects using the new Amplatzer muscular VSD occluder: results of a U.S. Registry. *Catheter Cardiovasc Interv*. 2004;61:196–201.

20. Feldman T, Wasserman HS, Herrmann HC, Gray W, Block PC, Whitlow P, et al. Percutaneous mitral valve repair using the edge-to-edge technique: six-month results of the EVEREST Phase I Clinical Trial. *J Am Coll Cardiol*. 2005;46:2134–2140.

21. Herrmann HC, Rohatgi S, Wasserman HS, Block P, Gray W, Hamilton A, et al. Mitral valve hemodynamic effects of percutaneous edge-to-edge repair with the MitraClip device for mitral regurgitation. *Catheter Cardiovasc Interv*. 2006;68:821–828.

22. Sugeng L, Shernan SK, Weinert L, Shook D, Raman J, Jeevanandam V, et al. Real-time three-dimensional transesophageal echocardiography in valve disease: comparison with surgical findings and evaluation of prosthetic valves. *J Am Soc Echocardiogr*. 2008;21:1347–1354.

23. Iung B, Cormier B, Ducimetiere P, et al. Immediate results of percutaneous mitral commissurotomy. A predictive model on a series of 1514 patients. *Circulation*. 1996;94:2124–2130.

24. Bonow RO, Carabello BA, Chatterjee K, et al. ACC/AHA 2006 guidelines for the management of patients with valvular heart disease: a report of the American College of Cardiology/American Heart Association Task Force on Practice Guidelines (Writing Committee to Revise the 1998 Guidelines or the Management of Patients With Valvular Heart Disease): developed in collaboration with the Society of Cardiovascular Anesthesiologists: endorsed by the Society for Cardiovascular Angiography and Interventions and The Society of Thoracic Surgeons. *J Am Coll Cardiol*. 2006;48:e1–148.

25. Fatkin D, Roy P, Morgan JJ, Feneley MP. Percutaneous balloon mitral valvotomy with the Inoue single-balloon catheter: commissural morphology as a determinant of outcome. *J Am Coll Cardiol*. 1993;21:390–397.

26. Messika-Zeitoun D, Blanc J, Iung B, et al. Impact of degree of commissural opening after percutaneous mitral commissurotomy on long-term outcome. *J Am Coll Cardiol Img*. 2009;2:1–7.

27. Gill EA, Kim MS, Carroll JD 3D TEE for evaluation of commissural opening before and during percutaneous mitral commissurotomy. *J Am Coll Cardiol Img*, 2009;2:1034–1035.

28. Hammermeister K, Sethi GK, Henderson WG, Grover FL, Oprian C, Rahimtoola SH. Outcomes 15 years after valve replacement with a mechanical versus a bioprosthetic valve: final report of the Veterans Affairs randomized trial. *J Am Coll Cardiol*. 2000;36:1152–1158.

29. Rothlin ME, Egloff L, Kugelmeier J, Turina M, Senning A. Reoperations after valvular heart surgery: indications and late results. *Thorac Cardiovasc Surg*. 1980;28:71–76.

30. Genoni M, Franzen D, Vogt P et al. Paravalvular leakage after mitral valve replacement: improved long-term survival with aggressive surgery? *Eur J Cardiothorac Surg*. 2000;17:14–19.

31. Pate G, Webb J, Thompson C et al. Percutaneous closure of a complex prosthetic mitral paravalvular leak using transesophageal echocardiographic guidance. *Can J Cardiol*. 2004;20:452–455.

32. Moneta A, Villa E, Donatelli F. An alternative technique for non-infective paraprosthetic leakage repair. *Eur J Cardiothorac Surg*. 2003;23:1074–1075.

33. Jindani A, Neville EM, Venn G, Williams BT. Paraprosthetic leak: a complication of cardiac valve replacement. *J Cardiovasc Surg (Torino)* 1991;32:503–508.

34. Hourihan M, Perry SB, Mandell VS et al. Transcatheter umbrella closure of valvular and paravalvular leaks. *J Am Coll Cardiol*. 1992;20:1371–1377.

35. Moscucci M, Deeb GM, Bach D, Eagle KA, Williams DM. Coil embolization of a periprosthetic mitral valve leak associated with severe hemolytic anemia. *Circulation*. 2001;104:E85–E86.

36. Cortes M, Garcia E, Garcia-Fernandez MA, Gomez JJ, Perez-David E, Fernandez F. Usefulness of transesophageal echocardiography in percutaneous transcatheter repairs of paravalvular mitral regurgitation. *Am J Cardiol*. 2008;101:382–386.

37. Perk G, Lang RM, Garcia-Fernandez MA, Lodato J, Sugeng L, Lopez J, Knight BP, Messika-Zeitoun D, Shah S, Slater J, Brochet E, Varkey M, Hijazi Z, Marino N, Ruiz C, Kronzon I. Use of real time three-dimensional transesophageal echocardiography in intracardiac catheter based interventions. *J Am Soc Echocardiogr*. 2009;22(8):865–882.

38. Kronzon I, Sugeng L, Perk G, Hirsh D, Weinert L, Garcia Fernandez MA, Lang RM. Real-time 3-dimensional transesophageal echocardiography in the evaluation of post-operative mitral annuloplasty ring and prosthetic valve dehiscence. *J Am Coll Cardiol*. 2009; 53(17):1543–1547.

39. Lindroos M, Kupari M, Heikkilä J, Tilvis R. Prevalence of aortic valve abnormalities in the elderly: an echocardiographic study of a random population sample. *J Am Coll Cardiol*. 1993;21: 1220–1225.

40. Freeman RV, Otto CM. Spectrum of calcific aortic valve disease: pathogenesis, disease progression and treatment strategies. *Circulation*. 2005;111:3316–3326.

41. Task Force on the Management of Valvular Heart Disease of the European Society of Cardiology. Guidelines on the management of valvular heart disease. *Eur Heart J*. 2007;28:230–268.

42. Webb JG, Pasupati S, Humphries K, Thompson C, Altwegg L, Moss R, et al. Percutaneous transarterial aortic valve replacement in selected high-risk patients with aortic stenosis. *Circulation*. 2007;116:755–763.

43. Zajarias, MD A G, Cribier, MD Outcomes and safety of percutaneous aortic valve replacement. *J Am Coll Cardiol*. 2009;53:1829–1836.

44. Zegdi R, Ciobotaru V, Noghin M, et al. Is it reasonable to treat all calcified aortic valves with a valved stent? Results from a human anatomical study in adults. *J Am Coll Cardiol*. 2008;51:579–584.

45. García-Fernández MA, Pérez-David E, Quiles J, Peralta J, García-Rojas I, Bermejo J, et al. Role of left atrial appendage obliteration in stroke reduction in patients with mitral valve prosthesis: a transesophageal echocardiographic study. *J Am Coll Cardiol*. 2003;42:1253–1258.

46. Crystal E, Lamy A, Connolly SJ, Kleine P, Hohnloser SH, Semelhago L, et al; Left Atrial Appendage Occlusion Study. Left Atrial Appendage Occlusion Study (LAAOS): a randomized clinical

trial of left atrial appendage occlusion during routine coronary artery bypass graft surgery for long-term stroke prevention. *Am Heart J.* 2003;145:174–178.

47. Blackshear JL, Johnson WD, Odell JA, Baker VS, Howard M, Pearce L, et al. Thoracoscopic extracardiac obliteration of the left atrial appendage for stroke risk reduction in atrial fibrillation. *J Am Coll Cardiol.* 2003;42:1249–1252.

48. Sick PB, Schuler G, Hauptmann KE, Grube E, Yakubov S, Turi ZG, et al. Initial worldwide experience with the WATCHMAN left atrial appendage system for stroke prevention in atrial fibrillation. *J Am Coll Cardiol.* 2007;49:1490–1495.

49. Möbius-Winkler S, Schuler GC, Sick PB. Interventional treatments for stroke prevention in atrial fibrillation with emphasis upon the WATCHMAN device. *Curr Opin Neurol.* 2008;21:64–69. Review.

50. Hanna IR, Kolm P, Martin R, Reisman M, Gray W, Block PC. Left atrial structure and function after percutaneous left atrial appendage transcatheter occlusion (PLAATO): six-month echocardiographic follow-up. *J Am Coll Cardiol.* 2004;43:1868–1872.

51. Ostermayer SH, Reisman M, Kramer PH, Matthews RV, Gray WA, Block PC, et al. Percutaneous left atrial appendage transcatheter occlusion (PLAATO system) to prevent stroke in high-risk patients with non-rheumatic atrial fibrillation: results from the international multi-center feasibility trials. *J Am Coll Cardiol.* 2005;46:9–14.

52. Feinberg WM, Blackshear JL, Laupacis A, Kronmal R, Hart RG. Prevalence, age distribution, and gender of patients with atrial fibrillation: analysis and implications. *Arch Intern Med.* 1995;155:469–473.

53. Benjamin EJ, Wolf PA, D'Agostino RB, Silbershatz H, Kannel WB, Levy D. Impact of atrial fibrillation on the risk of death: the Framingham Herat study. *Circulation.* 1998;98:946–952.

54. Haissaguerre M, Gencel L, Fischer B, et al. Successful catheter ablation of atrial fibrillation. *J Cardiovasc Electrophysiol.* 1994;5:1045–1052.

55. Pappone C, Rosanio S, Oreto G, et al. Circumferential radiofrequency ablation of pulmonary veins ostia: a new anatomic approach for curing atrial fibrillation. *Circulation.* 2000;102:2619–2628.

56. Calkins H, Brugada J, Packer DL, et al. HRS/EHRA/ECAS expert consensus statement on catheter and surgical ablation of atrial fibrillation: recommendations for personnel, policy, procedures and follow-up. A report of the Heart Rhythm Society (HRS) Task Force on Catheter and Surgical Ablation of Atrial Fibrillation. *Heart Rhythm.* 2007;4:816–861.

57. Chierchia G, Van Camp G, Sarkozy A, Asmundis C, Brugada P Double transseptal puncture guided by real-time three-dimensional transesophageal echocardiography during atrial fibrillation ablation. *Europace.* 2008;10:705–706.

58. Yang H, Srivathsan K, Wissner E, Chandrasekaran K. Atrial fibrillation ablation with a prosthetic mitral valve real-time 3-dimensional transesophageal echocardiography: novel utility. *Circulation.* 2008;117;e304–e305.

59. Balzer J, Kuhl H, Rassaf T, Hoffman R, Schauerte P, Kelm M, et al. Real-time transesophageal three-dimensional echocardiography for guidance of percutaneous cardiac interventions: first experience. *Clin Res Cardiol* 2008; [Epub ahead of print].

Future Developments of Three-Dimensional Echocardiography

13

Luigi P. Badano, Roberto M. Lang, Leopoldo Peres de Isla, and José Luis Zamorano

Recent advances in miniaturization, electronics, and computer technology have enabled the development of fully sampled matrix array transducers as well as the "on-line 3D display" of rendered images together with sophisticated software for post-processing and quantification of 3D images. The ease of data acquisition, the ability to image the entire heart nearly in real time, as well as the ability to focus on specific structures in a single beat has brought 3DE closer to routine clinical practice.

However, currently 3DE has become part of routine clinical practice only in a complementary role to 2DE. Most laboratories perform a complete 2DE study, followed by a focused 3DE, in patients with specific pathologies in which 3DE imaging could potentially provide additional diagnostic information.

In the near future, it can be anticipated that 3DE has the potential of assuming a prime role in the echocardiographic evaluation. However, in order to further augment the quality and expand the clinical applications of 3DE some of the current limitations will need to be overcome. First of all, significant improvements are required regarding the temporal resolution as well as the spatial resolution particularly in the the far field. Efforts should be made to enable the acquisition of a complete 3D datasets in a single heart beat, since this advancement will decrease acquisition time and artifacts created due to irregular heart rates, respiration and patient movement.

In addition to the new developments in hardware technology, advancements in dedicated software technology for processing, storage, display and analysis will be crucial for various clinical applications.

In the next paragraphs we will review the main future development of the 3DE technique that are required in order to make this technology usable in the routine echocardiogrphic practice.

13.1 Transducer Technology

3D transducer technology is one of the most active research fields for the main ultrasound companies. The ultimate goal is to develop a single transducer solution capable of switching from 2D to 3D mode with equal good quality which could also capture the entire full-volume dataset of the heart in a single heart beat. This important development will allow echocardiographers to incorporate 3D volume acquisition during (and not following) the routine 2D echocardiographic examination thus allowing a faster learning curve of the 3D technique as well as its incorporation into the clinical workflow. In this regard, the development of transesophageal 3D probe provide a good example of how combining the 3D volumetric data with the 2D data can provide immediate and often additional data without disruption of the 2D imaging workflow of the echocardiographic examination. To get to this point, transthoracic 3D transducers must provide higher resolution, sensitivity and frequency bandwidth. In addition, there is a need to improve the ergonomics of the 3D transducers by decreasing size (in particular the footprint) and weight. All these improvements will be driven by further miniaturization of the transducer electronics and the inter-connection technology. For example, the custom made integrated circuitry may be placed directly below the transducer material (acoustic stack), making the connection to the elements simpler. Improvements of the high-voltage transmit electronics will probably also be performed and 3D transducers with a higher number of piezoelectric elements and new piezoelectric materials will likely be introduced in the near future. Transducers will be smaller and versatile and capable of acquiring multiple modalities such as 2D, 3D, and Doppler echocardiography. With these advanced transducers, it will be possible to significantly reduce the number of steps required to complete an echocardiographic study, and thus reduce the time required for the acquisition of the study.

For example, all cut-planes required and all standard 2D views could theoretically be obtained from a single volumetric data set and used for diagnostic purposes, assuming that both spatial and temporal resolution are sufficiently high.

L.P. Badano (✉)
Head of Noninvasive Imaging Lab, Department of Cardiology, Vascular and Thoracic Sciences, University of Padua, Padua, Italy
email: lpbadano@gmail.com

L.P. Badano et al. (eds.), *Textbook of Real-Time Three Dimensional Echocardiography*, DOI: 10.1007/978-1-84996-495-1_13, © Springer-Verlag London Limited 2011

135

13.2 Data Set Navigation and Image Display

One of the main challenges that current 3D technologies poses to echocardiographers (especially to those grown with the M-mode and 2D modalities) is the need to navigate within the 3D data set to obtain the cut-planes or the 2D views required to solve a clinical problem. This navigation is time-consuming and current cropping and slicing tools are not readily intuitive. New generation 3D systems need to automatically orient the data set and automatically provide cut planes of potential clinical interest to the reader as well as sophisticated screen layouts to allow a comprehensive assessment of cardiac chambers using a multislice display (Fig. 13.1).[1]

Another area of active development is echocardiographic monitor technology. Currently, only flat screen 2D monitors are available on the 3D ultrasound systems and surface or volume rendering techniques have to be applied in order to provide the user with depth perception of 3D structures. However, the aim should be to have affordable stereoscopic monitor solutions to visualize the real 3D anatomy of cardiac structures. Up to now, the main problem with 3D monitors has been that image quality is significantly inferior to that of 2D ones. However, future technological progresses is expected to provide stereoscopic monitors on the next generation of 3D scanners. This will open the door to new applications using virtual dynamic systems, known as virtual reality, which can assist with the interpretation of 3D data of the heart in space and making it possible to "dive" into the 3D model of the heart. This display has the potential of becoming a unique resource for the assessment and evaluation of intracardiac anatomy in normal and diseased hearts. In addition, with the rapid growth of minimal invasive and robotic cardiac surgery, as well as interventional procedures, detailed knowledge of the complex dynamic intracardiac anatomy in 3D will become essential for interventionalists and surgeons to effectively perform procedures since they will be able to simulate surgeries and use heart holograms as training tools.[2]

Finally, researchers and industry alike are actively working to develop "fusion imaging," a technique which combines different imaging modalities (for instance, perfusion

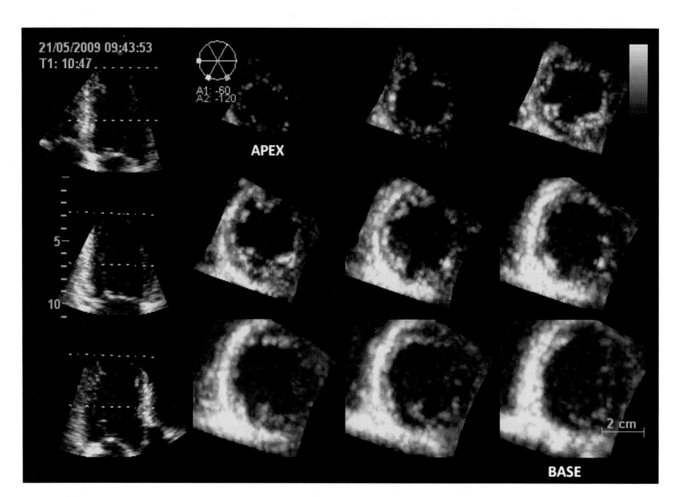

Fig. 13.1 Multislice display of a three-dimensional data set of the left ventricle acquired from the apical approach showing akinesia of the septal apical segment. On the left side, three apical views (from *top* to *bottom*: four-chamber, two-chamber and long-axis) are shown. The three columns of short axes show nine equidistant short-axis views of the left ventricle progressing from the apex (*upper left*) to the base (*lower right*) of the left ventricle. The accompanying video shows these images in real-time (Video 13.1)

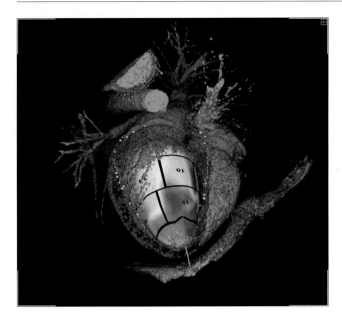

Fig. 13.2 Example of fusion imaging between 3D echocardiography and CT imaging. Registration of coronary venous anatomy to the site of latest mechanical contraction

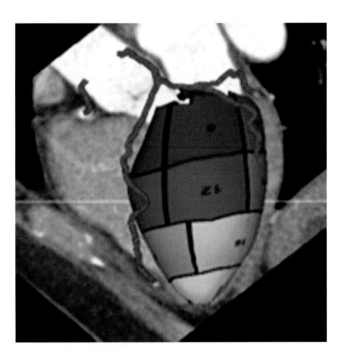

Fig. 13.3 Fusion Imaging of cardiac CT and 3D echocardiography. After registration of both images note the over-imposition of coronary arteries with LV endocardial reconstruction

from SPECT combined with anatomical information from 3DE in order to take advantage from both their individual diagnostic idiosyncrasies [Figs. 13.2 and 13.3]).[3]

Methods for registration and fusion of 3DE images with other imaging modalities such as MRI and computerized tomography are currently under investigation. Image registration is the process of transforming different image data sets into the same coordinate system in order to allow the examiner to compare data obtained from different imaging modalities. Fusion of 3DE images with either computerized tomography or MRI, thus combining the higher temporal resolution of the first with the exceptional spatial resolution of the latter, has the potential of impacting on cardiac imaging in a similar way that as PET-CT has done in oncology. For example, 3DE can be registered with pre-operative model segmentation from MRI and computerized tomography and used during interventions to track changes in cardiac function. Since 3DE is the only modality capable of acquiring cardiac 3D data in real-time during interventions, it is a natural complement to cardiac MRI and computerized tomography. In the future, fusion of 3DE with other imaging modalities will become available and clinical decision-making will be based on more comprehensive information.

13.3 Quantification

An important step forward will be the progression from semi-automated to fully automated border detection and chamber quantification methodologies, thus gradually eliminating the need for off-line analysis.[4]

This is of crucial importance, in particular in the interventional settings of the catheterization laboratory and the operating room, where immediate visual and quantitative feedback is particularly important. However, prerequisite for effective automated quantification tools is a significant improvement in image quality and temporal resolution of future 3DE systems. Furthermore, future 3DE should also provide measurements that are not routinely used today such as global and regional left ventricular shape and curvature.[5] Combining regional wall curvature with wall thickness and blood pressure may eventually provide regional wall stress estimates.

Additional clinical applications will likely include quantification of myocardial strain and strain-rate through 3DE speckle tracking,[6-8] assessment of myocardial perfusion using contrast agents (providing accurate detection of coronary artery disease without radiation exposure),[9-11] and selection of patients eligible for cardiac resynchronization parameters (fusion imaging between 3DE and CT venography to match the most delayed left ventricular wall segments with available cardiac vein of pace-maker wire implant sites).[3]

Improvements in quantification will, in turn, result in better patient management including better indications for heart failure medications, improved indications for defibrillator implantation and cardiac resynchronization therapy. In addition, 3DE will also improve the ability to detect the responses to these interventions. Patients receiving cardiotoxic chemotherapy will benefit from accurate detection of subtle decrements in myocardial function which may indicate the need to stop these medications.

Finally, the availability of data sets containing the entire heart will allow the echocardiographer to assess the relative contribution and interdependence of the various cardiac chambers to cardiac performance thereby improving our understanding of the function of the heart as an integrated system and not as the sum of multiple parts.

13.4 Connectivity

For the purposes of interpretation and storage, it is vital that the 3DE data sets are incorporated into digital information systems with full rendering and quantification capabilities. Prerequisite for reaching this goal is the extension of the DICOM standard to fully support digital 3D echocardiographic data in order to enable the review of 3D ultrasound data on third party DICOM viewers. In the long run, a well functioning 3D DICOM standard will spread the use of 3DE and enhance the clinician confidence with 3DE images.

References

1. Orderud F, Torp H, Rabben SI. Automatic alignment of standard views in 3D echocardiograms using real-time tracking. *SPIE Medical Imaging 2009: Ultrasonic Imaging and Signal Processing, Proceedings of SPIE*, Vol. 7265, 72650D-1-7.
2. van den Bosch AE, Koning AH, Meijboom FJ, McGhie JS, Simoons ML, van der Spek PJ, Bogers AJ. Dynamic 3D echocardiography in virtual reality. *Cardiovasc Ultrasound*. 2005;3:37.
3. Kanckstedt C, Muhlenbruch G, Mischke G, Schummers G, Becker M, Kuhl H, Franke A, Schmid M, Spuentrup E, Smahnken A, Lang RM, Kelm M, Gunther RW, Schauerte P. Registration of coronary venous anatmy to the site of latest mechanical contraction. Acta *Cardiol*. 2010; 65(2):161–170.
4. Walimbe V, Jaber WA, Garcia MA and Shekhar R. Multimodality cardiac stress testing: combining real-time 3-dimensional echocardiography and myocardial perfusion SPECT. *J Nucl Med*. 2009;50(2):226–230.
5. Orderud F, Hansegård J, Rabben SI. Real-time volume measurements real-time tracking of the left ventricle in 3D echocardiography using a state estimation approach. MICCAI 2007, Part I, LNCS 4791, pp. 858–865.
6. Mannaerts HF, van der Heide JA, Kamp O, Stoel MG, Twisk J, Visser CA. Early identification of left ventricular remodelling after myocardial infarction, assessed by transthoracic 3D echocardiography. *Eur Heart J*. 2004;25(8):680–687.
7. Tanaka H, Hara H, Saba S, Gorcsan J 3rd. Usefulness of three-dimensional speckle tracking strain to quantify dyssynchrony and the site of latest mechanical activation. *Am J Cardiol*. 2010; 105(2):235–242.
8. Seo Y, Ishizu T, Enomoto Y, Sugimori H, Yamamoto M, Machino T, Kawamura R, Aonuma K. Validation of 3-dimensional speckle tracking imaging to quantify regional myocardial deformation. *Circ Cardiovasc Imaging*. 2009;2(6):451–459.
9. Pérez de Isla L, Balcones DV, Fernández-Golfín C, Marcos-Alberca P, Almería C, Rodrigo JL, Macaya C, Zamorano J. Three-dimensional-wall motion tracking: a new and faster tool for myocardial strain assessment: comparison with two-dimensional-wall motion tracking. *J Am Soc Echocardiogr*. 2009;22(4):325–330.
10. Takeuchi M, Otani S, Weinert L, Spencer KT, Lang RM. Comparison of contrast-enhanced real-time live 3-dimensional dobutamine stress echocardiography with contrast 2 dimensional echocardiography for detecting stress-induced wall-motion abnormalities. *J Am Soc Echocardiogr*. 2006;19(3):294–299.
11. Toledo E, Lang RM, Collins KA, Lammertin G, Williams U, Weinert L, Bolotin G, Coon PD, Raman J, Jacobs LD, Mor-Avi V. Imaging and quantification of myocardial perfusion using real-time three-dimensional echocardiography. *J Am Coll Cardiol*. 2006;47(1): 146–154.

Real-Time Three-Dimensional Transesophageal Echocardiography

14

Pedro Marcos-Alberca and José Luis Zamorano

14.1 Overview

In the 1970s, pioneers explored the esophagus with ultrasound in patients with chronic lung disease. They obtained M-Mode recordings of the left ventricle, the aortic root, the mitral valve, and the left atrium. In 18 of 38 patients examined, recordings were of sufficient quality to allow precise measurements of linear dimensions.[1] Thirty years later, transesophageal echocardiography has become an essential diagnostic tool and has contributed to the understanding of the pathology, clinical diagnosis, management, and prognosis of many cardiovascular conditions such as aortic dissection, mitral valve disease, and ischemic stroke.[2,3] Transesophageal echocardiography provides, along with excellent spatial resolution, the possibility of obtaining views of anatomical structures of the heart that are not accessible by a transthoracic approach. For example, in the horizontal long axis view of the right cardiac chambers, we can visualize the opening of the caval veins in the right atrium. It was in the operating room and in the interventional lab where the development of three-dimensional capabilities for transesophageal imaging was carried out. The consolidation and expansion of reparative mitral valve surgery in patients with prolapse led to the involvement of top surgical and imaging groups to detail the anatomy of mitral prolapse using cardiac ultrasound.[4] Three-dimensional transesophageal echocardiography allows the operator to move from the practice of imagining the stereoscopic appearance of the mitral valve (largely based on his/her experience and skill) to visualizing the valve in its correct anatomical orientation (the so-called surgeon's view), providing newer, realistic views. As our approach with mitral valve prolapse and cardiac surgery, one can do the same with interventional cardiology and percutaneous procedures: *ostium secundum* atrial septal defect closure, partial or total periprosthetic leak closure, transcatheter aortic prosthesis implant, mitral clips, and left atrial appendage closure.

Since the operating room is the natural theater for transesophageal (3DE), obviously the visualization of innovative cardiac views from 3D dataset needs to be done in real time. Despite the advance planning of the surgical decision making, the surgeon asks for accurate and rapidly accessible information to adapt the surgical technique to particular operative findings. Moreover, the final result, especially in reparative surgery or percutaneous procedures, also needs to be easily and rapidly checked and showed to the surgeon or the interventionalist. It is necessary that a successful transesophageal 3DE needs to be a real-time one. The intraoperative or instrumentation scenario does not allow for complex and time consuming post-processing.[5]

In the following sections, we summarize the technological advances, clinical data, limitations, challenges, and future perspectives of real-time transesophageal 3DE.

14.2 Technology

14.2.1 First Developments: The Rotational Concept

The concept of 3D reconstructions in cross-sectional cardiac imaging comes from transthoracic echocardiography. Prototypes used specific transducers and hardware built with the purpose of obtaining sequential cross-sectional images using a predetermined rotational movement of the transducer. Thus, after a 180° turn around its central axis, a cone-shaped stack of sectorial scans can be processed to depict novel azimuthal cardiac views (the Z-Mode). The challenge in rotational echocardiography is to maintain fixed coordinates in both temporal and spatial dimensions for accurate reconstructions. The disappointing results with 3D rotational transthoracic echocardiography forced both engineers and cardiologists to find a different approach that could overcome these limitations. The esophagus is a relatively stable site for the imaging probe and, together with the superior

P. Marcos-Alberca (✉)
Cardiovascular Imaging Unit, Cardiology Department, Hospital Clínico San Carlos, Universidad Complutense, 28040 Madrid, Spain
e-mail: marcosal33@gmail.com

L.P. Badano et al. (eds.), *Textbook of Real-Time Three Dimensional Echocardiography,*
DOI: 10.1007/978-1-84996-495-1_14, © Springer-Verlag London Limited 2011

Fig. 14.1 Rotational-based transesophageal 3DE. (**a**) Cross-sectional images are sequentially acquired from a fixed location of the transducer in the mid-esophagus at 2° steps. (**b** and **c**) Original rotational stacks are resampled, and data converted in order to obtain axial stacks, moulding a 3D rendering of the heart (Adapted from Salustri and Roelandt.[7] Free access and reproduction when cited)

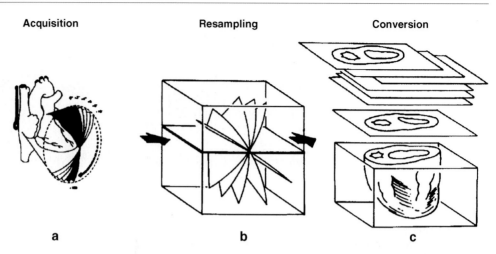

Acquisition   **Resampling**   **Conversion**

a   **b**   **c**

quality of the tomographic images, represents an ideal location for the exploration of the heart using rotational scan and 3D reconstructions.[6]

After the placement of a conventional multiplane transesophageal probe into the mid-esophagus, a dataset of cross-sectional views is obtained at 2° steps through the automatic computer-controlled rotation of the cross-sectional image around a central axis. For better results, the central axis is aligned with the structure of interest. Thus, taking into account the maximum spatial resolution in the X-axis, the highest quality images are located in the center of the acquired volume, according to the aim of the study (i.e., mitral valve for evaluation of prolapse or the interatrial septum in atrial septal defect). Reconstruction of rotational cross-sectional dataset needs to be ECG gated to synchronize the consecutive images acquired in several cardiac cycles in a final one-beat 3D reconstruction. The transducer position and its central axis of rotation must remain fixed during the full 180° arc sampling. In addition, the displacement of the diaphragm causes *stepstairs* artifacts, which have to be avoided through the sensing of the thoracic impedance using a specific software or navigator, together with optimal sedation of the patient in order to minimize deep breath, swallowing, or cough. It is extremely important that the first and the last images acquired are mirror images to avoid a mismatch between images in the conical volume, which will result in gross artifacts in the final display (Fig. 14.1).

Post-processing includes re-sampling and placement of cross-sectional images in their adequate position into the cardiac cycle, Cartesian conversion for slab stacking, interpolation to fill echo drop outs, edge enhancement, noise reductions, and final rendering. Data processing is performed off-line by robust specific software, so the visualization of the images in rotational transesophageal 3DE is not exactly real time and, often, time consuming and disappointing, especially due to the presence of artifacts from irregular rhythm or breathing anomalies.[7]

With advances in nanotechnology, both resolution and processing times have improved a lot. Current commercially

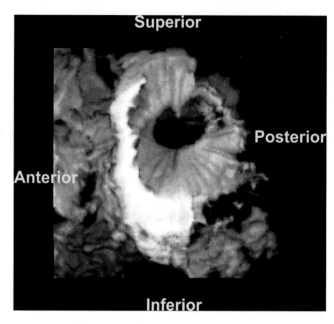

Fig. 14.2 Rotational acquisition of an *ostium secundum* atrial septal defect. The processing of the reformatted stack allows the visualization of the orifice from the left lateral side. The aorta lies ahead of the atrial septum (*anterior*) (Image courtesy of R. García-Orta and M.A. García-Fernández)

available rotational transesophageal 3DE equipment offers high-quality images. However, the need for the navigator, ECG gating, and post-processing still labels this approach as not actually real time (Fig. 14.2).[8]

14.2.2 Current Technology: The Azimuthal Revolution

A transesophageal probe able to generate 3DE imaging consists of a standard multiplane system operating at 5MHz[9]. Improvements in miniaturization, flexible circuits, and the impressive advances in high-density, non-coaxial, ribbon-based cabling have enabled matching 504 active channels in a 2-D array with a 6.3 mm by 6.3 mm aperture. So, the probe has the same size as a traditional multiplane transesophageal 2DE probe and comparable clinical functionality. One limitation in earlier models of the transesophageal 3DE probe was signal loss through the extensive cabling, which was overcome by incorporating preamps at the transducer end of the probe and by the addition of matching layers. As result, current commercially available transesophageal 3DE probes have improved signal-to-noise ratios, allowing better penetration.[10]

Similar to transthoracic 3DE, the processing of the received signal can be accomplished in several ways: (1) narrow angle or real-time display, (2) subsectorial narrow angle or *zoom* real-time display, (3) synchronic orthogonal biplane display or *X-Plane®*, (4) ECG-gated wide angle or *full volume* display, and (5) ECG-gated subsectorial color Doppler flow display. Indeed, only the first three modes are "real time" as the ECG-gated acquisitions, although brief, require some kind of post-processing.

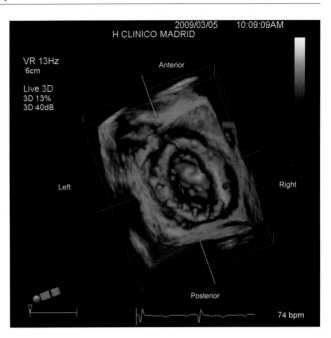

Fig. 14.3 The box and axes. Post-processing usually is accomplished using the software tool named as *the box*. Three axes going across the box: red, blue, and green. Axes are those of the coordinates system, that is, XYZ, and they define the three reference planes: coronal or frontal (XY), sagital or lateral (YZ), and axial or transversal (XZ). Planes can be displaced along the corresponding axis cutting the pyramidal acquisition

14.3 Relevant Cardiac Anatomy in Real-Time Transesophageal 3DE

The introduction of 3DE does not replace conventional tomographic imaging. Rather it adds value. Transesophageal 3DE examination provides tomographic views that are difficult or really impossible to obtain with the traditional transesophageal 2DE approach. In addition, the views are presented in a realistic, robust conic perspective. Therefore, with this notion of "add on" it is essential to know the elements and anatomical relationships displayed in the innovative views that 3DE provides.[11]

Imaging in 3D, one needs to keep in mind the correct position of the human body in any anatomic examination. 3D pyramids acquired using zoom real-time or full-volume displays are managed or post-processed to obtain sections or planes depicting normal or abnormal cardiac anatomy. Among the tools implemented in available software, the most popular is *the box*, which intuitively includes XYZ axes and standard planes: (1) sagittal plane (long axis or longitudinal), the vertical plane that divides volume acquisition into right and left portions; (2) coronal plane (frontal), the vertical plane that divides it into anterior and posterior portions; and (3) transverse plane (short axis), which runs parallel to the ground and divides the organ into superior and inferior portions (Fig. 14.3).

In transesophageal 3DE, these planes can be used to visualize the specific structures of the heart for examination purposes. Of all the structures of the heart that can be explored, transesophageal 3DE underscores the examination of the mitral valve and the atrial septum. This is due to their location in the area of optimal focus and their orientation

perpendicular or nearly perpendicular to the ultrasonic beam, characteristics that maximize their spatial resolution. Other structures particularly accessible by transesophageal 3DE are the aortic ring and the left ventricular outflow tract. However, the beam orientation parallel to the aortic leaflets often limits their optimal view. The openings of the pulmonary veins are located in the more lateral portions of the conical beam, and the intrinsic limitations of lateral resolution often prevent their accurate visualization. The entrance of the left atrial appendage, in proximity of the mitral valve, is easily visualized, although its distal portion is often excluded from the volume of acquisition.

The versatility of multiplane examination allows looking for the most appropriate cone beam orientation in order to achieve optimal resolution. In other words, we have to look for the maximal perpendicular incidence over the element of interest. For the mitral valve, a stable position at mid-oesophagus at 0° is adequate. For the atrial septum, the right vertical view at 90° (*caval plane*) offers fine acquisitions. The aortic ring and left ventricular outflow tract are best visualized as pyramidal stacks acquired from 120° to 135°, also in a mid-esophagus position left ventricle is best explored from a transgastric view, although sometimes air in the fornix prevents high-quality images.

For the mitral valve, volume acquisitions are processed as follows: atrial perspective is obtained from the transversal or axial planes, aorta is placed anteriorly, in the right superior quadrant of the monitor, mitral valve is located in the left inferior quadrant. To reproduce the surgical view, the anterior commissure is displayed above the posterior commissure. Close to the anterior leaflet, the entrance to the left atrial appendage is visualized. Anterior and posterior leaflets are easily identified and along the coaptation line, the different scallops can be visualized. By turning the dataset 180° around the X-axis, the valve is visualized from its ventricular perspective. Subvalvular structures (chordae tendineae and papillary muscles) and the edge of the leaflets are displayed. Fine color Doppler examinations require a progressive cutting of the valvular coaptation line, usually using the sagittal or longitudinal plane, from "commissure to commissure" (Fig. 14.4).

For the atrial septum, two innovative cut planes can be obtained. First, the stack is reoriented as a left lateral dissection. So, the aorta lays anteriorly, in the left part of the image, and immediately below, the mitro-aortic continuity and A2 and A3 scallops of the anterior mitral leaflet. The posterior commissure and the posterior wall of the left atrium are visualized in the right part of the image. The left side of the atrial septum and the opening of the right pulmonary veins lie in the background (Fig. 14.5). A 180° turn of the volume around its axis allows the visualization of the right atria and the right side of the interatrial wall. Now, the aorta will be located at the right side of the screen and the posterior wall of the right atrium in the left. The perspective is very similar to a right anterior oblique projection in fluoroscopy. The superior and inferior cava vein are visualized in the upper and lower parts, respectively. The insertion of the septal tricuspid leaflet, the tricuspid ring, and Todaro's tendon are visualized

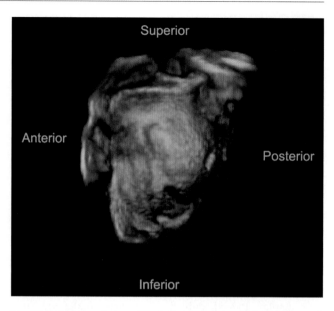

Fig. 14.5 Left lateral view of the left atria showing, in the background, the normal interatrial septum. The aorta is anterior and the bifurcation of the pulmonary artery behind it, forming the roof of the cropped pyramid. This amazing perspective offers visualization of unique anatomic elements. Note the footprint of the *fossa ovalis* and the limbus at the center of the septum (atrial fibrillation) running in the base of the left atria

immediately below the aortic valve. Immediately posterior to it, is the orifice of the coronary sinus. These elements mark the limits of Koch's triangle. In the background, the right side of the atrial septum, the limbus of the *fossa ovalis* and the *fossa ovalis* itself can be visualized. (Fig 14.6).

Finally, the visualization of the left ventricular outflow tract and the aortic ring with transesophageal 3DE implies the

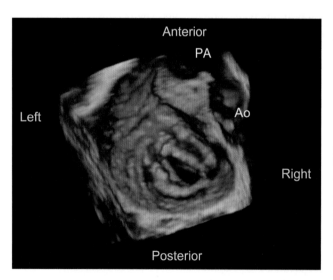

Fig. 14.4 Mitral stenosis. The mitral valve is examined from the atrial roof (the surgeon view). With this type of processing, the great vessels are placed anteriorly and the left atrial appendage in the upper left corner. The atrial ring is heavily calcified. The gross leaflet due to the rheumatic process enhances spatial Z-resolution. Both commissures, anterolateral and posteromedial, are fused. *PA* pulmonary artery, *O* aorta

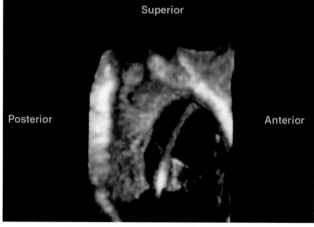

Fig. 14.6 Right lateral view of an *ostium secundum* atrial septal defect type. The processing of the zoom real-time 3D display includes rotation and cutting of the pyramidal acquisition so that an innovative and intuitive plane is achieved, maintaining the attitudinal perspective for an anatomic position. In the background, the right side of the septal defect can be seen. The catheter originates from the inferior caval vein and enters through the defect into the left atrium

Fig. 14.7 Aortic valve and aortic ring visualized from the aortic root, similar to the surgical view after aortotomy. This area is best acquired and processed using zoom real-time 3D display starting from a standard view at 135° in the mid-esophagus. Thus, the aortic valve is at the center of the Z-axis to improve its resolution. (**a**) diastole, (**b**) systole

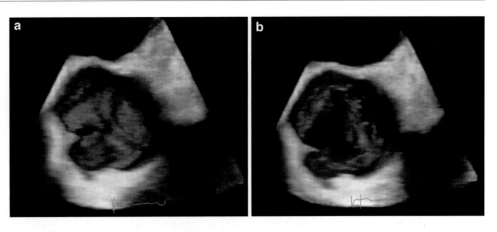

processing of volume acquisitions with the coronal or frontal plane. Slight rotations or tilting around the Z-axis allows the atrial or ventricular visualization of the mitro-aortic junction, a frequent location of abscess in infective endocarditis. With progressive and meticulous cutting of the left ventricular outflow tract using the sagittal plane, we can examine the upper interventricular septum and the ventricular side of the aortic ring. A 180° turn around the Y-axis allows depicting the aortic root and with sagittal cutting, the aortic side of the aortic valve ring can be depicted. Sometimes, particularly when the aortic leaflets are thickened or calcified, very realistic images of the valve can be obtained. However, echo dropouts due to parallel beam incidence are frequently responsible for suboptimal visualization in normal leaflets (Fig. 14.7).

14.4 Clinical Applications

Real-time transesophageal 3DE is a recently developed clinical tool. It is therefore not surprising that clinical experience is currently limited. However, ease of use and the high-quality images it provides has fueled its rapid deployment.

14.4.1 Intraoperative Echocardiography

Shortly after the development of pioneering rotational transesophageal 3DE systems, cardiologists sought to implement them in routine clinical intraoperative echocardiography. Preliminary reports indicate transesophageal 3DE as feasible, accurate, and able to provide additional and complementary valvular morphologic information compared with conventional transesophageal 2DE. Transesophageal 3DE detected most of the major valvular morphologic abnormalities (leaflet perforations, fenestrations, and masses) confirmed on pathologic examination. In around 25% of intraoperative echo studies, transesophageal 3DE yields new additional information

that sometimes resulting in a change in the decision to perform repair rather than replacement. However, the limitations of rotational systems, the unacceptable time consumed to afford 3D exams, and concerns about their reproducibility prevented a wide and unconditional acceptance of earlier systems.[12]

Conversely, real-time transesophageal 3DE offers high-quality images that mirror the details perceived by the surgeon in the operating room. The planning, optimization, and postoperative surveillance of mitral valve repair techniques and devices are the most frequent indication for intraoperative echocardiography. Using data obtained from real-time 3DE images, computerized rendering of the prolapsing mitral valve, mitral annulus, and subvalvular apparatus can be obtained. Important measurements to maximize the surgical result are easily realized. Such tools will allow the surgeon to design operations that thoroughly analyze valve geometry and stress distribution before opening the chest (Fig. 14.8).[13] In a real scenario, the increasing importance of transesophageal 3DE in the operating room is highlighted by an increasing number of papers published. Volumetric acquisition allows accurate and fast comprehensive 3D visualization of the mitral and aortic valves, revealing the mechanism of regurgitation, systolic anterior motion, the width of the hypertrophic ventricular septum for myectomy, and intraoperative measurement of left ventricular ejection fraction and aortic valve area.

Recently, transesophageal 3DE has gained a pivotal role in transcatheter-based transapical aortic valve implantation (Fig. 14.9).[14–17]

14.4.2 Percutaneous Catheter and Device-Based Procedures

Non-coronary therapeutic procedures through percutaneous vascular access have gained increasing importance in the last two decades. In their early days, device-based procedures sought to repair congenital cardiac defects preventing the need

Fig. 14.8 Rendering of a prolapsing mitral valve. Advanced processing tools offer precise measurements of potential utility in surgical decision making. Exact results demand time-consuming off-line image post-processing. Further developments will guarantee actual real-time intraoperative display

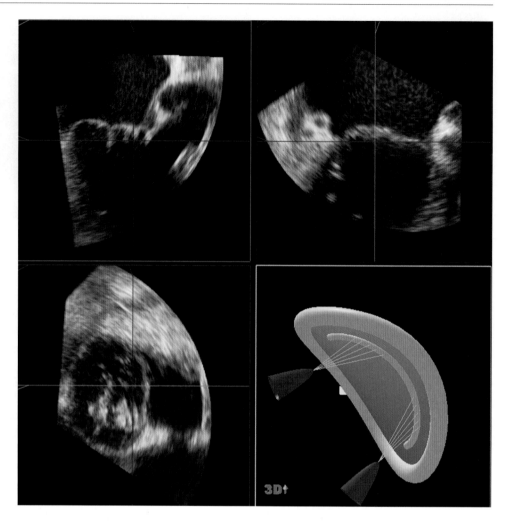

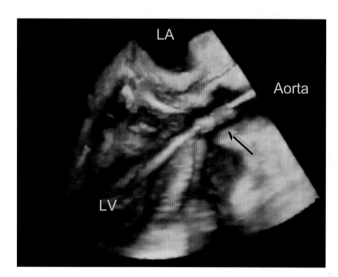

Fig. 14.9 Intraoperative real-time transesophageal 3DE in transcatheter transapical aortic prosthetic valve implantation. The pyramid is acquired starting from a standard plane at 135°. The sheath into the left ventricle and the catheter with the mounted non-inflated prostheses across the aortic valve are clearly depicted (*green arrow*)

for surgery: persistence of ductus arteriosus, aortic coarctation, pulmonary stenosis, atrial septal defects, and patent foramen ovalis. Pioneers used intravascular ultrasound as a guide for the deployment of devices to close atrial septal defects. Thereafter, commercial intracardiac ultrasound catheters were introduced for this purpose, with better spatial and deep resolution, and with the addition of color Doppler capabilities to assess the success of the procedure by excluding significant leaks.[18, 19]

Nowadays, percutaneous-device-based closure of atrial septal defect and patent foramen oval is well established in routine clinical practice, and there is not much discussion regarding the importance of transesophageal echocardiography examination before, during and after the procedure. In this scenario, transesophageal 3DE improves some aspects of very highly protocolized interventions, which are subject to few blockbuster innovations.[20] For instance, the quantification of the size of the atrial septal defect, the dynamic change of the orifice during cardiac cycle, or the measurement of the rims that may influence the choice of the device size and the feasibility of its placement, can be best checked with real-time transesophageal 3DE.[21,22] In addition, in the last few years, new technologies and techniques have allowed to cover the treatment of more pathologies using percutaneous access, avoiding prohibitive or very high-risk cardiac surgeries: transcatheter aortic valve implantation, device- based closure of periprosthetic mitral and aortic leaks (see also Chapter 12), septal alcohol ablation in obstructive severe hypertrophic cardiomyopathy, left atrial appendage exclusion, mitral valve prolapse or flail correction, and postmyocardial infarction ventricular septal defect. Therefore, the number of indications are expected to increase and so will the time spent in the use of transesophageal echocardiography in the cath lab.[23]

Preliminary reports reveal how the innovative and high-quality images provided with transesophageal 3DE have been of great value in supporting new percutaneous therapeutic procedures and monitoring the entire procedure. Septal puncture, insertion of wires and their placement, insertion of balloons and devices and their correct placement and, above all, the evaluation of the final result is better assessed with transesophageal 3DE. Occlusion with devices of the left atrial appendage in patients with atrial fibrillation would avoid anticoagulation in patients in whom it is contraindicated. Transesophageal 3DE is feasible for the visualization and quantitative analysis of the left atrial appendage orifice area and correlates better than 2D echo with measurements obtained with 64-slice cardiac computerized tomography. Thus, transesophageal 2DE systematically underestimated the left atrial appendage orifice area compared with transesophageal 3DE.[24] Other applications of transesophageal 3DE include the visualization of paravalvular regurgitation of mitral prostheses and their closure with dual umbrella or specifically designed devices, and the correction of severe mitral valve prolapse or mitral flail secondary to chordae rupture.[25,26] The visualization of masses, infected or not, located in atrial or ventricular leads of defibrillators or pacemakers are facilitated with transesophageal 3DE.[27] Of all the available display modes, simultaneous dual-plane visualization and subsectorial narrow angle or zoom real-time display seem to be the two most accurate, reproducible, and feasible modes in order to provide real time and useful information to the operator. These benefits may accelerate the learning curve and improve the confidence level of the interventional cardiologist in order to increase safety, accuracy, and efficacy of interventional cardiac procedures.[28]

14.4.3 Radiofrequency Catheter Ablation of Atrial Tachyarrhythmias

The advent of catheter ablation of left-sided atrial tachyarrhythmias introduced the echo-guided puncture of the interatrial septum. Transesophageal 3DE permits fast and safe transatrial access with a single puncture attempt through the direct visualization of the *fossa ovalis*.[29] The implementation of the ablation of the pulmonary veins to treat atrial fibrillation widened indications for echocardiography in the cath lab including not only atrial septum puncture but also the placement of specifically designed catheters (i.e., *lasso* catheter) over the pulmonary vein opening and the monitoring of spontaneous bubble formation to indicate excessive myocardial heating and the danger of carbonization and cardiac perforation. Experience gathered using transesophageal monitoring in successful cryoablation of left side accessory pathways suggests a potential role in pulmonary vein ablation, especially reducing the need of fluoroscopy and radiation exposure of both patients and operators. In the electrophysiology lab, the realistic anatomic information provide fast and complete information about the underlying pathomorphology, improving spatial orientation and monitoring the procedure online without loss of image quality.[30]

14.5 Challenges and Future Perspectives

Current hardware technology and the demanding requirements of graphics processing do not allow sufficient resolution of images when the structure to be visualized is located laterally or is too deep. This is the case when attempting to visualize the orifices of the pulmonary veins, which are of interest in ablative procedures, and both the left and right ventricles. Although the transgastric view sometimes obtains good images of the ventricles, foreshortening decreases the likelihood to obtaining accurate volumetric calculations and visualization of ventricular lesions, for instance, free-wall ventricular rupture or a pseudoaneurysm. For the same reasons, low temporal resolution limits the examination of fast moving structures or accurate and reproducible analysis of regional contractility. Real-time examinations with narrow angle or real-time display, or subsectorial narrow angle or zoom real-time display noticeably increases temporal resolution. Nonetheless, it constitutes a clear limitation with regard to full-volume acquisitions, including 3D color Doppler acquisitions. High-performance hardware and software will increase both spatial (lateral and in-depth) and temporal (volume rate) resolutions in the coming years.[31]

On the other hand, specifically designed ring-array transducers mounted over conventional 8.5 French vascular catheters with real-time 3DE capabilities will be soon commercially available.[32] They are expected to replace transesophageal 3DE examination in interventional procedures, since, at present, the lengthy duration of the procedures requires anesthesia for transesophageal 3DE monitoring in order to warrant patient tolerance. Anesthesia will not be required for intracardiac echocardiographic examination.

References

1. Frazin L, Talano JV, Stephanides L, Loeb HS, Kopel L, Gunnar RM. Esophageal echocardiography. *Circulation*. 1976;54(1): 102–108.
2. Kuhl HP, Hanrath P. The impact of transesophageal echocardiography on daily clinical practice. *Eur J Echocardiogr*. 2004;5(6): 455–468.
3. Sengupta PP, Khandheria BK. Transesophageal echocardiography. *Heart*. 2005;91(4):541–547.
4. Levine RA, Weyman AE, Handschumacher MD. Three-dimensional echocardiography: techniques and applications. *Am J Cardiol*. 1992;69(20):121H–130H; discussion 131H-134H.
5. Salgo IS. 3D echocardiographic visualization for intracardiac beating heart surgery and intervention. *Semin Thorac Cardiovasc Surg*. 2007;19(4):325–329.
6. Salustri A, Roelandt JR. Ultrasonic three-dimensional reconstruction of the heart. *Ultrasound Med Biol*. 1995;21(3):281–293.
7. Salustri A, Roelandt J. Three dimensional reconstruction of the heart with rotational acquisition: methods and clinical applications. *Br Heart J*. 1995;73(5 Suppl 2):10–15.
8. Garcia-Orta R, Moreno E, Vidal M, Ruiz-Lopez F, Oyonarte JM, Lara J, Moreno T, Garcia-Fernandezd MA, Azpitarte J. Three-dimensional versus two-dimensional transesophageal echocardiography in mitral valve repair. *J Am Soc Echocardiogr*. 2007;20(1):4–12.
9. Xie MX, Wang XF, Cheng TO, Lu Q, Yuan L, Liu X. Real-time 3-dimensional echocardiography: a review of the development of the technology and its clinical application. *Prog Cardiovasc Dis*. 2005;48(3):209–225.
10. Pua EC, Idriss SF, Wolf PD, Smith SW. Real-time 3D transesophageal echocardiography. *Ultrason Imaging*. 2004;26(4):217–232.
11. Nanda NC, Kisslo J, Lang R, Pandian N, Marwick T, Shirali G, Kelly G. Examination protocol for three-dimensional echocardiography. *Echocardiography*. 2004;21(8):763–768.
12. Abraham TP, Warner JG, Jr., Kon ND, Lantz PE, Fowle KM, Brooker RF, Ge S, Nomeir AM, Kitzman DW. Feasibility, accuracy, and incremental value of intraoperative three-dimensional transesophageal echocardiography in valve surgery. *Am J Cardiol*. 1997;80(12):1577–1582.
13. Ryan LP, Salgo IS, Gorman RC, Gorman JH, 3rd. The emerging role of three-dimensional echocardiography in mitral valve repair. *Semin Thorac Cardiovasc Surg*. 2006;18(2):126–134.
14. Sugeng L, Shernan SK, Weinert L, Shook D, Raman J, Jeevanandam V, DuPont F, Fox J, Mor-Avi V, Lang RM. Real-time three-dimensional transesophageal echocardiography in valve disease: comparison with surgical findings and evaluation of prosthetic valves. *J Am Soc Echocardiogr*. 2008;21(12):1347–1354.
15. Grewal J, Mankad S, Freeman WK, Click RL, Suri RM, Abel MD, Oh JK, Pellikka PA, Nesbitt GC, Syed I, Mulvagh SL, Miller FA. Real-time three-dimensional transesophageal echocardiography in the intraoperative assessment of mitral valve disease. *J Am Soc Echocardiogr*. 2009;22(1):34–41.
16. Scohy TV, Ten Cate FJ, Lecomte PV, McGhie J, de Jong PL, Hofland J, Bogers AJ. Usefulness of intraoperative real-time 3D transesophageal echocardiography in cardiac surgery. *J Card Surg*. 2008;23(6):784–786.
17. Scohy TV, Soliman OI, Lecomte PV, McGhie J, Kappetein AP, Hofland J, Ten Cate FJ. Intraoperative real time three-dimensional transesophageal echocardiographic measurement of hemodynamic, anatomic and functional changes after aortic valve replacement. *Echocardiography*. 2009;26(1):96–99.
18. Vazquez de Prada JA, Jiang L, Chen MH, Padial LR, Guerrero JL, Schwammenthal E, King ME, Weyman AE, Chen C, Levine RA. Intracardiac ultrasonographic assessment of atrial septal defect area: in vitro validation and technical considerations. *Am Heart J*. 1995;130(2):302–306.
19. Bartel T, Konorza T, Arjumand J, Ebradlidze T, Eggebrecht H, Caspari G, Neudorf U, Erbel R. Intracardiac echocardiography is superior to conventional monitoring for guiding device closure of interatrial communications. *Circulation*. 2003;107(6):795–797.
20. Boutin C, Musewe NN, Smallhorn JF, Dyck JD, Kobayashi T, Benson LN. Echocardiographic follow-up of atrial septal defect after catheter closure by double-umbrella device. *Circulation*. 1993;88(2):621–627.
21. Acar P, Saliba Z, Bonhoeffer P, Aggoun Y, Bonnet D, Sidi D, Kachaner J. Influence of atrial septal defect anatomy in patient selection and assessment of closure with the Cardioseal device; a three-dimensional transesophageal echocardiographic reconstruction. *Eur Heart J*. 2000;21(7):573–581.
22. Maeno YV, Benson LN, McLaughlin PR, Boutin C. Dynamic morphology of the secundum atrial septal defect evaluated by three dimensional transesophageal echocardiography. *Heart*. 2000;83(6):673–677.
23. Garg P, Walton AS. The new world of cardiac interventions: a brief review of the recent advances in non-coronary percutaneous interventions. *Heart Lung Circ*. 2008;17(3):186–199.
24. Shah SJ, Bardo DM, Sugeng L, Weinert L, Lodato JA, Knight BP, Lopez JJ, Lang RM. Real-time three-dimensional transesophageal echocardiography of the left atrial appendage: initial experience in the clinical setting. *J Am Soc Echocardiogr*. 2008;21(12):1362–1368.
25. Manda J, Kesanolla SK, Hsuing MC, Nanda NC, Abo-Salem E, Dutta R, Laney CA, Wei J, Chang CY, Tsai SK, Hansalia S, Yin WH, Young MS. Comparison of real time two-dimensional with live/real time three-dimensional transesophageal echocardiography in the evaluation of mitral valve prolapse and chordae rupture. *Echocardiography*. 2008;25(10):1131–1137.
26. Yavari A, Spyropoulos A, Khawaja MZ, McWilliams ET. Paravalvular regurgitation of a Starr-Edwards mitral prosthesis depicted by real time three-dimensional transesophageal echocardiography. *Echocardiography*. 2008;25(10):1145–1146.
27. Paley AJ, Kronzon I. A defibrillator wire vegetation: the contribution of 3D real time transesophageal echocardiography. *Echocardiography*. 2008;25(9):1014–1015.
28. Balzer J, Kuhl H, Rassaf T, Hoffmann R, Schauerte P, Kelm M, Franke A. Real-time transesophageal three-dimensional echocardiography for guidance of percutaneous cardiac interventions: first experience. *Clin Res Cardiol*. 2008;97(9):565–574.
29. Chierchia GB, Capulzini L, de Asmundis C, Sarkozy A, Roos M, Paparella G, Boussy T, Van Camp G, Kerkhove D, Brugada P. First experience with real-time three-dimensional transesophageal echocardiography-guided transseptal in patients undergoing atrial fibrillation ablation. *Europace*. 2008;10(11):1325–1328.
30. Clark J, Bockoven JR, Lane J, Patel CR, Smith G. Use of three-dimensional catheter guidance and trans-esophageal echocardiography to eliminate fluoroscopy in catheter ablation of left-sided accessory pathways. *Pacing Clin Electrophysiol*. 2008;31(3): 283–289.
31. Kuo J, Bredthauer GR, Castellucci JB, von Ramm OT. Interactive volume rendering of real-time three-dimensional ultrasound images. *IEEE Trans Ultrason Ferroelectr Freq Control*. 2007;54(2): 313–318.
32. Light ED, Angle JF, Smith SW. Real-time 3-D ultrasound guidance of interventional devices. *IEEE Trans Ultrason Ferroelectr Freq Control*. 2008;55(9):2066–2078.

Benjamin H. Freed, Lissa Sugeng,
David H. Adams, and Roberto Lang

15.1 Mitral Valve Anatomy

The mitral valve has a complicated 3D structure made up
multiple, distinct anatomical components. The entire unit is
situated in the left atrioventricular groove allowing blood to
move freely from the left atrium into a relaxed left ventricle
during diastole. In order to correctly identify lesions and
describe dysfunction of the mitral valve unit, it is important
to understand the complex physiology of each component.
The following paragraphs will, therefore, explore in detail
the mitral valve annulus, leaflets, commissures, chordae,
papillary muscles, and left ventricle.

15.1.1 Mitral Annulus

The mitral annulus is a fibromuscular ring to which the anterior and posterior mitral valve leaflets attach.[1] The opening
motion of the leaflets hinges at their insertion site on the annulus. The normal mitral valve annulus has a 3D saddle shape
with the "lowest points" at the level of the commissures.[2] This
allows proper leaflet apposition during systole. The annulus
can be divided into the anterior and posterior annulus based
on the insertion of the corresponding leaflet. In order to repli-
cate the surgeon's intraoperative view of the mitral valve, it is
useful to consider the hands of a clock when describing locations on the annulus, in which 12 o'clock corresponds to the
midpoint of the anterior annulus. The anterior portion of the
annulus attaches to the right and left fibrous trigone. The right
trigone is a fibrous area situated between the mitral, tricuspid,
and non-coronary cusp of the aortic valve and membranous
septum. The left trigone is a fibrous area located between
the left and non-coronary cusps of the aortic annuli which is

commonly referred to as the aortic-mitral curtain. The posterior portion of the annulus is less well developed due to the
discontinuity of the fibrous skeleton of the heart in this region.
This explains why the posterior portion of the mitral annulus
is more prone to pathologic dilatation while the anterior portion is relatively resistant (Fig. 15.1).[3]

15.1.2 Mitral Valve Leaflets

The mitral valve has both an anterior and posterior leaflet.
The posterior mitral leaflet has a quadrangular shape and is
attached to approximately three-fifths of the annular circumference. The anterior mitral leaflet has a semi-circular shape
and is attached to approximately two-fifths of the annular circumference.[4] Although the posterior mitral leaflet attaches to
a larger portion of the circumference of the annulus than the

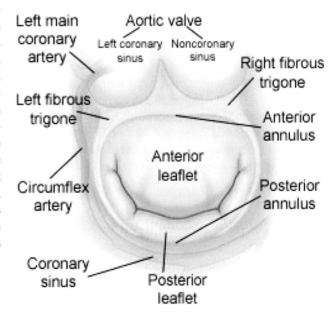

Fig. 15.1 Illustration of the mitral valve annulus (Reproduced with
permission from www.mitralvalverepair.org; courtesy of The Mitral
Valve Reference Center at Mount Sinai Hospital, New York)

R. Lang, (✉)
From the Department of Surgery, Section of Cardiothoracic Surgery,
Mount Sinai Hospital, New York, New York and The Department of
Medicine, Section of Cardiology, The University of Chicago Medical
Center, Chicago, Illinois
e-mail: rlang@medicine.bsd.uchicago.edu

L.P. Badano et al. (eds.), *Textbook of Real-Time Three Dimensional Echocardiography*,
DOI: 10.1007/978-1-84996-495-1_15, © Springer-Verlag London Limited 2011

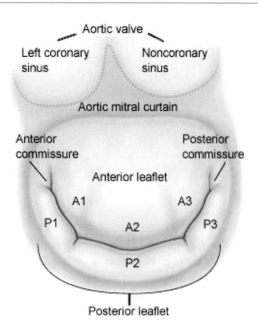

Fig. 15.2 Illustration of the mitral valve leaflets (Reproduced with permission from www.mitralvalverepair.org; courtesy of The Mitral Valve Reference Center at Mount Sinai Hospital, New York)

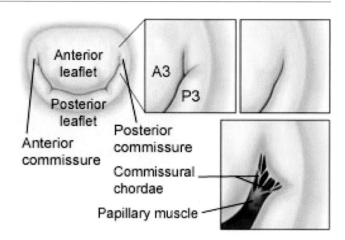

Fig. 15.3 Illustration of the mitral valve commissures (Reproduced with permission from www.mitralvalverepair.org; courtesy of The Mitral Valve Reference Center at Mount Sinai Hospital, New York)

anterior mitral leaflet, the posterior leaflet is shorter. Carpentier et al. proposed a useful nomenclature for segmental anatomy of each leaflet which makes it easier to identify specific mitral valve lesions.[5] The posterior mitral leaflet has two well-defined indentations which divides it into three separate sections or "scallops". The anterior or medial scallop is defined as P1, the middle scallop is defined as P2, and the posterior or lateral scallop is defined as P3. The three opposing segments of the anterior leaflet are designated as A1 (anterior segment), A2 (middle segment), and A3 (posterior segment), respectively. During systole, the margins of both mitral leaflets oppose each other for several millimeters to ensure valve competency against normal left ventricular end-systolic pressure. The length of opposition during systole is the difference between the total mitral leaflet length and the exposed mitral leaflet length during systole and is commonly referred to as the "coaptation zone".[1] It is best visualized in the transesophageal 2DE views of the mitral valve seen in the mid-esophageal position or from a zoomed acquisition of the mitral valve when using real time 3DE (Fig. 15.2).

15.1.3 Mitral Valve Commissures

The commissures define a distinct area where the anterior and posterior mitral leaflets appose each other during systole. Carpentier divides the commissures into anterior-lateral and posterior-medial.[5] The amount of tissue devoted to this area varies from several millimeters of leaflet tissue to distinct leaflet segments (Fig. 15.3).

15.1.4 Mitral Valve Chordae

The chordae tendinae are responsible for determining the position and tension on the anterior and posterior leaflets at left ventricular end-systole. The chordae are fibrous extensions from the heads of the papillary muscles and are named according to their insertion site on the mitral leaflets. Marginal or primary chordae insert on the free margin of the mitral leaflets and prevent marginal prolapse. Intermediate or secondary chordae insert on the ventricular surface of the leaflets and prevent billowing and reduce tension on the leaflet tissue. These chords may also play a role in determining dynamic ventricular shape and function due to their contribution to ventricular-valve continuity.[6,7] Basal or tertiary chordae insert on the posterior leaflet base and mitral annulus and connect it to the papillary muscle. It is unclear if they have any other function.

15.1.5 Mitral Valve Papillary Muscle and the Left Ventricle

There are two papillary muscles – the anterolateral and the posteromedial – which originate from the area between the apical and middle thirds of the left ventricular free wall. The anterolateral papillary muscle is composed of an anterior and posterior head while the posteromedial papillary muscle is composed of an anterior, intermediate, and posterior heads.[8] Each papillary muscle provides chordae to both leaflets and the axial relationship of the chordae prevents chordal abrasion or dyssynchrony. The anterolateral papillary muscle has a dual blood supply from both the left anterior descending and left circumflex arteries while the posteromedial papillary muscle receives its single blood supply from either the left circumflex or right coronary artery. Since the posteromedial papillary muscle receives blood from only one artery, it is more prone to disruption during a myocardial infarction. Since the papillary muscles connect directly to the left ventricle, any change in ventricular shape in this area can change the axial relationship of the chordae and leaflets, resulting in poor coaptation.

15.2 Quantitation of Mitral Regurgitation

Echocardiography is the standard modality used to assess the severity of mitral regurgitation. The ACC/AHA guidelines recommend that patients with symptomatic, severe mitral regurgitation should be referred for surgery, but not all patients with asymptomatic, severe mitral regurgitation require intervention.[9] Only a certain percentage of this population, based largely on certain echocardiographic data, will require surgery. This is why it is crucial to understand the new criteria that make up the now standardized guidelines for different grades of mitral regurgitation. Transthoracic echocardiography is usually sufficient in providing the necessary data. However, other types of modalities including cardiac MRI or transesophageal echocardiography might be needed in cases where there is a discrepancy in data or if the patient has poor acoustic windows.

The various criteria that are required for properly assessing mitral valve regurgitation severity include structural, qualitative Doppler, and quantitative Doppler parameters. Zoghbi et al. combined these parameters into specific signs, supportive signs, and quantitative data.[10] Reporting of mitral regurgitation severity should be consistent with the American Society of Echocardiography criteria for descriptive and semi-quantitative grading as described by Zoghbi et al. (Table 15.1)

The qualitative parameters that distinguish mild from severe mitral regurgitation include color flow jet width and area, the intensity of the continuous-wave Doppler signal, the pulmonary venous flow contour, the peak early mitral inflow velocity, the left atrial and left ventricle size, and the mitral valve apparatus. According to Zoghbi et al., a color flow jet occupying less than 20% of the left atrial area is considered a specific sign for mild MR whereas a jet occupying greater than 40% of the left atrium is considered specific for severe MR. In addition, a vena contracta width less than 0.3 cm is a specific finding for mild MR and greater than 0.7 cm is more likely to be severe mitral regurgitation. Other specific qualitative findings include amount of color flow convergence, presence of systolic flow reversal in pulmonary veins using pulsed wave Doppler, and identification of severe disruption of mitral valve apparatus (i.e., flail leaflet or ruptured papillary muscle).

Supportive qualitative findings require the examination of the density of continuous wave Doppler, the size of the left atrium and left ventricle, and the velocity of the peak transmittal inflow using pulsed wave Doppler. A low density continuous wave Doppler is more consistent with mild mitral regurgitation whereas a dense, well-defined envelope is more likely to constitute severe mitral regurgitation. Moderate to severe left atrial enlargement with some degree of left ventricular dilatation, particularly in the presence of normal left ventricular function, supports severe mitral regurgitation as opposed to mild mitral regurgitation. Lastly, a peak velocity

Table 15.1 Grading MR by Doppler echocardiography

	Mitral regurgitation		
	Mild	Moderate	Severe
Qualitative			
Angiographic grade	1+	2+	3–4+
Color Doppler jet area	small, central jet (less than 4 cm² or less than 20% LA area)	Signs of MR greater than mild present but no criteria for severe MR	Vena contracta width greater than 0.7 cm with large central MR jet (area greater than 40% of LA area) or with a wall-impinging jet of any size, swirling in LA
Doppler vena contracta width (cm)	Less than 0.3	0.3–0.69	Greater than or equal to 0.70
Quantitative (cath or echo)			
Regurgitant volume (ml per beat)	Less than 30	30–59	Greater than or equal to 60
Regurgitant fraction (%)	Less than 30	30–49	Greater than or equal to 50
Regurgitant orifice area (cm²)	Less than 0.20	0.2–0.39	Greater than or equal to 0.40
Additional essential criteria			
Left atrial size			Enlarged
Left ventricular size			Enlarged

Valve gradients are flow dependent and when used as estimates of severity of valve stenosis should be assessed with knowledge of cardiac output or forward flow across the valve. Modified from Zoghbi et al.[10], Copyright 2003. With permission from American Society of Echocardiography.

of mitral inflow greater than 1.2 m/s with E-wave dominance is suggestive of severe mitral regurgitation whereas an A-wave dominant inflow supports mild mitral regurgitation.

Although qualitative findings are helpful for differentiating mild from moderate mitral regurgitation, they can be highly subjective. In addition, there are no specific or supportive signs for moderate mitral regurgitation and even the specific signs lack sensitivity for identifying severe mitral regurgitation.[10] Therefore, there are several quantitative parameters that have been developed to aid in the detection of mitral regurgitation severity. These parameters include the regurgitant volume which measures absolute volume, the regurgitant fraction which measures relative volume overload, and the effective regurgitation orifice area which measures lesion severity.[10]

Measuring these parameters can be performed by pulsed wave Doppler, quantitative 2DE, and proximal isovelocity surface area method. Using pulsed wave Doppler, the area of the mitral and aortic annulus is multiplied by their respective tissue velocity integral. This calculation provides the mitral and aortic stroke volume for which the difference between these two volumes is the regurgitant volume. Regurgitant fraction is the ratio of regurgitant volume to mitral (total) stroke volume, and effective regurgitant orifice area is the ratio of regurgitant volume to the regurgitant jet time-velocity integral. Using quantitative 2DE is similar to the pulsed wave Doppler method except that mitral stroke volume is replaced by that of left ventricular stroke volume. Using color flow imaging, proximal isovelocity surface area is seen as concentric series of hemispheric rings of alternating colors on the ventricular side of the regurgitant valve.[11] The diameter of the ring closest to the regurgitant orifice is used to calculate the area of the regurgitant valve which is then multiplied by the aliasing velocity. Effective regurgitant orifice area is calculated as the ratio of flow to peak regurgitant velocity and regurgitant volume is calculated as the product of effective regurgitant orifice area and the regurgitant time-velocity integral.[12]

15.3 Mitral Valve Imaging

In order to identify all lesions and resultant dysfunctions and help determine the etiology of the disease, the mitral valve's various anatomical components should be assessed in a systematic manner using both transthoracic and transesophageal echocardiography. Usually, transthoracic should be used initially. Although this modality may provide sufficient visualization of the mitral valve apparatus, in most cases, transesophageal (2D or 3D) is required for a more complete assessment of mitral degenerative disease.

Irrespective of the modality used, the orientation of the mitral valve apparatus needs to be defined in order to correctly describe the anatomy and ensure proper communication between the surgeon and the operator. The mitral valve can be displayed in three different ways – the anatomical view, the transesophageal view, and the surgical view.[1] The *anatomical view* displays the valve from the base of the heart as if the imager were positioned in the left atrium looking down towards the left ventricle. In this view, the patient's left and right side correspond to the imagers left and right side while the anterior and posterior mitral valve leaflets are to the left and right, respectively. The *transesophageal view* corresponds to the orientation of the mitral valve seen in the transgastric basal short axis view; as if the imager were positioned in the left ventricle and looking up at the mitral valve. This view, used in all ultrasound platforms, results from rotating the anatomical view 180°. Therefore, in the transesophageal view, the operator's left and right side is reversed relative to the patient (Fig. 15.4). Lastly, the *surgeon's view* is similar to the first view but standing to the right of the patient so that the anatomical view is rotated counterclockwise almost 90° (Fig. 15.5).

When examining the mitral valve using transesophageal 2DE, the operator should examine the mitral valve from the four-chamber, bi-commissural, two-chamber, long axis, and transgastric basal short axis views (Fig. 15.6). The classification of the mitral valve scallops in any given view may vary according to the individual anatomy. In addition, foreshortening the left ventricle may lead to misidentification of the mitral valve scallops. Accordingly, orientation to internal landmarks such as the mitral valve commissures is paramount to enhance the accuracy of the scallop's diagnosis. This systematic approach is also useful in identifying the regurgitating segment. A regurgitation jet arising from the left coaptation point indicates involvement of P3/A3 whereas a jet arising from the right suggests involvement of A1/P1 scallops.

15.3.1 Mid-esophageal Four-Chamber View

This view is obtained by advancing the endoscope tip to the mid-esophageal position (about 30–35 cm from the incisors) and slightly retroflexing to direct the imaging sector towards the left ventricular apex. At 0°, the coaptation line of the mitral valve is transected perpendicularly, showing both commissures and the A2-P2 scallops. Using the transesophageal transducer in a monoplane approach from a superior to caudal motion, the mitral valve can be viewed from medial (A3-P3) to lateral (A1-P1).

15.3.2 Mid-esophageal Bi-commissural View

From the mid-esophageal 4-chamber view, this view can be obtained by rotating the imaging angle to about 60°. The

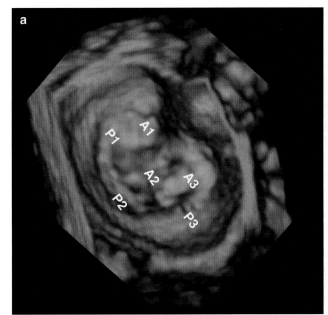

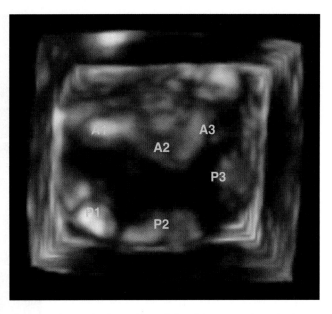

Fig. 15.5 Surgeon's view using real-time 3D transesophageal echocardiography (Reproduced with permission from O'Gara et al.[4])

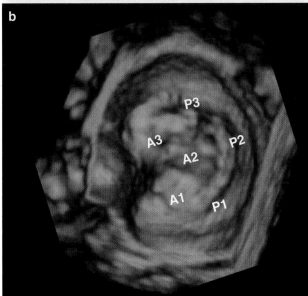

Fig. 15.4 (**a**) Anatomical view. (**b**) Transesophageal view. (Mitral valve view as visualized in the transgastric basal short axis view). All these examples were obtained with the use of real-time 3D transesophageal echocardiography volume rendering using zoomed views (Modified from O'Gara et al.[4])

15.3.3 Mid-esophageal Two-Chamber View

By further rotating the transducer angle to 90°, it is possible to visualize the leaflets so that the medial scallop (P3) is on the left of the image and all three segments of the anterior leaflet (A1, A2, A3) are on the right. This view provides excellent visualization of the entire anterior mitral leaflet and particularly the posteromedial (P3/A3) coaptation segments.

15.3.4 Mid-esophageal Long-Axis View

As the image is rotated further to an angle of 120°, the mitral and aortic valves come into view but it is difficult to visualize the papillary muscles. The imaging plane transects the coaptation line perpendicularly so that the middle posterior scallop (P2) is on the left and the middle anterior leaflet (A2) is on the right. Since P2 is most frequently affected in myxomatous degeneration, this is one of the most useful views.

15.3.5 Transgastric Basal Short-Axis View

This view is obtained by advancing the probe into the stomach (35–40 cm from the incisors) and anteflexing the probe tip against the stomach's fundus. This imaging plane allows for visualization of all six segments of the mitral valve leaflets with the posteromedial commissure closest to the apex of the sector and the anterolateral commissure farthest away from the transducer.

imaging plane now passes through the intercommissural plane transecting both leaflets to view both commissures with the medial scallop (P3) to the left, the middle anterior leaflet (A2) in the middle, and the lateral scallop (P1) to the right. The length of the P1 and P3 segments should be measured in this view because a length of either segment of over 1.5 cm suggests the likelihood of systolic anterior motion of the anterior leaflet post-repair and, therefore, a more complex mitral valve repair to avoid this complication. This view is also helpful in identifying the regurgitating segment.

Fig. 15.6 (**a**) Four-chamber view obtained at 0° depicting A2 on the left and P2 on the right. (**b**) Bicommissural view by electronically rotating the transducer tip to 55° showing P3 on the left, A2 in the middle, and P1 on the right. (**c**) Two-chamber view obtained by rotating the transducer to 90° to visualize P3 on the left and the three scallops of the anterior mitral valve leaflet on the right. (**d**) Long-axis view obtained by further rotating the transducer to 120° to view P2 on the left and A2 on the right. The left column corresponds to MV images (as visualized from the left atrial perspective) obtained with the use of real-time 3D-TEE volume rendering. Red lines represent the approximate cut planes from which the respective 2D TEE images were obtained. *Ao* aorta, *Lat* lateral aspect of MV, *Med* medial aspect of MV, *MV* mitral valve, *TEE* transesophageal echocardiography (Reproduced with permission from O'Gara et al.[4])

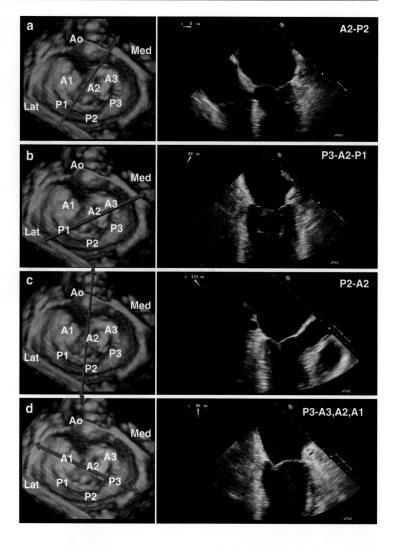

15.4 Real Time Transesophageal 3D Echocardiogram

The recent use of a transesophageal 3D transducer permits excellent visualization of the mitral valve apparatus with real-time acquisition and on-line display of images of the mitral valve and ventricle (Fig. 15.7).[13] This probe combines novel electronic circuitry with miniaturized beam-forming technology in the tip of an otherwise conventional transesophageal probe (Fig. 15.8). Prior gated transesophageal 3DE acquisition methods display the mitral valve from both atrial and ventricular perspectives that are unique to 3D imaging. What distinguishes the fully sampled matrix array transesophageal 3DE from rotational 3D acquisition is the consistency of superb quality of the mitral valve, devoid of rotational artifacts. Whereas rotational transesophageal has allowed only 80% image quality, the new transesophageal 3DE has proven to have excellent visualization scores for the mitral valve leaflets; in the range of 85%–91% for all scallops, as recently reported.[14] In addition, recent literature suggests a correlation of 96% between pre-operative transesophageal 3DE assessment of mitral valve scallop involvement and surgical findings.[15]

The mitral valve annulus, leaflets, commissures, and subvalvular structures are best displayed when obtained in zoom mode to avoid stitch artifacts due to respiration and arrhythmias that may occur in a wide-angled acquisition. This mode displays a small, magnified pyramidal volume of the mitral valve, which may vary from a 20° by 20° up to 90° × 90° depending on the density setting. To simulate a surgeon's view of the valve (from left atrium to left ventricle while standing to the right of the patient), the transesophageal 3DE image is positioned with the aortic valve at the 11-o'clock position. To visualize the submitral structures or left ventricle, a wide-angled acquisition consisting of four smaller wedges of volume obtained

Fig. 15.7 Examples of 3D renderings of the mitral valve obtained from 3D-MTEE data set using software designed for quantitative analysis of the mitral apparatus. **Top**, **left**: antero-posterior diameter is shown in green. **Top**, **right**: Annular height. **Bottom**, **left**: Anterior mitral leaflet surface area (hatched) with posterior middle scallop leaflet prolapse. **Bottom**, **right**: Angle between the mitral and aortic annuli. *A* anterior, *P* posterior, *AL* anterolateral, *PM* posteromedial, *Ao* aorta (Reproduced with permission from O'Gara et al.[4])

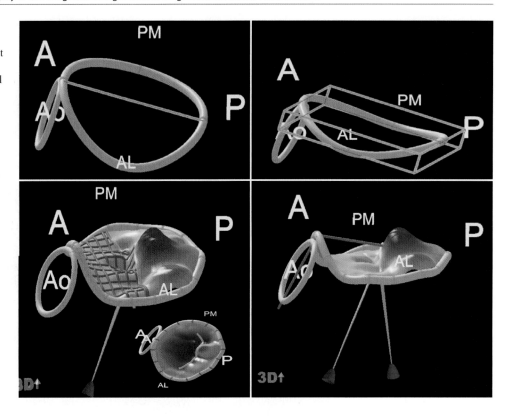

over four cardiac cycles should be obtained in order to assess papillary muscle location or quantitate left ventricular function.

While visualization of anatomy in its true 3D state is important, many physicians believe that the most significant value 3DE has for adult echocardiography is the ability to perform accurate and reproducible quantification. True myocardial motion occurs in 3D, and traditional 2D scanning planes do not capture the entire motion, or else move or "slip" while scanning. Quantifying implies segmenting structures of interest from the 3D voxel set[13]. This interface is typically constructed as a mesh of points and lines and displayed in a process known as surface rendering. This also allows the mitral apparatus to be segmented at end-systole with great accuracy. The true 3D nature of the mitral annulus, leaflets and chordal apparatus can be measured. This further allows sophisticated analyses of the nonplanar shape of the mitral annulus. These 3D measurements include: annular diameters, annular nonplanarity, commissural lengths, leaflet surface areas, and aortic to mitral annular orientation. These measurements of the mitral valve apparatus may aid in better defining the pathophysiologic triad of mitral valve disease and planning mitral valve surgery. In addition, it is likely to give a more detailed understanding of annular and annuloplasty ring dynamics before and after surgery.

15.5 The Pathophysiologic Triad of Mitral Valve Disease

Diseases that affect the mitral valve are best described by defining the *etiology* of the disease, the specific *lesions* caused by it, and the *dysfunction* it causes the mitral valve apparatus. This "pathophysiologic triad" was first described by Carpentier et al. in the early 1980s and is still extremely useful today in characterizing degenerative mitral valve regurgitation.[5,16]

Degenerative mitral valve disease is commonly caused by two very distinct entities called Barlow's disease and fibroelastic deficiency (Fig. 15.9).[17,18] Barlow's disease results in an excess of myxomatous tissue which leads to multisegmental prolapse. It is typically diagnosed in young adulthood. Patients with this disease are often followed for many decades with well-preserved left ventricular size until surgery is indicated usually in the fourth or fifth decade of life. In contrast, fibroelastic deficiency results from loss of mechanical integrity due to abnormalities of connective tissue structure and/or function. It usually causes a localized or unisegmental flail leaflet due to ruptured chordae. Patients most commonly present in the sixth decade of life with a relatively short history of mitral valve regurgitation. It is the most common form of organic mitral valve disease for which

Fig. 15.8 Multiplane acquisition equipment included transducers (*right*) and locating devices (*left*). The imaging plane could be sequentially changed either by rotating the transducer mechanically or internally (*top right*), by linear sweep (*right, center*) or by step-wise tilting resulting in a fan-like sweep (*bottom right*). For each imaging plane, transducer position and orientation is registered using either acoustic (*left, top* and *center*) or electromagnetic (*bottom left*) locator devices (Reproduced with permission from Lang et al.[21])

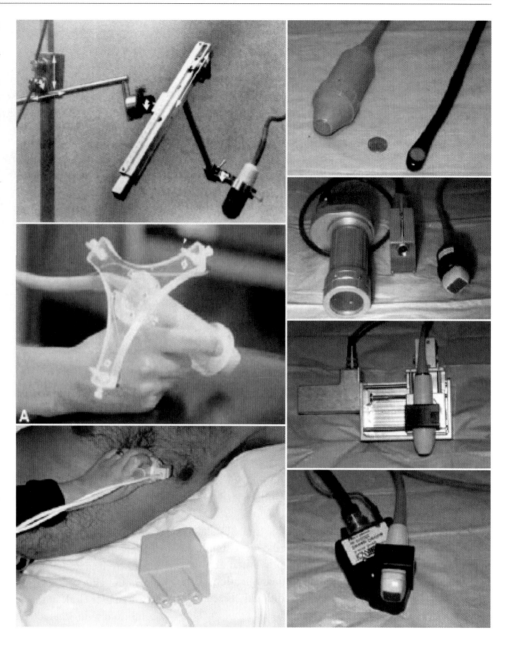

surgery is required. Form Fruste defines some combination of both Barlow's Disease and fibroelastic deficiency.

The lesions resulting from these diseases include chordal elongation or rupture, leaflet distension, annular dilatation, and annular, leaflet, and/or papillary muscle calcification (Fig. 15.10). Barlow's disease, for example, commonly results in chordal elongation, thickened leaflets with excess tissue, billowing of the leaflets, annular dilatation and calcification of the annulus or anterior papillary muscle. The timing of the regurgitant jet can help differentiate the lesions in Barlow's disease. If the regurgitant jet occurs in mid-to-late systole, it is usually due to chordal elongation resulting in prolapse as opposed to chordal rupture, which tends to cause holosystolic,

early regurgitation. Chordal rupture from Barlow's disease is relatively uncommon. Fibroelastic deficiency, on the other hand, leads to chordal thinning, elongation, and/or rupture, with classic findings of flail and mitral regurgitation of varying severity (Fig. 15.11).[19] In these individuals, rupture of a single chord is the most common cause of leaflet dysfunction. In most cases, the remaining leaflet segments have a normal appearance with the posterior annulus being mildly dilated (Table 15.2).

The last section of the triad is the dysfunction of the mitral valve that the above lesions cause. Carpentier et al. classified the mitral valve dysfunction based on the systolic position of the leaflet margins in relation to the annular plane.[18] Type I dysfunction

Fig. 15.9 Real-time 3D transesophageal echocardiogram volume rendering (*left*) and corresponding QLAB 3D parametric image (*right*) of a normal mitral valve (*top row*), mitral valve with Barlow's disease (*center row*), and mitral valve with fibroelastic deficiency (*bottom row*). The red area on the parametric images represents prolapse. Note the multisegmental prolapse of Barlow's disease versus the unisegmental prolapse of fibroelastic deficiency. *A* anterior, *P* posterior, *AL* anterolateral, *PM* posteromedial, *Ao* aorta (Reproduced with permission from Lang et al.[13])

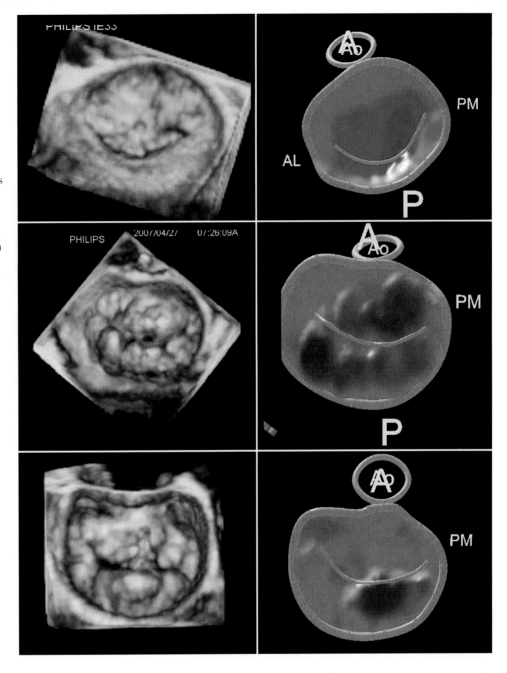

is normal leaflet motion while type II dysfunction describes excess motion of the leaflet margin above the plane of the annulus. Type II dysfunction is the most common dysfunction in degenerative disease. Type III dysfunction is restricted leaflet motion resulting in coaptation below the annular plane. This dysfunction can be further subdivided into type IIIa (restricted leaflet motion in systole and diastole) and type IIIb (predominantly restricted leaflet motion in systole only) (Fig. 15.12).

It is important to emphasize that the different components of the pathophysiologic triad are not mutually exclusive and can be combined in any number of ways. For example, patients with chronic atrial fibrillation commonly develop

annular dilatation which would be categorized as a type I dysfunction. Type II dysfunction is commonly caused by chordal elongation or rupture which, as mentioned above, can be secondary to Barlow's Disease or fibroelastic deficiency. The typical lesions seen in type IIIa dysfunction, which may occur in conjunction with type II dysfunction in degenerative patients with Barlow's disease, are chordal or papillary retraction, fusion, and thickening, usually involving the anterior subvalvular apparatus. Type IIIb dysfunction is the result of ventricular remodeling, with the primary lesion being leaflet tethering due to papillary muscle displacement as occurs in ischemic mitral regurgitation. It may coexist

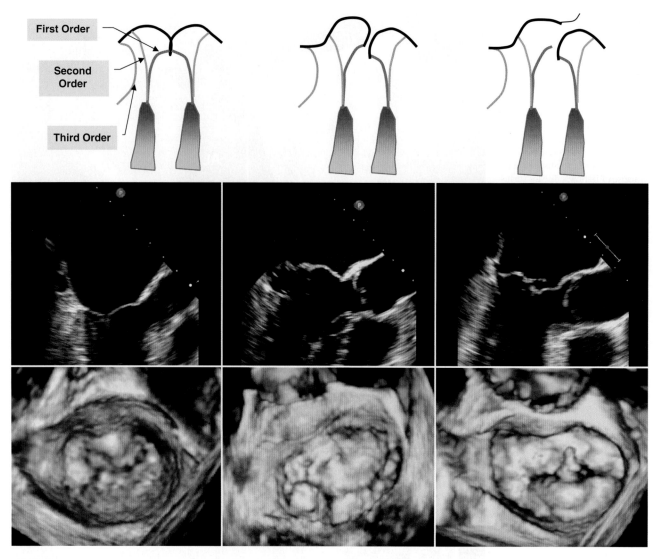

Fig. 15.10 Schematic (*upper row*) and 2D as well as 3D echocardiographic examples of patient with a normal mitral valve (*left panels*), mitral valve prolapse (*P1, middle panels*) and a flail mitral valve (*P2, right panels*) as visualized with 2D TEE long-axis mid esophageal TEE views (*middle row*) and real-time 3D TEE volume rendering from the left atrial perspective (*bottom row*). The surgical views obtained with real-time 3D TEE provide unique visualization and better understanding of the anatomic relationships of the mitral valve annulus, commissures, and leaflets (Reproduced with permission from O'Gara et al.[4])

with prolapse (type II dysfunction) in patients with degenerative mitral regurgitation with long-standing severe regurgitation that has resulted in pronounced left ventricular dilatation. Associated annular dilatation is a common finding in patients with chronic degenerative mitral regurgitation, but the classification of dysfunction should differentiate the primary lesion causing the regurgitation (i.e., chordal rupture) from secondary lesions (i.e., annular dilatation) (Table 15.3).

15.6 Post-Repair Assessment

At the completion of the mitral valve repair, before leaving the operating room, it is imperative that the echocardiographer examine the mitral valve apparatus to rule out any complications that would lead to early reoperation.[20] These complications include residual valvular or para-ring regurgitation, significant transmitral gradients, and systolic anterior motion. Residual mitral regurgitation can occur when the depth of coaptation is less than 5 mm in a 2D long axis view. A segmental analysis of the entire coaptation surface, including the commissures, must be performed to rule out significant regurgitation (≥2+). If a residual leak is identified, the lesion responsible and the dysfunction it causes must be determined and reported in a segmental fashion. The most common causes of residual leaks include uncorrected segmental prolapse or restriction, residual restricted leaflet indentation, incorrectly sized or positioned ring that distorts the zone of coaptation, leaflet perforation from an annuloplasty suture, or a defect in a leaflet closure line. Once the cause is identified,

Fig. 15.11 Echocardiographic differentiation of Carpentier type II dysfunction. (**a**): Upper panel shows chordal rupture due to fibroelastic deficiency with a flail leaflet segment but otherwise normal-sized leaflets resulting in posterior leaflet prolapse. The corresponding surgical view is shown in the lower panel. (**b**): Upper panel shows chordal elongation resulting in posterior leaflet prolapse: leaflets are tall with excess leaflet tissue, typical of Barlow's disease; note that although the body of the anterior leaflet billows above the annular plane, the margin of the anterior leaflet does not prolapse. These tall leaflets place the patient at risk for systolic anterior motion after repair. The corresponding surgical view is shown in the lower panel. Arrows indicate the regurgitant jet. Dotted lines represent the annular plane (Reproduced with permission from Adams et al.[1])

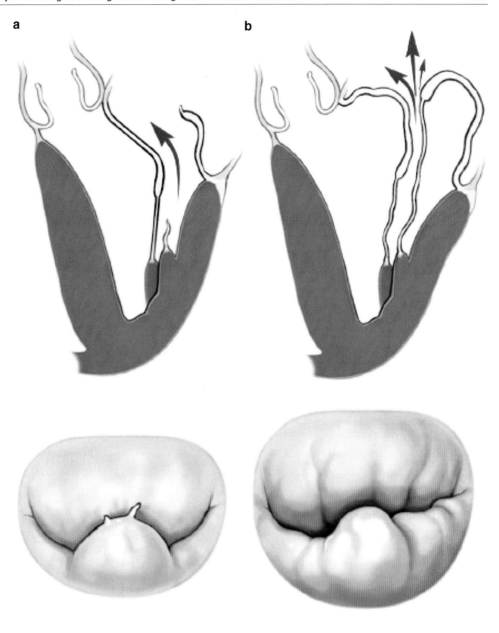

Table 15.2 Key differences between Barlow's disease and fibroelastic deficiency

Etiology of mitral valve degenerative disease	Barlow's disease	Fibroelastic deficiency
Pathophysiology	Excess of myxomatous tissue	Abnormal connective tissue structure/function
Valve involvement	Multisegmental	Unisegmental
Age of presentation	Younger	Older
Associated lesions	Chordal elongation, thickened leaflets, annular dilatation and calcification	Chordal thinning, elongation, and rupture
Most common dysfunction	Prolapse	Flail

a prompt return to cardiopulmonary bypass and subsequent valve re-exploration should be performed.

Another complication post-repair that must be ruled out is systolic anterior motion causing left ventricular obstruction. Systolic anterior motion is a phenomenon that is almost unique to mitral valve repair. It results from a mismatch of annular septolateral dimension and the residual combined leaflet height causing the margin of the anterior leaflet to fall into the left ventricular outflow tract. This causes a significant outflow tract gradient as well as varying degrees of mitral regurgitation. The mid-esophageal long axis view is best for identifying this phenomenon. Sometimes it is possible to reposition the anterior leaflet out of the outflow tract by increasing preload or afterload. However, if these maneuvers are not successful, valve re-exploration and placement

Fig. 15.12 Carpentier's classification system of mitral regurgitation mechanisms. Each type describes the specific mitral valve dysfunction and gives several examples of the lesions that cause it (Modified from Carpentier[5])

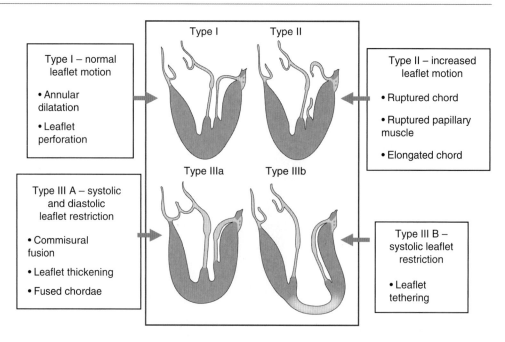

Type I – normal leaflet motion

• Annular dilatation

• Leaflet perforation

Type II – increased leaflet motion

• Ruptured chord

• Ruptured papillary muscle

• Elongated chord

Type III A – systolic and diastolic leaflet restriction

• Commisural fusion

• Leaflet thickening

• Fused chordae

Type III B – systolic leaflet restriction

• Leaflet tethering

Table15.3 Key differences in the specific types of dysfunction according to Carpentier's classification for mitral valve degeneration

Dysfunction	Type I	Type II	Type IIIa	Type IIIb
Motion of leaflet margin	Normal	Excess motion above plane of annulus	Restricted motion in systole and diastole	Restricted motion in systole only
Specific disease processes	Chronic atrial fibrillation	Barlow's disease or fibroelastic deficiency	Barlow's disease or fibroelastic deficiency	Ventricular remodeling
Associated lesions	Annular dilation only	Chordal elongation or rupture	Chordal or papillary retraction, fusion, and thickening	Leaflet tethering due to papillary muscle displacement

of a larger ring, shortening of leaflet height, or even valve replacement is necessary.

Surgical techniques have progressed significantly so that even some of the most complex cases of degenerative mitral valve regurgitation can be repaired rather than replaced. The echocardiogram has a critical role in the management algorithm for this disease because it defines parameters for guideline intervention and also serves as the gatekeeper for the patient's access to appropriate level surgical expertise. Once severe mitral regurgitation is determined by transthoracic echocardiogram and surgery is decided on as an acceptable therapy, transesophageal echocardiogram can be used to strategize how best to proceed. Preoperative assessment with transesophageal echocardiography dictates how extensive the disease is by detailing each part of the mitral valve apparatus, defining the etiology of the disease, locating the specific lesion, and identifying the type of dysfunction. While standard transesophageal 2DE is useful in this assessment, the increasing use of real-time transesophageal 3DE will facilitate both lesion identification and localization. The intraoperative assessment of the mitral valve procedure is no less important a role. The echocardiographer provides a clear demonstration of the lesions and dysfunctions that must be confirmed by surgical analysis in the operating room and

also permits the immediate result of the valve repair, guiding the surgeon to either accept the result or return to cardiopulmonary bypass to correct a residual concern.

References

1. Adams DH, Anyanwu AC, Sugeng L, Lang RM. Degenerative mitral valve regurgitation: surgical echocardiography. *Curr Cardiol Rep*. 2008;10:226–232.
2. Muresian H. The clinical anatomy of the mitral valve. *Clin Anat*. 2008;22:85–98.
3. Isnard R, Acar C. The mitral annulus area: a useful tool for the surgeon. *J Heart Valve Dis*. 2008;17:243–250.
4. O'Gara P, Sugeng L, Lang R, et al. The role of imaging in chronic degenerative mitral regurgitation. *J Am Coll Cardiol Img*. 2008; 1:221–237.
5. Carpentier A. Cardiac valve surgery – the "french correction". *J Thorac Cardiovasc Surg*. 1983;86:323–337.
6. Rodriguez F, Langer F, Harrington KB, et al. Importance of mitral valve second-order chordae for left ventricular geometry, wall thickening mechanics, and global systolic function. *Circulation*. 2004;110:115–122.
7. Rodriguez F, Langer F, Harrington KB, et al. Effect of cutting second-order chordai on in-vivo anterior mitral leaflet compound curvature. *J Heart Valve Dis*. 2005;14:592–601.

8. Dreyfus GD, Bahrami T, Alayle N, et al. Repair of anterior leaflet prolapse by papillary muscle repositioning: a new surgical option. *Ann Thorac Surg.* 2001;71:1464–1470.

9. Bonow RO, Carabello BA, Chatterjee K, et al. ACC/AHA 2006 Guidelines for the management of patients with valvular heart disease: a report of the American College of Cardiology/American Heart Association Task Force on Practice Guidelines (Writing Committee to Revise the 1998 Guidelines for the Management of Patients With Valvular Heart Disease): developed in collaboration with the Society of Cardiovascular Anesthesiologists: endorsed by the Society for Cardiovascular Angiography and Interventions and the Society of Thoracic Surgeons. *Circulation.* 2006;114; e84–e231.

10. Zoghbi WA, Enriquez-Sarano M, Foster E, Grayburn PA, Kraft CD, Levine RA, Nihoyannopoulos P, Otto CM, Quinones MA, Rakowski H, Stewart WJ, Waggoner A, Weissman NJ. Recommendations for evaluation of the severity of native valvular regurgitation with two-dimensional and Doppler echocardiography. *J Am Soc Echocardiogr.* 2003;16:777–802.

11. Vandervoort PM, Rivera JM, Mele D, Palacios IF, Dinsmore RE, Weyman AE, Levine RA, Thomas JD. Application of color Doppler flow mapping to calculate effective regurgitant orifice area. An in vitro study and initial clinical observations. *Circulation.* 1993; 88:1150–1156.

12. Enriquez-Sarano M, Miller FA Jr, Hayes SN, Bailey KR, Tajik AJ, Seward JB. Effective mitral regurgitant orifice area: clinical use and pitfalls of the proximal isovelocity surface area method. *J Am Coll Cardiol.* 1995;25:703–709.

13. Lang RM, Salgo IS, Anyanwu AC, Adams DH. The road to mitral valve repair with live 3D transesophageal echocardiography. *Medicamundi.* 2008;52:37–42.

14. Sugeng L, Shernan SK, Salgo IS, Weinert L, Shook D, Raman J, Jeevanandam V, DuPont F, Settlemier S, Savord B, Fox J, Mor-Avi V, Lang RM. Live 3-Dimensional transesophageal echocardiography initial experience using the fully-sampled matrix array probe. *J Am Coll Cardiol.* 2008;52:446–449.

15. Sugeng L, Shernan SK, Weinert L, Shook D, Raman J, Jeevanandam V, DuPont F, Fox J, Mor-Avi V, Lang RM. Real-time 3D transesophageal echocardiography in valve disease: comparison with surgical findings and evaluation of prosthetic valves. *J Am Soc Echocardiogr.* 2008;21:1347–1354.

16. Carpentier AF, Lessana A, Relland JY et al. The "physio-ring": an advanced concept in mitral valve annuloplasty. *Ann Thorac Surg.* 1995;60:1177–1185.

17. Anyanwu AC, Adams DH. Etiologic classification of degenerative mitral valve disease: Barlow's disease and fibroelastic deficiency. *Semin Thorac Cardiovasc Surg.* 2007;19:90–96.

18. Carpentier AF, Chauvaud S, Fabiani JN et al. Reconstructive surgery of mitral valve incompetence: ten-year appraisal. *J Thorac Cardiovasc Surg.* 1980;79:338–348.

19. Flameng W, Meuris B, Herijgers P, Herregods MC. Durability of mitral valve repair in Barlow disease versus fibroelastic deficiency. *J Thorac Cardiovasc Surg.* 2008;135:274–282.

20. Adams DH, Anyanwu AC. The cardiologist's role in increasing the rate of mitral valve repair in degenerative disease. *Curr Opin Cardiol.* 2008;23:105–110.

21 Lang RM, Mor-Avi V, Sugeng L, Nieman PS, Sahn DJ. Three-dimensional echocardiography: the benefits of the additional dimension. *J Am Coll Cardiol.* 2006;48:2053–2069.

Visualization and Assessment of Coronary Arteries with Three-Dimensional Echocardiography

16

Andreas Hagendorff

16.1 Introduction

Conventional echocardiography is still the most important imaging modality for detecting ischemic heart disease in clinical practice and is well established in the diagnostic scenario of coronary artery disease. Ischemic heart disease, however, is normally detected by regional wall motion defects induced by severe hypoperfusion at rest or stress-induced myocardial ischemia. Thus, coronary artery disease is usually assumed, if hypo- or akinesis is present at rest or can be provoked by stress-induced ischemia. Thus, coronary artery disease is indirectly detected by the assessment of volume and shape of the left ventricular cavity, and by the global as well regional motion and thickness of the left ventricular wall. This conventional approach to detect the functional sequelae of hypoperfusion on the myocardium underestimates the methodological possibilities of echocardiography to diagnose coronary artery disease.

Whereas imaging of several portions of the coronary artery tree is possible by conventional (2DE), the direct visualization of coronary arteries by echocardiography, however, has not been generally introduced into clinical practice. Improvements in ultrasound technology – especially the new transducers – enable new dimensions for the detection of cardiac morphology – especially in patients with good acoustic window – with a better achievable visualization of the coronary arteries.

Whereas the conventional 2DE of coronary arteries is rarely described, mainly by case reports documenting the right coronary artery,[1-3] imaging of coronary artery flow by transthoracic color-coded Doppler echocardiography is more common, especially for detection of the medial and distal proportion of the left anterior descending artery. In combination with the administration of adenosine, transthoracic color-coded Doppler echocardiography with the acquisition of Doppler spectra of coronary flow enables the noninvasive estimation of coronary flow reserve. Because the distal parts of the left anterior descending artery can be well visualized in almost all patients, the measurement of coronary artery flow reserve has been introduced in clinical practice in some hospitals and medical offices.[4-10] The noninvasive analysis of coronary flow reserve determined in the distal portions of the left anterior descending artery using adenosine can be recommended in all patients after percutaneous coronary interventions performed in the left anterior descending artery instead of routine follow-up angiography. If normal coronary flow reserve is detected, it has been shown that "control angiography" is not necessary. The coronary flow within the distal parts of posterolateral branches of the right coronary artery is also suitable for estimation of coronary flow reserve in most patients by using transthoracic Doppler echocardiography.[11,12,7,10] The detection of the marginal branches and the circumflex artery, however, remains still a problem with transthoracic color-coded echocardiography. This problem can be solved by using transesophageal echocardiography fragment reconstruction. Large proximal portions of the right coronary artery and of the circumflex artery as well as the complete left main stem and the proximal proportion of the left anterior descending artery can be visualized using transesophageal echocardiography, but this method is actually not established in clinical practice.[13]

Thus, the direct visualization of coronary arteries and coronary artery flow – as well as perfusion analysis of the myocardium by myocardial contrast echocardiography – will enhance the diagnostic armamentarium of echocardiography in patients with ischemic heart disease and will become increasingly important. Furthermore, it is encouraging to evaluate the possibilities of real-time multidimensional imaging for the visualization of the coronary arteries and the detection of coronary artery disease, and to balance the advantages and disadvantages of this new coronary imaging method. With regard to other methods of coronary imaging like cardiac magnetic resonance imaging and cardiac computed tomography, the capabilities of echocardiography have to be emphasized. Therefore, it is surprising that many cardiologists do not know how to visualize coronary arteries by

A. Hagendorff
Department of Cardiology – Angiology,
University of Leipzig, Germany
e-mail: andreas.hagendorff@medizin.uni-leipzig.de

L.P. Badano et al. (eds.), *Textbook of Real-Time Three Dimensional Echocardiography*,
DOI: 10.1007/978-1-84996-495-1_16, © Springer-Verlag London Limited 2011

echocardiography despite the potential of combined morphological and functional imaging – especially because the spatial resolution of echocardiography is comparable or better than the other imaging modalities in patients with good acoustic window, and the temporal resolution of echocardiography is per se the highest. In this context, it is also important to recognize that echocardiography is an attractive, noninvasive, and harmless alternative in comparison to methods with x-ray exposure and with the risks of side effects due to angiographic contrast agents. The only problem of the visualization of coronary arteries by echocardiography is the prerequisite of methodological knowledge and training.

Multidimensional echocardiography is a new modality for imaging cardiac structures with a less spatial resolution than 2DE. Therefore, spatial resolution of multidimensional imaging is yet thought to be too poor for imaging small cardiac structures like the coronary arteries. Nevertheless, ultrasound settings can be adjusted, to offer new approaches for the multidimensional visualization of coronary arteries using conventional, color-coded and contrast echocardiography.

16.2 The Detection of Coronary Arteries and Coronary Artery Flow by Conventional Echocardiography

Two-dimensional transthoracic imaging of the native proximal portions of the right coronary artery, and the left main stem and the proximal circumflex artery, and the left anterior descending artery is possible almost in all patients using parasternal short axis views[14]. In patients with good acoustic window, the proximal and middle portions of the left anterior descending artery and the right coronary artery can be visualized by oblique parasternal views within the anterior and posterior interventricular grooves. Sometimes parts of the circumflex artery and the marginal branches can be visualized within the coronary groove by an oblique view dorsal to the standardized four-chamber view, whereas the proximal parts of the right coronary artery and the left anterior descending branch can be imaged by an oblique view ventral to the standardized four-chamber view. However, the apical approach is uncommon for visualizing native coronaries.

In contrast, color-coded 2D imaging of coronaries as well as transthoracic Doppler echocardiography of coronary flow is an established tool used in specialized institutions to assess coronary flow reserve. Methods to detect color signals from the left anterior descending artery, the right coronary artery, as well as the circumflex artery are well described in the literature.[4–10] It is easier to detect the color flow signal within the distal portions of the left anterior descending artery by scanning the apical four-chamber view. Then, the vessel is normally cut vertically within the apical anterior

interventricular groove. By turning and tilting the transducer into an oblique apical long axis view, the longitudinal portions of the left anterior descending artery can be visualized. The middle portions of the left anterior descending artery can be visualized with an oblique caudal short axis view. The proximal part of the left anterior descending artery can be visualized by a cranial short axis view. The distal portions of right coronary artery – mostly the posterolateral perforator branches – are visualized by an oblique apical two-chamber view ventral to the standardized two-chamber view. The middle parts of the right coronary artery are rarely detected by the subcostal approach; the proximal part of the right coronary artery, however, is nearly always detectable using the parasternal long and short axis views. The circumflex artery and the marginal branches remain a challenge for transthoracic imaging. These branches can normally be visualized by an oblique four-chamber view within the lateral regions of the left ventricle. Using this approach these vessels are cut vertically, which impairs the recording of good Doppler spectra. It is obvious that multidimensional imaging will facilitate the detection of multidimensional structures like coronary arteries and detection of coronary artery flow modern technology helps visualize these structures with the same image quality.

The 2D imaging of coronary arteries with ultrasound contrast agents has not shown any advantages in comparison to native and color-coded imaging.

The main advantage of 2D scanning of coronary arteries is the high temporal resolution with frame rates up to 200 frames/s using gray scale imaging and up to 40 frames using the color-coded approach.

16.3 The Detection of Coronary Arteries and Coronary Artery Flow by 3D Echocardiography: Methodological Aspects

The detection of coronary arteries and coronary artery flow do not differ between the 2D and 3D techniques.

However, there are some additional aspects to discuss.

The 3D imaging of native vessels is feasible using the parasternal approach. The proximal portion of the right coronary artery seems to be the major focus of 3D imaging (Fig. 16.1). Because this portion of the vessel is highly visible in nearly all patients, calcification and narrowing of the right coronary ostium can be detected (Fig. 16.2). If the left anterior descending artery is detectable using 2DE from parasternal views, it is also possible to have a 3D approach to visualize these portions of the vessel. In contrast to 2D imaging, which shows a scanned slice of about 2–3 mm thickness, a complete 3D data set will show the complete course

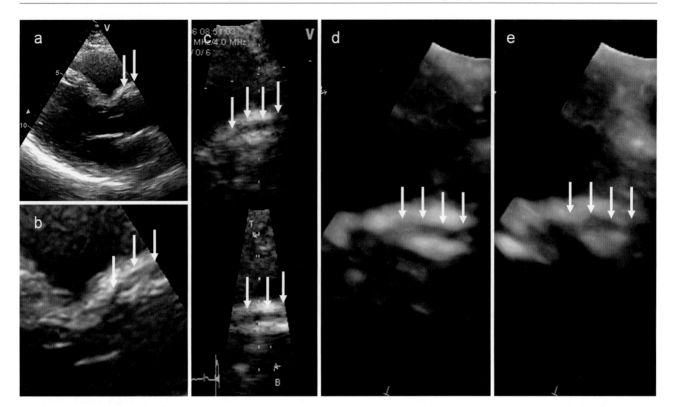

Fig. 16.1 3D visualization of the proximal portion of the right coronary artery using the parasternal approach. The ostium of the right coronary artery and the proximal portion of the right coronary artery shown in the parasternal long axis view (**a**) and after zooming (**b**). The region of interest using the volume probe by biplane scanning (**c**). Two diastolic frames of the multidimensional visualized right coronary artery (**d,e**). *Arrows* mark the right coronary artery. (video1a: Two-dimensional echocardiography of the proximal proportion of the right coronary artery; video1b: Native 3D-echocardiography: Visualization of the proximal proportion of the right coronary artery)

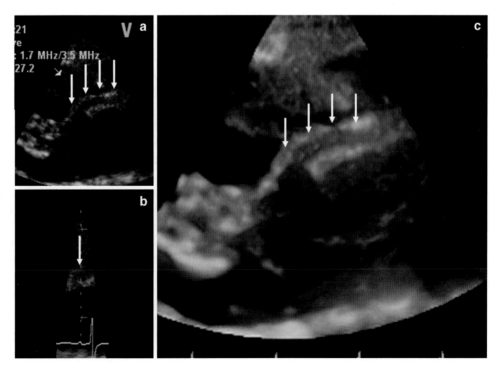

Fig. 16.2 3D visualization of the proximal portion of the right coronary artery. Using a small 3D sector, often longer parts of the vessel can be visualized. Using the biplane approach for scanning the region of interest, the long axis view is documented by a broader sector (**a**), the short axis view by a small sector (**b**). Exclusion of ostial narrowing by multidimensional imaging of the right coronary artery (**c**). *Arrows* mark the right coronary artery. (video 2: native 3D-echocardiography - visualization of the proximal proportion of the right coronary artery using a monochrome color map)

Fig. 16.3 3D imaging of the ostium and the proximal proportion of the right coronary artery by inverting the gray scale of the multidimensional data set in two different patients (**a**, **b**). The lumen of the right coronary artery is completely visualized from its origin at the aortic root for more than 3 (**a**) to 7 cm (**b**). *Arrows* mark the right coronary artery. (video3a: Native 3D-echocardiography: Visualization of a normal proximal proportion of the right coronary artery using an invert color function. video3b: Native 3D-echocardiography: Visualization of a crook-like looking proximal proportion of the right coronary artery using an invert color function)

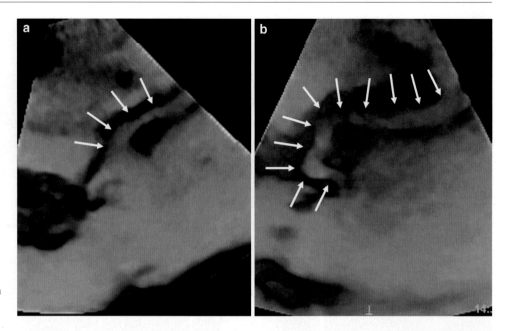

of the vessel. Thus, it is possible to visualize the first 6–8 cm of the right coronary artery. The right coronary artery can be analyzed much better by inverting the color of the multidimensional data set (Fig. 16.3). Using this application, the lumen of the right coronary artery is directly visualized as a bright tube. Narrowing of the vessel can be visualized by postprocessing using the six- or nine-slice application through the vessel.

To improve the image quality for 3D imaging of the right coronary artery, the following tips may be helpful. First, the target region has to be enlarged using the zoom function and the frame rate should be increased to the maximum. Second, to increase temporal resolution a near real-time full-volume data set with the maximum volume size has to be acquired. Using these settings, it is possible to visualize the ostium of the right coronary artery as well as the proximal portion of the right coronary artery with a temporal resolution up to 160 frames/s (Fig. 16.4).

If the target vessel is large, the vessel can be imaged in real time by using a broad sector in a longitudinal direction to the vessel and by a small sector perpendicular to the vessel.

The 3D color-coded imaging of coronary artery flow is possible using the same approaches described for 2D coronary imaging (Fig. 16.5). Since the 3D course of the coronary can be followed within the volumetric data set, a larger portion of coronary artery – especially of the left anterior descending artery – can usually be visualized by 3D imaging than by 2D imaging (Fig. 16.6). The 3D imaging of the distal portions of the left anterior descending artery is easier than visualizing it in a 2D scan plan. For practical aspects, the target region has to be selected using the color-coded biplane mode, which prepares the acquisition of a near real-time full-volume data set. Then, the angle of the surrounding gray scale sector has to be minimized to increase temporal resolution of the color-coded sector. If the position of the vessel is difficult to visualize, i.e., if only a small portion of the coronary flow within the distal left anterior descending artery is visualized within the anterior interventricular groove, a small pyramidal square sector has to be chosen to ensure that the largest portion of the vessel will be acquired in the volumetric data set. After adjusting for pulse repetition rate, tissue transparency, and depth, the pyramidal space around the target vessel has to be acquired using a full-volume color-coded 3D data set to visualize the coronary flow of the distal portions of the left anterior descending artery. If possible, a full-volume data set should be acquired over seven heart cycles to increase the spatial as well as temporal resolutions. In this way, frame rates

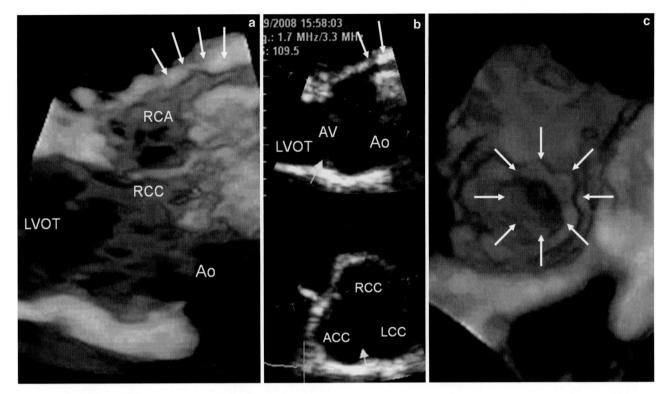

Fig. 16.4 3D imaging of the ostium of the right coronary artery. The ostium and the proximal portion of the right coronary artery can be visualized in a near real-time full-volume data set acquired for a heartbeat with a temporal resolution of 110 frames/s (see (**b**)) by zooming the region of interest. The longitudinal view of the proximal portion of the right coronary artery is shown in (**a**). The en-face view into the right coronary artery ostium from the lumen of the aorta is shown in (**c**).

Arrows mark the right coronary artery. *LVOT* left ventricular outflow tract, *RCC* right coronary cusp, *Ao* aorta ascendens, *LCC* left coronary cusp, *ACC* acoronary cusp. (video4a: Native 3D-echocardiography: long axis view of the proximal proportion of the right coronary artery (frame rate 110/s) - video 4b: Native 3D-echocardiography: en-face view into the ostium of the right coronary artery (frame rate 110/s)

up to 17 frames/s of multidimensional color-coded flow imaging can be achieved (Fig. 16.7). Even if the vessel is not properly visualized within the anterior interventricular groove during acquisition, it can be visualized by postprocessing the data set and increasing tissue transparency. The six- or nine-slice technique facilitates the analysis of the color-coded flow signals because narrowing or enlargements of the vessel can be estimated by scan planes showing the longitudinal course of the vessel. Using 3D color-coded flow imaging, septal branches in patients with hypertrophy or hypertrophic cardiomyopathy can easily be visualized (Fig. 16.9). Furthermore, changes in vessel diameter during a stress test can be estimated by comparing images acquired during resting and hyperemic states, e.g., during adenosine infusion (Fig. 16.8). Despite feasibility, the quantification of vessel narrowing by 3D color-coded flow signals, however, has to be evaluated in further studies compared to flow data obtained from transthoracic Doppler echocardiography and angiography.

The quality of the full-volume data sets depends on their acquisition methods and patient characteristics. It is obvious that a good acoustic window, sinus rhythm, and breath-holding is necessary for a good image quality. The most important limitation of single-shot real-time acquisition of coronary flow is temporal resolution.

The 3D imaging of coronaries using contrast agents is a promising tool (Fig. 16.10). The main challenge of coronary artery imaging with contrast is the acquisition at the optimal time point of contrast wash-in. If the coronary artery tree has to be visualized, the time frame during which the coronaries are filled with contrast without

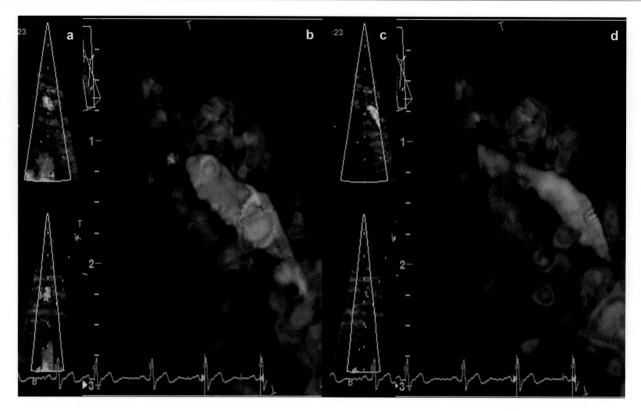

Fig. 16.5 3D visualization of coronary artery flow determined in a distal portion of the left anterior descending artery. The distal anterior interventricular groove as the region of interest is focused by biplane scanning within a small sector (**a**) and (**c**). Using acquisition of color-coded near real-time full-volume data set, a portion of 10 to 40 mm of the distal anterior descending artery can be visualized. Two diastolic frames of the vessel are shown in (**b**) and (**d**). (video5: Fig. 16.5: Color-coded 3D-echocardiography: Visualization of coronary flow in the distal left anterior descending artery - ZOOM-mode)

opacification of the myocardium has to be selected. Therefore, a fast bolus administration with sufficient cardiac opacification are filled with contrast without shadowing and blooming artifacts is necessary. If the bolus administration of the contrast is too slow, the detection of coronaries has to be performed during the time interval of the replenishment after a long flush during a continuous contrast infusion. Both techniques require knowledge about contrast applications and training regarding contrast imaging. In addition, it has to be emphasized that only a small amount of contrast (few resonating bubbles) is sufficient to obtain an enhancement of the vessel lumen.

16.4 Limitations

At present, the 3D imaging of coronary arteries is not introduced into clinical routine. The feasibility and potential of this new method have to be evaluated in further studies. It is obvious that expertise in echocardiography and training in specific methodological aspects are prerequisites to evaluate if this attractive method of 3D imaging of coronary arteries is possible and feasible with commercially available transducers and ultrasound settings. Furthermore, this new method has to be introduced to physicians and popularized among patients as a possible diagnostic alternative to methods involving x-ray exposure like cardiac computerized tomography.

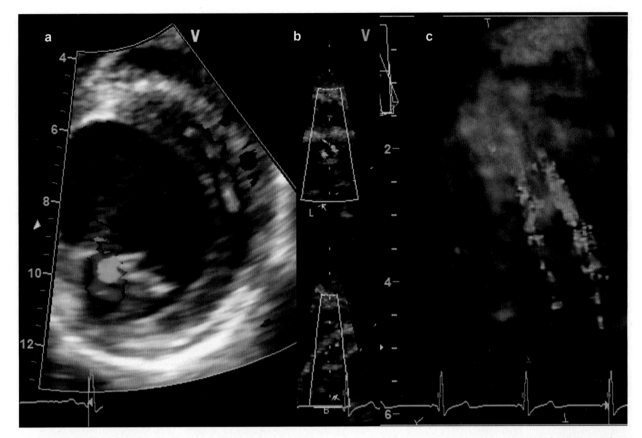

Fig. 16.6 Monoplane color-coded documentation of coronary artery flow within septal branches using a subcostal view (**a**). Biplane scanning of the region of interest using the color-coded application (**b**) is performed prior to the acquisition of the near real-time color-coded full-volume data set. 3D visualization of the coronary artery flow of two large septal branches is shown using increasing tissue transparency (**c**). (video6a: Two-dimensional color coded imaging of coronary flow in septal branches - short axis view; video6b: Color-coded 3D-echocardiography: Visualization of coronary flow in septal branches)

16.5 Summary

The detection of ischemic heart disease by echocardiography is usually performed by wall motion analysis at rest and during stress-induced ischemia. Whereas the direct visualization of coronary arteries by 2DE is not an established clinical tool, the color-coded imaging and the detection of coronary flow by transthoracic Doppler echocardiography is established in many institutions for the estimation of coronary flow reserve. Multidimensional echocardiography provides new options for the noninvasive imaging of cardiac arteries. The ostium and the proximal portion of the right coronary artery seem to be an optimal target for this new approach because this portion of the vessel can be visualized and acquired by echocardiography. The multidimensional color-coded imaging of distinct portions of all three main coronary arteries can be performed as well. The multidimensional contrast imaging of coronaries enables further possibilities, but it is limited by many methodological factors. In summary, multidimensional imaging of the coronary arteries by echocardiography is feasible and possible. However – especially in patients with limited acoustic window – it is still a diagnostic challenge and needs methodological expertise along with practical education and training.

16.6 Conclusions

Multidimensional imaging of the coronary arteries by echocardiography is a new, noninvasive and harmless method, which should be introduced, in addition to the two-dimensional approach, into the clinical diagnostic scenario. It will be an interesting alternative to methods involving x-ray as well as angiographic contrast exposure.

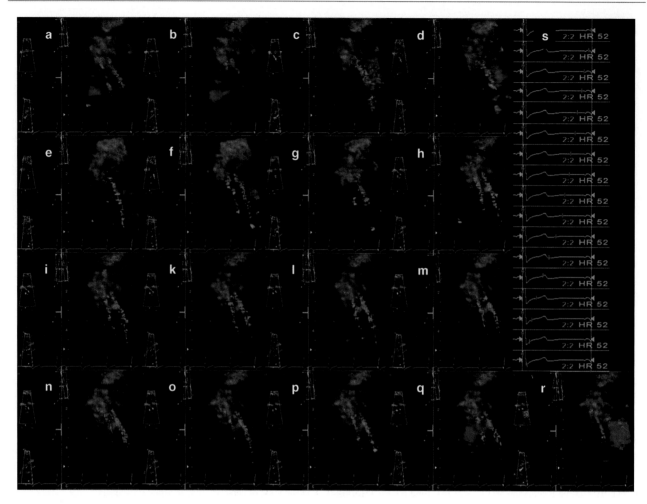

Fig. 16.7 Documentation of the high temporal resolution of the 3D visualization of coronary artery flow. At a heart rate of 52 beat/s, 17 frames can be acquired ((**a**)–(**r**)). The corresponding markers and the ECG can be seen in the figure (video7=video6b: Color-coded 3D-echocardiography: Fig 16.7 shows the single frames of the cineloop to document the time resolution)

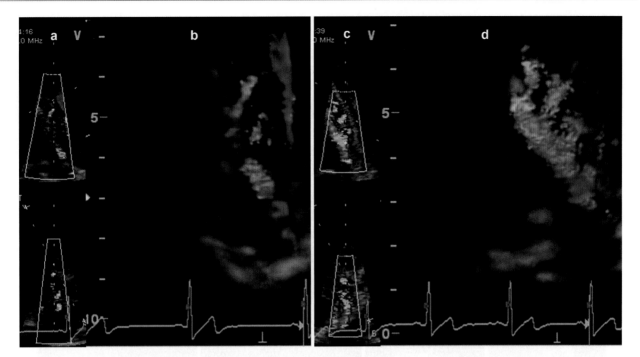

Fig. 16.8 3D visualization of coronary artery flow in small septal branches in a patient with hypertrophic cardiomyopathy. The region of interest is focussed by biplane scanning (**a**, **c**) prior to the acquisition of the near real-time full-volume color-coded data set. Two different views of the flow determined within the septal branches are shown (**b**, **d**).

(video8a: Color-coded 3D-echocardiography - Visualization of coronary flow in the distal right coronary artery and posterolateral branches at rest; video8b: Color-coded 3D-echocardiography - Visualization of coronary flow in the distal right coronary artery and posterolateral branches during adenosine stress)

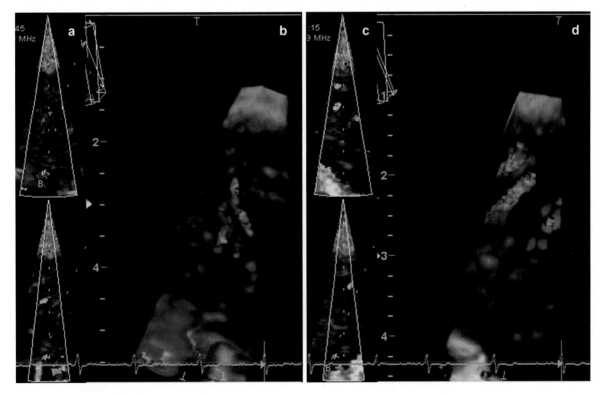

Fig. 16.9 3D visualization of coronary artery flow determined in the distal right coronary artery at rest (**a**, **b**) and during adenosine stress (**c**, **d**). Before acquisition the region of interest is focused by biplane scanning as shown in (**a**) and (**c**). Using the same settings for color-coded flow visualization, the vessel at rest is visualized in (**b**). The significant dilatation of the vessel and the increase of flow is documented by the color intensity and the enlargement of the color-coded signals of the vessel in (**d**). (video9a and 9b: Color-coded 3D-echocardiography - Visualization of coronary flow in septal branches in a patient with hypertrophic cardiomyopathy)

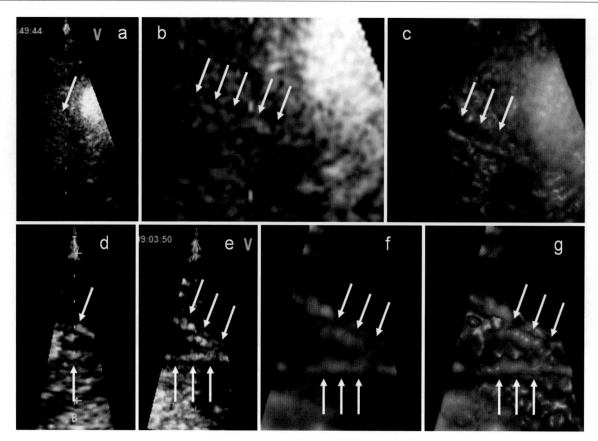

Fig. 16.10 3D visualization of septal branches using contrast application. Figures (**a–c**) show a monoplane visualization of the vessel within the interventricular septum in (**a**) and using the zooming function in (**b**). The 3D visualization of the same proportion of the vessel is shown in (**c**). Figures (**d–g**) show a bifurcation of a septal branch. In (**d**) and (**e**), the region of interest is shown by the biplane approach during the inflow of the contrast agent. Figures (**f**) and (**g**) show the same vessel by 3D visualization using different postprocessing. (video10a: Fig.16.10: Contrast 3D-echocardiography- Visualization of small septal branches during the early wash-in of the microbubbles; video10b: Contrast 3D-echocardiography - Visualization of a vessel bifurcation in the septal left ventricular regions during the early wash-in of the microbubbles)

References

1. Dimitrow PP, Krzanowski M. Coronary flow reserve assessment. *Eur Heart J.* 2005;26:849.
2. Holte E, Vegsundvåg J, Wiseth R Direct visualization of a significant stenosis of the right coronary artery by transthoracic echocardiography. A case report. *Cardiovasc Ultrasound.* 2007;5:33.
3. Hiraishi S, Misawa H, Takeda N, Horiguchi Y, Fujino N, Ogawa N, Hirota H. Transthoracic ultrasonic visualisation of coronary aneurysm, stenosis, and occlusion in Kawasaki disease. *Heart.* 2000; 83:400–405.
4. Dimitrow PP. Transthoracic Doppler echocardiography – noninvasive diagnostic window for coronary flow reserve assessment. *Cardiovasc Ultrasound.* 2003;1:4.
5. Hagendorff A, Werner A, Pfeiffer D, Becher H. Estimation of vasodilator response by analysis of Doppler intensity kinetics with myocardial contrast echocardiography using an intravenous standardized bolus administration. *Eur J Echocardiogr.* 2004;5:272–283.
6. Iwata S, Hozumi T, Matsumura Y, Sugioka K, Yoshitani H, Murata E, Takemoto Y, Kobayashi Y, Yoshiyama M, Yoshikawa J. Cut-off value of coronary flow velocity reserve by transthoracic Doppler echocardiography for the assessment of significant donor left anterior descending artery stenosis in patients with spontaneously visible collaterals. *Am J Cardiol.* 2006;98:298–302.
7. Murata E, Hozumi T, Matsumura Y, Fujimoto K, Sugioka K, Takemoto Y, Watanabe H, Yamagishi H, Yoshiyama M, Iwao H, Yoshikawa J. Coronary flow velocity reserve measurement in three major coronary arteries using transthoracic Doppler echocardiography. *Echocardiography.* 2006;23:279–286.
8. Pizzuto F, Voci P, Mariano E, Puddu PE, Sardella G, Nigri A. Assessment of flow velocity reserve by transthoracic Doppler echocardiography and venous adenosine infusion before and after left anterior descending coronary artery stenting. *J Am Coll Cardiol.* 2001;38:155–162.
9. Ruscazio M, Montisci R, Colonna P, Caiati C, Chen L, Lai G, Cadeddu M, Pirisi R, Iliceto S. Detection of coronary restenosis after coronary angioplasty by contrast-enhanced transthoracic echocardiographic Doppler assessment of coronary flow velocity reserve. *J Am Coll Cardiol.* 2002;40:896–903.
10. Watanabe H, Hozumi T, Hirata K, Otsuka R, Tokai K, Muro T, Shimada K, Yoshiyama M, Takeuchi K, Yoshikawa J. Noninvasive coronary flow velocity reserve measurement in the posterior descending coronary artery for detecting coronary stenosis in the

right coronary artery using contrast-enhanced transthoracic Doppler echocardiography. *Echocardiography*. 2004;21:225–233.

11. Krzanowski M, Bodzo W, Dimitrow PP. Imaging of all three coronary arteries by transthoracic echocardiography. An illustrated guide. *Cardiovasc Ultrasound*. 2003;1:16.

12. Tries HP, Lambertz H, Lethen H. Transthoracic echocardiographic visualization of coronary artery blood flow and assessment of coronary flow reserve in the right coronary artery: a first report of 3 patients. *J Am Soc Echocardiogr*. 2002;15:739–742.

13. Wild PS, Zotz R. Fragment reconstruction of coronary arteries by transesophageal echocardiography. A method for visualizing coronary arteries with ultrasound. *Circulation*. 2002;105:1579–1584.

14. Lambertz H, Tries HP, Stein T, Lethen H. Noninvasive assessment of coronary flow reserve with transthoracic signal-enhanced Doppler echocardiography. *J Am Soc Echocardiogr*. 1999;12: 186–195.

Assessment of Tricuspid Valve Morphology and Function

17

Denisa Muraru and Luigi P. Badano

17.1 Introduction

The tricuspid valve (TV) is a complex structure, and its function plays an important role in several heart diseases, including left-sided valve disease and heart failure. The development of functional tricuspid regurgitation is directly associated with increased morbidity and mortality.[1–5] These data have increased the motivation to repair functional tricuspid regurgitation, especially at the time of concomitant surgery for left-sided disease.[3] However, the unsatisfactory results of current approaches suggest an incomplete understanding of the anatomy and underlying mechanisms.[3,6] As in the case of mitral regurgitation, a better understanding of the pathophysiological mechanisms underlying functional tricuspid regurgitation could potentially suggest more effective surgical treatment.

Routine assessment of the TV is mostly done by standard two-dimensional echocardiography (2DE) despite the unique configuration of tricuspid leaflets and annulus, and anatomic complexity of the right ventricle. However, simultaneous visualization of the three TV leaflets cannot be achieved routinely from standard 2DE imaging views. Usually, only two leaflets can be imaged in one 2DE view and determination of individual leaflet involvement (especially the posterior leaflet) is challenging when a disease process is present (Fig. 17.1).[7] This limitation can be partially overcome with an anterior to posterior sweep to see both the anterior and the posterior leaflets using the apical four-chamber or subcostal view. Afterwards, the echocardiographer starts a difficult mental process to reconstruct a stereoscopic image of the TV based on the interpretation of the multiple tomographic images obtained with the sweep. Sometimes, the mental exercise of reconstruction may be inadequate to obtain a precise diagnosis even for an experienced observer, particularly when dealing with complex valvular abnormalities.

The advent of three-dimensional echocardiography (3DE) may obviate for this exercise by allowing a more objective and quantitative evaluation of TV anatomy and function (Table 17.1) that would reduce the subjectivity in the interpretation of the images.[8–10]

17.2 Anatomy of Tricuspid Valve

The TV is a complex anatomic structure composed of leaflet tissue, chordae tendineae, papillary muscles, and the supporting annular ring, right atrium and ventricular myocardium. It is the most apically placed cardiac valve and it has the largest orifice area (Fig. 17.2).

The TV leaflets (anterior, posterior, and septal) are attached to a fibrous annulus and are unequal in size: the anterior leaflet is usually the largest and extends from the infundibular region anteriorly to the inferolateral wall posteriorly; the septal leaflet extends from the interventricular septum of the infundibulum to the posterior ventricular border; the posterior leaflet attaches along the posterior margin of the annulus from the septum to the inferolateral wall. The insertion of the septal leaflet of the TV is characteristically apical relative to the septal insertion of the anterior mitral leaflet.

The tricuspid annulus shows a non-planar structure with an elliptical saddle-shaped pattern, having two high points (superiorly oriented toward the right atrium) and two low points inferiorly oriented towards the right ventricle, which is best seen in mid-systole.[11]

Three papillary muscle groups usually support the TV leaflets and lie beneath each of the three commissures.

17.3 Approaches to 3D Imaging of the Tricuspid Valve

3DE with its unique capability of obtaining an "en face" view of the TV allows simultaneous visualization of the three leaflets in motion during the cardiac cycle and their attachment to the tricuspid annulus (Fig. 17.2). 3DE allows

L.P. Badano (✉)
Department of Cardiology, Vascular and Thoracic Sciences,
University of Padua, Padua, Italy
e-mail: lpbadano@gmail.com

L.P. Badano et al. (eds.), *Textbook of Real-Time Three Dimensional Echocardiography*,
DOI: 10.1007/978-1-84996-495-1_17, © Springer-Verlag London Limited 2011

Fig. 17.1 Visualization of the tricuspid valve leaflets by two-dimensional echocardiography. The lines on the anatomical drawing show the range of the two-dimensional tomographic planes for each corresponding view. Below the two-dimensional images has been reported the percentage of leaflet identification in each standard two-dimensional view (Reproduced with permission from Badano et al.[9])

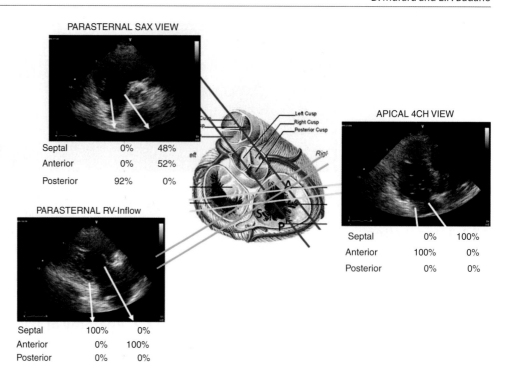

Table 17.1 Summary of the additive diagnostic value of three-dimensional echocardiography over current two-dimensional technique in various diseases of the tricuspid valve

Tricuspid valve disease	Additive diagnostic value of 3DE
Organic tricuspid regurgitation	Precise morphology of the TV leaflets, leaflet coaptation, annulus size. Chordae rupture. Regurgitation mechanism
Ebstein anomaly[29–31]	Precise morphology of the TV leaflets, extent of development their formation, level of their attachment, and their degree of coaptation. Visualization of the mechanism of regurgitation or stenosis. Visualization of subvalvular apparatus
Rheumatic valve disease[27,32,33]	Detailed leaflet anatomy, commissural fusion degree, leaflet shortening and thickening. Tricuspid annulus dilatation. Direct planimetry of residual orifice.
Carcinoid heart disease[34]	Comprehensive assessment of TV anatomy. Identification of the regions of ineffective leaflet coaptation and the lack of commissural fusion. Better assessment of regurgitation severity
Infective endocarditis[35,36]	Comprehensive assessment of TV anatomy. Vegetation characteristics and size. Regurgitation mechanism
Interference from pacemaker lead[13]	Identification of regurgitation mechanism
Functional tricuspid regurgitation[11,20,24,25]	Measurement of tenting volume. Extent of dilatation and shape of TV annulus. Better estimation of regurgitation severity
Traumatic tricuspid regurgitation[19]	Visualization of papillary muscle and/or chordal rupture

the echocardiographer to visualize leaflet coaptation and separation of the commissures. A detailed anatomical description of the TV including unique analysis of tricuspid annulus shape and size, TV leaflets shape and mobility, and TV commissural width has been reported by Anwar and colleagues.[7]

Like 2DE, there are three main approaches to be used with 3DE: parasternal, apical and subcostal. However, when trying to image a cardiac structure with 3DE we should take into account the different spatial resolution we can obtain by using the different approaches (Chapter 4). According to resolution capabilities of current 3DE transducers, the best approach to obtain an *en face* view of the TV from the right atrium (the so-called "surgical view") is the parasternal short axis, in which structures are imaged by the axial and lateral dimensions. Conversely, the worst result is expected to be obtained by the apical approach which uses the lateral and elevation dimensions. An intermediate result will be obtained by using the parasternal right ventricular inflow in which the axial and elevation dimensions are used.

An additional feature of matrix array 3DE transducer is that they can acquire both in actual real-time (particularly in real-time zoom mode), and in stitched 3D mode (i.e., two or more consecutive cardiac cycles merged together). Both of these acquisition modalities are useful for imaging the TV. The real-time zoom mode has several advantages over the full-volume acquisition: (1) image resolution is much higher than that of full-volume mode, (2) since we do not need either suspended respiration or acquisition of multiple cardiac cycles, it is feasible also in dyspnoic patients and in patients with atrial fibrillation, (3) the possibility to

Fig. 17.2 Three-dimensional acquisition of a full-volume data set from apical approach allows a complete assessment of the cardiac structures which are part of the tricuspid complex. Sagittal view of the right side of the heart allowing the analysis of spatial relationships between TV leaflets, papillary muscles, and right ventricular anatomy (*upper panel*, video); normal tricuspid valve leaflets visualized from atrial (*mid-left panel*, video) and ventricular side (*mid-right panel*, video); quantitative analysis and surface rendering of right ventricle (*lower-left panel*, video); and quantitative analysis and surface rendering of the right atrium (*lower-right panel*). *ATL* anterior tricuspid leaflet, *Ao* aorta, *MB* moderator band, *MV* mitral valve, *PTL* posterior tricuspid leaflet, *RA* right atrium, *RV* right ventricle, *RVOT* right ventricular outflow tract, *STL* septal tricuspid leaflet, *TV* tricuspid valve

Video 17.2.1 Sagittal view of the the right side of the heart obtained from three-dimensional acquisition of a full-volume data set from apical approach. This view allows the analysis of spatial relationships between TV leaflets, papillary muscles, and right ventricular anatomy

Video 17.2.2 Normal tricuspid valve leaflets visualized from right atrial side

Video 17.2.3 Normal tricuspid valve leaflets visualized from right ventricular side

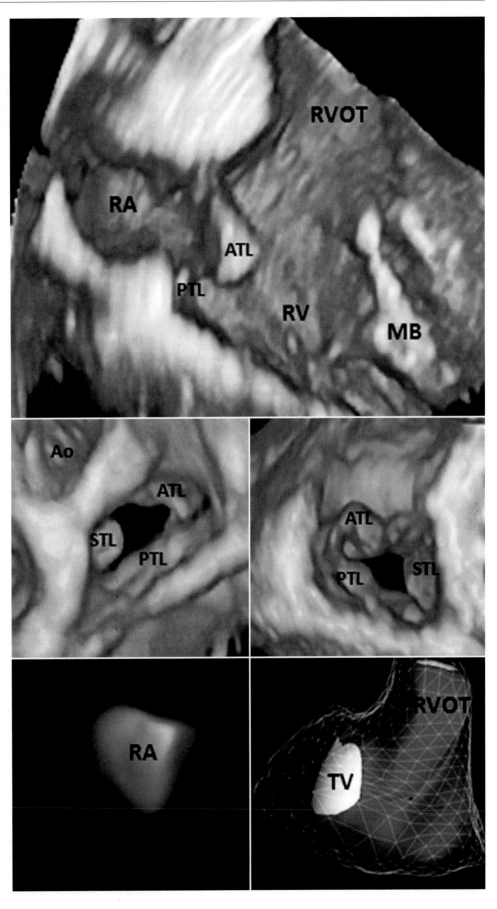

electronically steer the 3D beam by rotating the "track ball", with no need of moving the transducer, may be a major advantage for the purpose of imaging the TV from the parasternal approach, because this approach often requires a very acute angle between the transducer and the skin combined with the need to fit a large transducer footprint into a narrow intercostal space, (4) by steering the 3D beam in order to place the long axis of the TV along the y-axis, the visualization of the three leaflets and the full shape of the valve orifice from both atrial or ventricular side is enabled. Use of full-volume acquisition allows a wider coverage of the region of interest. Therefore, most relevant structures and their spatial relationships (e.g., leaflets, chordae and papillary muscles) can be more realistically delineated, and anatomic continuity can be assessed. But this approach has at least two major limitations: (1) a reduced spatial resolution of the structures with respect to the real-time zoom mode, and (2) the possible presence of artifacts due to rhythm disturbances and respiratory movements.

From the practical point of view, in order to acquire a 3DE data set of the TV, it is recommended to place the transducer in a modified parasternal long-axis position to visualize the right ventricular inflow, set the overall gain control higher than normal, centre the TV in the 3D volume, steer the 3D beam, or manually adjust the transducer, to optimize the image in order to simultaneously view all three leaflets and finally acquire. From the apex, the TV can be imaged in a similar way as for 2D imaging. Acquisition of a full-volume data set or real-time zoom mode from the apical approach optimized for right heart structures will yield the widest field of visualization for the TV complex (e.g., leaflets, annulus, chordae, papillary muscles, and right ventricle, Fig. 17.2) allowing the assessment of their spatial relationships and anatomic continuity. After acquisition, cropping from the apex toward the base, or from the atrial roof towards the apex will display the "en face" view of the TV both from the ventricular and from atrial ("surgical view") side, respectively (Fig. 17.2). Frequently, it is possible to visualize TV and mitral valve side-by-side using full volume modality. The subcostal approach can be used in some patients to obtain adequate views of the TV. Beam steering is very useful when using this approach because an acute angle between the abdomen surface and the transducer is frequently required to place the transducer close to the liver and below the costochondral junction.

In patients with good 2DE images, assessment of TV anatomy and function with RT3DE is feasible in around 90% of normal subjects.[7] However, in our experience complete visualization of the TV seems to be more frequent in patients with dilated right ventricles and atria than in normal subjects. The visualization of the TV seems to be facilitated in these patients because there is an enhanced ultrasound reflection due to larger and thicker leaflets, distended annulus, and enlarged right side cavities.

17.4 Tricuspid Regurgitation

The most common cause of tricuspid regurgitation is not an organic disease affecting the TV but rather an impaired valve coaptation caused by a dilation of the right ventricle and/or of the tricuspid annulus.[12] However, a variety of primary disease processes can directly affect the TV complex and lead to valve incompetence: infective endocarditis, congenital disease, like Ebstein anomaly or atrioventricular canal, rheumatic fever, carcinoid syndrome, endomyocardial fibrosis, myxomatous degeneration of the TV leading to prolapse, penetrating and non-penetrating trauma, and iatrogenic damages during cardiac surgery, biopsies, catheter placement in right heart chambers (Figs. 17.3 and 17.4).[13–19]

As in the case of mitral regurgitation, a complete understanding of the leaflet morphology and of the pathophysiological mechanisms underlying tricuspid regurgitation could potentially lead to improved techniques for valve repair and to design physiologically suitable annular rings.

Even though primary valve diseases are uncommon causes of TV regurgitation, 3DE can be useful for a better characterization of valve lesions in different etiologies (Fig. 17.3). Rheumatic involvement of the TV is less common than that of left-sided valves. Regurgitation is a consequence of deformity, shortening and retraction of one or more leaflets of the TV, as well as of shortening and fusion of the chordae tendinee and papillary muscles. 2DE usually detects both tickening and distortion of the leaflets, but it cannot provide a comprehensive assessment of the extension of valve apparatus involvement. The full-volume data set from apical approach usually provides a comprehensive assessment of the whole TV apparatus which can be examined from different perspectives. The "en face" view of the TV from the ventricle allows the visualization of the commissural fusion, which is helpful to establish a correct diagnosis of rheumatic etiology of TV regurgitation (Fig. 17.3, panel F). TV leaflet involvement in degenerative myxomatous disease is visualized by 3DE as a bulging or protrusion of one or more segments from a single or multiple TV leaflets (Fig. 17.3, panel A). In addition, the presence of chordal rupture and extent of the concomitant annular dilation can be assessed in the same view (Fig. 17.3, panel A). In the carcinoid disease, the valve appears thickened, fibrotic with markedly restricted motion during cardiac cycle; 3DE can show the regions of ineffective leaflet coaptation and the lack of commissural fusion (Fig. 17.3, panel C).

Tricuspid annular dilatation seems to be the underlying mechanism of functional TV regurgitation. The extent of TV annulus dilatation may be a more reliable indicator of tricuspid valve pathology than the degree of regurgitation itself.[3]

Using 3DE, two independent groups[11,20] were able to demonstrate that, similar to the mitral annulus, the normal TV annulus is saddle-shaped, with the highest points located in an anterior-posterior orientation and the lowest points in a

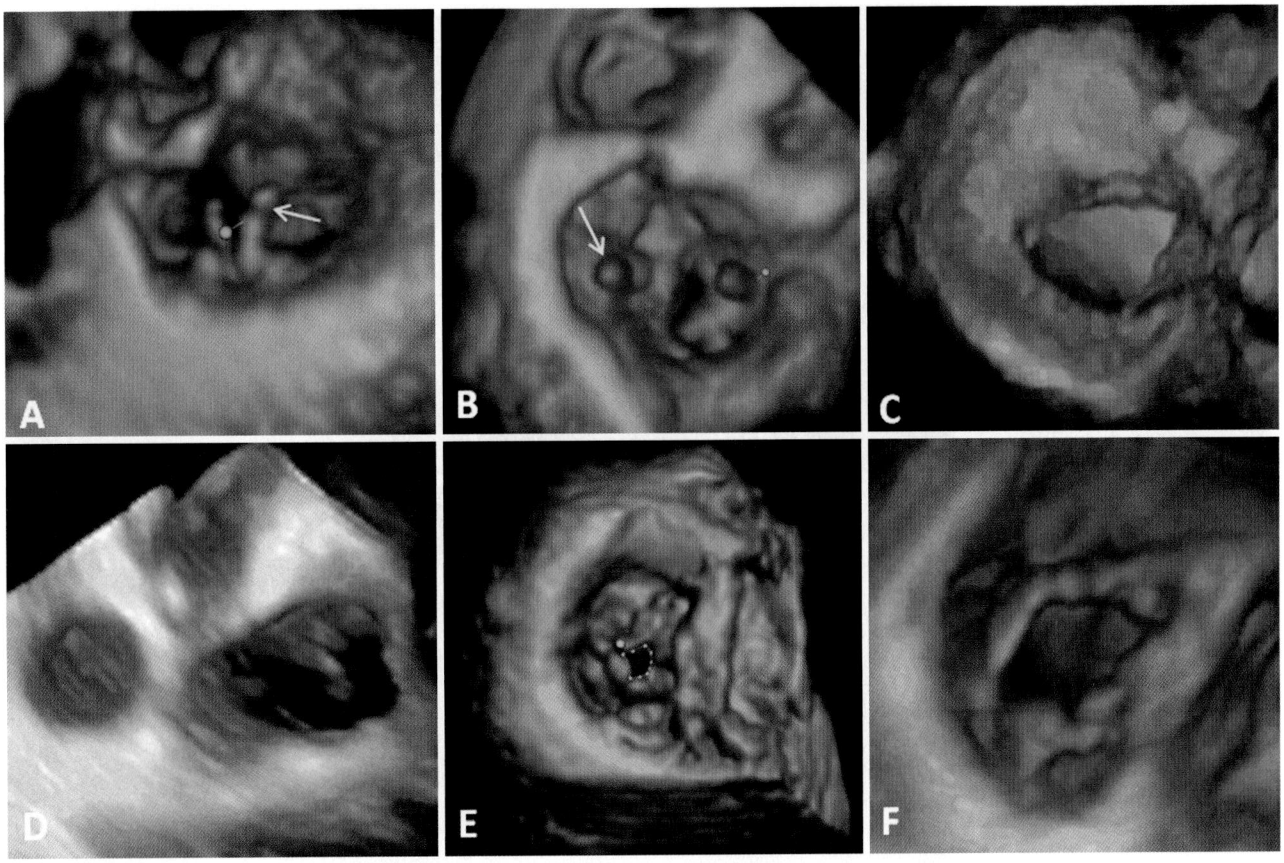

Fig. 17.3 Three-dimensional assessment of the mechanism of regurgitation in various tricuspid valve disease: anterior tricuspid leaflet with ruptured chordae (*arrow*) and prolapse (*Panel A*, right atrial "surgical" view); pacemaker lead (*arrow*) interference causing immobilization of the septal leaflet (*Panel B*, right atrial view); carcinoid tricuspid valvulopaty with adhesion of the valve leaflets to right ventricular walls that prevent the valve to close during systole (*Panel C*, right ventricular view, video. Courtesy by Andreas Hagendorff, Leipzig, Germany); nearly complete detachment of the posterior tricuspid leaflet during biopsy in a heart transplant patient (*Panel D*, right atrial view, video); functional tricuspid regurgitation, dilated annulus and tenting of the three leaflets with loss of systolic coaptation and delineation of regurgitant orifice (*Panel E*, right ventricular view); rheumatic tricuspid valve steno-insufficiency (*Panel F*, right ventricular view, video)

Video 17.3.C Carcinoid tricuspid valvulopathy with adhesion of the valve leaflets to right ventricular walls that prevent the valve to close during systole

Video 17.3.D Nearly complete detachment of the posterior tricuspid leaflet during biopsy in a heart transplant patient

Video 17.3.F Ventricular view of a rheumatic tricuspid valve steno-insufficiency

medio-lateral orientation (Fig. 17.5). They also elucidated the mechanism of functional tricuspid regurgitation by showing that, with the development of functional TR, the tricuspid annulus not only dilates, but also it becomes flatter and more circular. In addition, they showed that as the annulus becomes more circular with tricuspid regurgitation, the increase of the anterior-posterior distance was greater than that of the medio-lateral distance. This may result from the dilation of the tricuspid annulus preferentially along its free-wall distance. This latter finding has an important clinical implication.

Matsunaga and colleagues[21] demonstrated that preoperative tricuspid annular dilation was associated with the development of late postoperative tricuspid regurgitation after repair of ischemic mitral regurgitation. Dreyfus and colleagues[3] reported that the long-term outcome of patients was improved when the decision to perform tricuspid annuloplasty was based on the extent of tricuspid annular dilation rather than the degree of tricuspid regurgitation at the time of surgery. Reference measures for TV repair include tricuspid annulus size >2.1 cm/m^2 and tricuspid annulus fractional shortening <25%.[22] However, both Matsunaga and Dreyfus used 2DE for decision making surgery and this may have led to some inaccuracies in measuring the true annular size.

Anwar and colleagues[23] demonstrated that the tricuspid annulus shape is not circular, but oval, with a minor and a major diameter, both in normally sized and in dilated annulus. In addition, they showed that the currently used tricuspid annulus diameters

Fig. 17.4 Ebstein's anomaly. Anatomical specimen of classical Ebstein's anomaly demonstrating the attachments (*arrows*) of the posterior tricuspid leaflet to the underlying right ventricular (RV) free wall and the large atrialized portion of the RV (ARV) (*Panel A*, reproduced with permission from Attenhofer Jost CH et al.) with the corresponding 3D view (panel B, video). Ventricular (*Panel C*, video) and atrial (*Panel D*, video) view of the TV showing the large sail-like anterior leaflet (ATL) and the septal (STL) and posterior (PTL) leaflets attached to RV wall (*arrows*). The deformed leaflets are clearly visible. The characteristic bubble-like aspect of ATL represents the effect of leaflet tethering by fibrous attachments to the RV wall. The regions of ineffective leaflet coaptation can also be easily identified

Video 17.4.B Ebstein's anomaly. 3D view reproducing the anatomical specimen of classical Ebstein's anomaly shown in the text. We can appreciate the attachments of the posterior tricuspid leaflet to the underlying right ventricular free wall and the large atrialized portion of the right ventricle

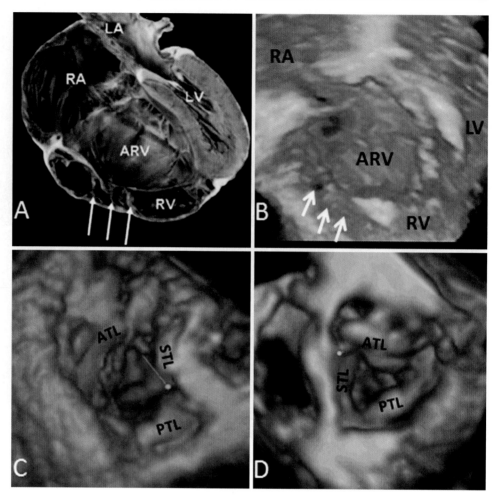

Video 17.4.C Ebstein's anomaly. Ventricular view of the tricuspid valve showing the large sail-like anterior leaflet, and the septal and posterior leaflets attached to RV wall. The deformed leaflets are clearly visible. The characteristic bubble-like aspect of anterior tricuspid valve represents the effect of leaflet tethering by fibrous attachments to the right ventricular wall. The regions of ineffective leaflet coaptation can also be easily identified

Video 17.4.D Ebstein anomaly. Same structures as in previous videos seen from the atrial perspective

Video 17.5 Right atrial view of the tricuspid valve in a normal subject with a clear delineation of the tricuspid annulus and its spatial relationships with mitral and aortic valves

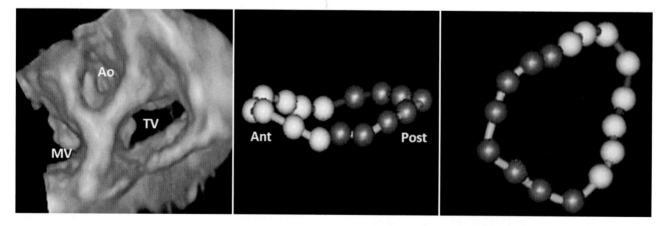

Fig. 17.5 Left panel: right atrial view of the tricuspid valve (TV) in a normal subject with a clear delineation of the tricuspid annulus and its spatial relationships with mitral (MV) and aortic (Ao) valves (video). **Central panel**: reconstructed tricuspid annulus viewed from profile and showing its saddle shape, with the highest points located in an anterior-posterior orientation and the lowest points in a medio-lateral orientation. **Right panel**: reconstructed tricuspid annulus viewed from the right atrium

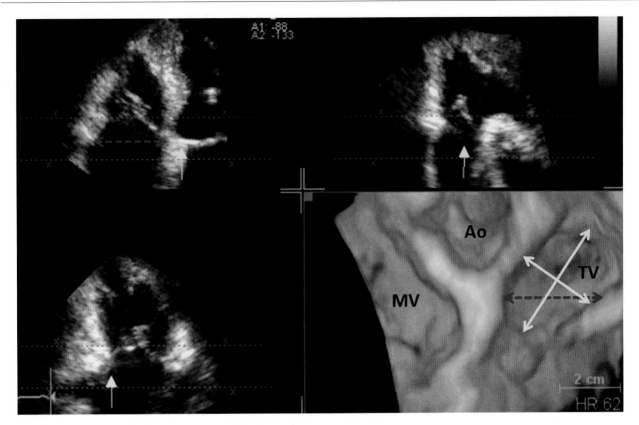

Fig. 17.6 Comparison of tricuspid annulus diameter measurements by two-dimensional (*red dashed arrow*) and three-dimensional echocardiography (*double headed yellow arrows*). When the measurement performed with two-dimensional echo is reported on the three-dimensional rendering of the tricuspid annulus viewed from the right atrium, one can realize that the two-dimensional measure taken in four-chamber view does represent nor the minor neither the major diameter of the actual annulus

measured with 2DE (both measured in apical four chamber view and in parasternal short-axis view) systematically underestimated the actual tricuspid annulus size (Fig. 17.6). As a consequence, 65% of patients with normal tricuspid annulus diameter at 2DE showed grade 1–2 tricuspid regurgitation compared with 30% of patients with normal tricuspid annulus size at 3DE.[23] Conversely, calculation of tricuspid annulus fractional shortening yielded the same results using 2DE and 3DE.[23] This is because the extent of underestimation of tricuspid annulus diameter made by 2DE is comparable in diastole and in systole.

In addition to tricuspid annulus shape, size and function, 3DE allows to assess TV leaflet geometry in functional tricuspid regurgitation. In patients with pulmonary hypertension (i.e., right ventricular to right atrium gradient ≥30 mm Hg), Sukmawan et al.[24] reported that patients with tricuspid regurgitation showed a tethering of tricuspid leaflets into the right ventricle. The measured TV tenting volume was linearly correlated with right ventricular volume and with TV regurgitant jet area.

At the moment there are no data supporting the use of 3DE to select patients to be addressed to surgical repair of functional tricuspid regurgitation. However, as for mitral regurgitation, an improved assessment of valve anatomy and understanding of the pathophysiological mechanisms underlying the TV regurgitation could suggest new and more effective techniques for TV repair.

Finally, 3DE can help in estimating the severity of TV regurgitation using color flow. Velayudhan et al.[25] demonstrated the feasibility of obtaining the area of the vena contracta of the tricuspid regurgitant jet by cropping the 3DE color Doppler data set with imaging planes exactly parallel to the TV orifice (Fig. 17.7). The authors found a poor correlation between the area of the vena contracta obtained by 3DE and its width measured by 2DE supporting the concept that, similar to mitral regurgitation, the vena contracta of the regurgitant tricuspid jet has a complex geometry. However, they found reasonable relationships between the area of the vena contracta measured with 3DE and conventional estimates of tricuspid regurgitation severity by 2DE color Doppler (i.e., regurgitant jet area and its ratio with right atrial area) and proposed new criteria for estimating tricuspid regurgitation severity based on vena contracta area: <0.5 cm^2 for mild; 0.5–0.75 cm^2 for moderate; >0.75 cm^2 for severe.

17.5 Tricuspid Stenosis

Tricuspid stenosis is uncommon in adult patients. In nearly all cases it is due to rheumatic disease in association with rheumatic mitral and/or aortic valve involvement. However,

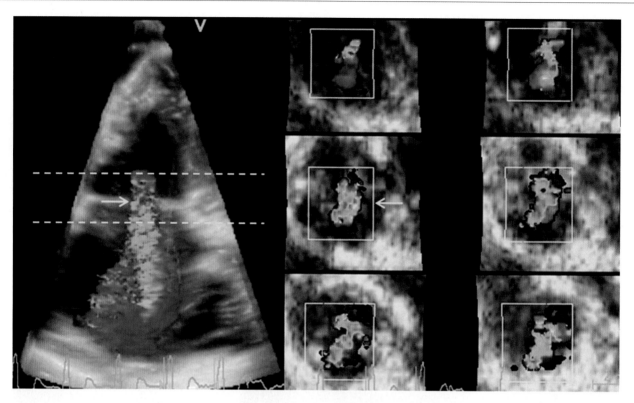

Fig. 17.7 Three-dimensional visualization of the tricuspid regurgitant jet and vena contracta (*arrow*) obtained by cropping a 3D data set acquired from apical approach (*left panel*, video); paraplane slicing of the proximal part of the jet allows the identification and the measurement of the jet area (*arrow*) at the level of vena contracta (*right panel*)

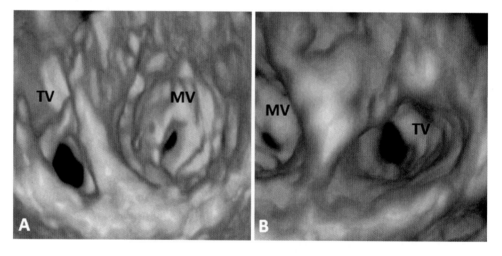

Fig. 17.8 Rheumatic tricuspid valve (TV) stenosis seen from the right ventricle (*Panel A*, video) and from the right atrium (*Panel B*, video). The deformed and thickened leaflets are clearly visualized as well as fused commissures and the stenotic orifice of the valve. Stenotic TV orifice can easily and accurately be planimetered to obtain an objective measure of stenosis severity. MV, mitral valve

Video 17.7 Three-dimensional visualization of the tricuspid regurgitant jet and vena contract obtained by cropping a 3D data set acquired from apical approach

Video 17.8 Rheumatic tricuspid valve stenosis seen from the right ventricle. The deformed and thickened leaflets are clearly visualized as well as fused commissures and the stenotic orifice of the valve

carinoid heart disease can lead to tricuspid stenosis as well.

2DE images show thickening and shortening of the TV leaflets. Doppler recordings of trans-tricuspid flow velocity allow calculation of mean gradient and pressure half time valve area as described for the mitral valve.[26] However, unlike what it is routinely done for mitral stenosis, neither transthoracic nor transesophageal 2DE can provide an "*en face*" view of the stenotic orifice and visualize commissural fusion of the TV. Using 3DE, the stenotic orifice of the TV can be clearly visualized from the ventricular side and planimetered (Fig. 17.3, panel F, and Fig. 17.8).[27]

17.6 Infective Endocarditis of the Tricuspid Valve

In patients with TV endocarditis, 3DE may show the stereoscopic morphology and attachments of vegetations, mobility of vegetations with blood flow, and possible complications such as leaflet prolapse or perforation (Fig. 17.9).

The size of a vegetation is an important predictor for embolic events and for response to treatment. Maximum diameter measurements from 2DE are routinely used to determine mass size. However, most vegetations are irregularly shaped, making it difficult to accurately image or select the largest diameter. The selection of a diameter that is not truly the largest may lead to underestimation of the true size of the vegetation and to the misinterpretation of patient prognosis. 3DE images the entire volume of a vegetation allowing for accurate measurements in multiple planes.[28]

17.7 Congenital

Ebstein's anomaly is a congenital defect of the tricuspid valve in which the origins of the septal or posterior leaflets, or both, are displaced downward into the right ventricle, with a large sail-like anterior leaflet that results in atrialization of the right ventricular inflow (Fig. 17.4). There is a wide spectrum of

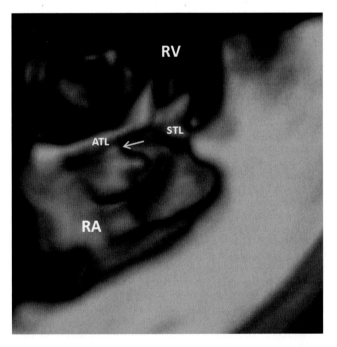

Fig. 17.9 Tricuspid valve endocarditis in a young intravenous drug addict (video). Non-tomographic view allows to visualize the actual shape and attachment point of the vegetation (*arrow*). *ATL* anterior tricuspid leaflet, *STL* septal tricuspid leaflet, *RA* right atrium, *RV* right ventricle

Video 17.9 Tricuspid valve endocarditis in a young intravenous drug addict. Non-tomographic view allows to visualize the actual shape and attachment point of the vegetation

severity. Although 2DE can show the characteristic displacement of the septal leaflet and the redundant and elongated anterior leaflet, the complex anatomy of the disease and the mechanisms of valve regurgitation are very difficult to assess. In adult patients with Ebstein anomaly of the TV, Patel and colleagues[29] have reported that 3DE was particularly useful in delineating the chordal attachment of the three leaflets of the TV. This was accomplished by multiple systematic cropping and sectioning of the 3DE data sets, that show the characteristic bubble-like appearance resulting from bulging of the non-tethered areas of the TV leaflets (Fig. 17.4). In addition, an *en face* view of the valve obtained with 3DE can be used to measure the leaflet surface areas, and to visualize the regions of ineffective leaflet coaptation (Fig. 17.4). Moreover, 3DE can be useful in evaluating the size of the functional right ventricle, and to obtain an *en face* view of the vena contracta to estimate the severity of tricuspid regurgitation.

17.8 Present Limitations and Future Perspectives

Despite all the data supporting the use of 3DE to assess TV morphology and function, especially in patients who are candidates to cardiac surgery for left-sided diseases, this technique has not been integrated into the clinical routine. There are several reasons to explain this: some pertaining the 3D technique per se, and they have been discussed in Chapter 4, and two others are related to the application of the technique to the study of the TV.

The first reason is a clinical one. At the moment, there is no evidence that 3D assessment of TV anatomy and function may improve surgical results. However, clinical research is active in this field and results are expected soon.

The second reason is the lack of standardized measures and specific software to be used to quantitate tricuspid annulus and leaflet size and shape, as they have been developed for the mitral valve. The increasing interest for the TV from both echocardiographers and surgeons will fuel development and implementation of such a tool.

17.9 Conclusions

Imaging of the TV by 2DE is hampered by its inability to visualize all three leaflets simultaneously. Conversely, 3DE provides a unique tool for a comprehensive assessment of morphology and function of the TV complex preoperatively. Understanding the anatomy and the pathophysiological mechanisms underlying the various TV diseases will provide the basis for surgical planning in order to tailor the intervention to patient's individual needs.

References

1. Behm CZ, Nath J, Foster E. Clinical correlates and mortality of hemodynamically significant tricuspid regurgitation. *J Heart Valve Dis*. 2004;3:784–789.
2. Hung J, Koelling T, Semigran MJ, Dec GW, Levine RA, Di Salvo TG. Usefulness of echocardiographic determined tricuspid regurgitation in predicting event-free survival in severe heart failure secondary to idiopathic-dilated cardiomyopathy or to ischemic cardiomyopathy. *Am J Cardiol*. 1998;82:1301–1303, A10.
3. Dreyfus GD, Corbi PJ, Chan KM, Bahrami T. Secondary tricuspid regurgitation or dilatation: which should be the criteria for surgical repair? *Ann Thorac Surg*. 2005;79:127–132.
4. Nath J, Foster E, Heidenreich PA. Impact of tricuspid regurgitation on long-term survival. *J Am Coll Cardiol*. 2004;43:405–409.
5. Sagie A, Schwammenthal E, Newell JB et al. Significant tricuspid regurgitation is a marker for adverse outcome in patients undergoing percutaneous balloon mitral valvuloplasty. *J Am Coll Cardiol*. 1994;24:696–702.
6. McCarthy PM, Bhudia SK, Rajeswaran J et al. Tricuspid valve repair: durability and risk factors for failure. *J Thorac Cardiovasc Surg*. 2004;127:674–685.
7. Anwar AM, Geleijnse ML, Soliman OI et al. Assessment of normal tricuspid valve anatomy in adults by real-time three-dimensional echocardiography. *Int J Cardiovasc Imaging*. 2007;23:717–724.
8. Lang RM, Mor-Avi V, Sugeng L, Nieman PS, Sahn DJ. Three-dimensional echocardiography. The benefits of the additional dimension. *J Am Coll Cardiol*. 2006;48:2053–2069.
9. Badano LP, Dall'Armellina E, Monaghan MJ et al. Real-time three-dimensional echocardiography: tehnological gadget or clinical tool? *J Cardiovasc Med*. 2007;8:144–162.
10. Badano LP, Agricola E, Perez de Isla L, Gianfagna P, Zamorano JL. Evaluation of the tricuspid valve morphology and function by transthoracic real-time three-dimensional echocardiography. *Eur J Echocardiogr*. 2009;10:477–484.
11. Ton-Nu TT, Levine RA, Handschumacher MD et al. Geometric determinants of functional tricuspid regurgitation: insights from 3-dimensional echocardiography. *Circulation*. 2006;114: 143–149.
12. Sagie A, Schwammenthal E, Padial LR, Vazquez de Prada JA, Weyman AE, Levine RA. Determinants of functional tricuspid regurgitation in incomplete tricuspid valve closure: Doppler color flow study of 109 patients. *J Am Coll Cardiol*. 1994;446–453.
13. Nucifora G, Badano LP, Allocca G et al. Severe tricuspid regurgitation due to entrapment of the anterior leaflet of the valve by a permanent pacemaker lead: role of real time three-dimensional echocardiography. *Echocardiography*. 2007;24:649–652.
14. Schnabel R, Khaw AV, von Bardeleben RS et al. Assessment of the tricuspid valve morphology by transthoracic real-time-3D-echocardiography. *Echocardiography*. 2005;22:15–23.
15. Ahlgrim AA, Nanda NC, Berther E, Gill EA. Three-dimensional echocardiography: an alternative imaging choice for evaluation of tricuspid valve disorders. *Cardiol Clin*. 2007;25:305–309.
16. Pothineni KR, Duncan K, Yelamanchili P et al. Live/real-time three-dimensional transthoracic echocardiographic assessment of tricuspid valve pathology: incremental value over the two-dimensional technique. *Echocardiography*. 2007;24:541–552.
17. Parranon S, Abadir S, Acar P. New insight into the tricuspid valve in Ebstein anomaly using three-dimensional echocardiography. *Heart*. 2006;92:1627.
18. Anwar AM, Attia WM, Nosir YF, El-Amin AM. Unusual bileaflet tricuspid valve by real time three-dimensional echocardiography. *Echocardiography*. 2008;25:534–536.
19. Reddy VK, Nanda S, Bandarupalli N, Pothineni KR, Nanda NC. Traumatic tricuspid papillary muscle and chordae rupture: emerging role of three-dimensional echocardiography. *Echocardiography*. 2008;25:653–657.
20. Fukuda S, Saracino G, Matsumura Y et al. Three-dimensional geometry of the tricuspid annulus in healthy subjects and in patients with functional tricuspid regurgitation: a real-time, 3-dimensional echocardiographic study. *Circulation*. 2006;114:I492–I498.
21. Matsunaga A, Duran CM. Progression of TR after repaired functional ischemic mitral regurgitation. *Circulation*. 2005;112 (suppl:I-453–I-457.
22. Colombo T, Russo C, Ciliberto GR et al. Tricuspid regurgitation secondary to mitral valve disease: tricuspid annulus function as guide to tricuspid valve repair. *Cardiovasc Surg*. 2001;9:369–377.
23. Anwar AM, Geleijnse ML, Ten Cate FJ, Meijboom FJ. Assessment of tricuspid valve annulus size, shape and function using real-time three-dimensional echocardiography. *Interact Cardiovasc Thorac Surg*. 2006;5:683–687.
24. Sukmawan R, Watanabe N, Ogasawara Y et al. Geometric changes of tricuspid valve tenting in tricuspid regurgitation secondary to pulmonary hypertension quantified by novel system with transthoracic real-time 3-dimensional echocardiography. *J Am Soc Echocardiogr*. 2007;20:470–476.
25. Velayudhan DE, Brown TM, Nanda NC et al. Quantification of tricuspid regurgitation by live three-dimensional transthoracic echocardiographic measurements of vena contracta area. *Echocardiography*. 2006;23:793–800.
26. Pearlman AS. Role of echocardiography in the diagnosis and evaluation of severity of mitral and tricuspid stenosis. *Circulation*. 1991;84(Suppl):I-193–I-197.
27. Faletra F, La Marchesina U, Bragato R, De Chiara F. Three dimensional transthoracic echocardiography images of tricuspid stenosis. *Heart*. 2005;91:499.
28. Asch FP, Bieganski PM, Panza JA, Weissman NJ. Real-time 3-dimensional echocardiography evaluation of intracardiac masses. *Echocardiography*. 2006;23:218–224.
29. Patel V, Nanda NC, Rajdev S et al. Live/real time three-dimensional transthoracic echocardiographic assessment of Ebstein's anomaly. *Echocardiography*. 2005;22:847–854.
30. Vettukattil JJ, Bharucha T, Anderson RH. Defining Ebstein's malformation using three-dimensional echocardiography. *Interact Cardiovasc Thorac Surg*. 2007;6(6):685–690.
31. Acar P, Abadir S, Roux D et al. Ebstein's anomaly assessed by real-time 3-D echocardiography. *Ann Thorac Surg*. 2006;82:731–733.
32. Henein MY, O'sullivan CA, Li W et al. Evidence for rheumatic valve disease in patients with severe tricuspid regurgitation long after mitral valve surgery: the role of 3D echo reconstruction. *J Heart Valve Dis*. 2003;12:566–572.
33. Anwar AM, Geleijnse ML, Soliman OI, McGhie JS, Nemes A, Ten Cate FJ. Evaluation of rheumatic tricuspid valve stenosis by real-time three-dimensional echocardiography. *Heart*. 2007;93:363–364.
34. Shakur R, Becher H. Three-dimensional echocardiogram of severe tricuspid regurgitation from carcinoid syndrome. *Echocardiography*. 2009;24(3):274–275.
35. Allocca G, Slavich G, Nucifora G, Slavich M, Frassani R, Crapis M, Badano L. Successful treatment of polymicrobial multivalve infective endocarditis. Multivalve infective endocarditis. *Int J Cardiovasc Imaging*. 2007;23(4):501–505.
36. Liu YW, Tsai WC, Lin CC, Hsu CH, Li WT, Lin LJ, Chen JH. Usefulness of real-time three-dimensional echocardiography for diagnosis of infective endocarditis. *Scand Cardiovasc J*. 2009;6:1–6.

Role of Three-Dimensional Echocardiography in Drug Trials

18

Fausto Rigo, Maurizio Galderisi, Denisa Muraru, and Luigi P. Badano

18.1 Introduction

There are two main typologies of clinical trials in whom echocardiography may be used. The first one is represented by studies in which echocardiography is used as part of the assessment, but does not contribute substantially to the end-points. This is the case of trials using echo parameters to define a given study population, a use accepted and supported also by the regulatory authorities. The second one, more ambitious for echocardiography, corresponds to studies involving echocardiographic measurements (e.g., chamber volume and/or shape and LV mass) as primary or secondary efficacy and safety end-points. This second use of echocardiography is debated, at least when the effect of a therapy is concerned. In fact, for phase II trials echo parameters are considered acceptable to prove a concept of a treatment, while the use of echo measures as primary end-points in phase III (purpose of registering a drug) remains controversial. In this case it is necessary to demonstrate that a given echo measure is a real surrogate of clinical events. In this view, the prognostic value alone is not sufficient and should be combined with the demonstration that modifications of the echo measures correspond (better if proportionally) to changes in outcome events. By analyzing the existing notes for guidance of regulatory authorities, echo parameters are not established end-points of pivotal trials designed in order to approve new drugs in conditions like heart failure, post-myocardial infarction dysfunction and arterial hypertension.

However, the role of echocardiography in clinical trials has substantially changed in the last decade because of two main reasons:

1. The accuracy (validation) of echocardiographic tools and measurements does not refer to post-mortem autopsy anymore, but to cardiac magnetic resonance which is considered the gold standard of noninvasive imaging of the heart.

In interventional trials, cardiac magnetic resonance allows to reduce substantially the sample size of a given study population because of the small variability (i.e., reduced standard deviation of the average) of its measurements.

2. New echo technologies – mainly 3DE and Speckle Tracking Echocardiography – have been developed in order to be technologically competitive (feasibility, accuracy, reproducibility) with cardiac magnetic resonance but less expensive, more available and feasible also in patients with devices.

The application of echocardiography remained substantially unchanged in the first typology of clinical trials, in which also surrogates of the best available tools and measurements can be used (e.g., chamber volumes by 2DE, and even some linear measurements) provided that 2DE views are acquired in the proper way. In this kind of studies, in particular in those using echo parameters to define a given study population, the procedure of inclusion can be performed peripherally or, better, by an echo core laboratory, able to provide criteria confirmation in a very short time (<3 days). Conversely, the use of new ultrasound technologies is becoming imperative in trials in which echocardiography should provide measurements as possible study end-points. The improvement in feasibility, accuracy and reproducibility means, in fact, that in group studies, much smaller sample size can be used to detect the same change of a given measurement or parameter. Alternatively, using the same sample size, smaller degrees of change can be identified (Table 18.1). Indeed, the sample size is directly related to the square of the standard deviation (variability) of the measurement employed and inversely to the square of the extent of change in the parameter (e.g., left ventricular volume or mass according to the formula:

$$n = \frac{SD^2(t_1 \text{-} t_2)^2}{change^2}$$

where n is the number of patients needed, $t_1 - t_2$ is 2.8 to obtain a power of 80%, and change is the extent of change to detect in a given measure.

The need of core lab measurements is absolutely mandatory in the latter study typology, in order to further minimize

F. Rigo (✉)
Non Invasive Cardiology Department,
Dell'Angelo Hospital, Venice, Italy
e-mail: faustorigo@alice.it

Table 18.1 Sample size needed to detect a significant decrease of LV mass in hypertensive patients

Echo technique	Weeks	SD of the decrease in LV mass (g)	Patients needed at 80% power
3DE	12	±23.23	42
2DE	12	±68.10	364
M-mode	12	±43.4	148

2DE two dimensional echocardiography, *3DE* three-dimensional echocardiography, *LV* left ventricular, *SD* standard deviation.

the variability of measurements. In general the level of clinical relevance of a given echo parameter, even irrespective of the statistical significance of the average values, should be considered with attention. For instance, the relevance of left ventricular ejection fraction changes after a certain treatment should be taken into account much more in relation with the measurements variability (standard deviations) than in relation with the mere statistical significance of these changes. A change of 1–1.5 points in EF average could be not so clinically relevant in a context of 5 point variability.

18.2 Left Ventricular Geometry and Function

18.2.1 Left Ventricular Size, Wall Thickness and LV Volumes

The calculation of left ventricular (LV) volumes is imperative in patients with cardiac diseases other than hypertension and aortic stenosis and in particular in those with distorted ventricles and/or with wall motion abnormalities (coronary artery disease and/or acute myocardial infarction).[1,2] 2DE-derived LV volumes are among the best predictors of post-acute myocardial infarction outcome and mortality.[1] Among the various algorithm used to calculate left ventricular volumes form 2D tomographic views, the biplane method of disc summation is the most accurate in abnormally shaped ventricles.[1] When compared to MRI, 2DE LV volumes show constant underestimation[3] and higher inter-study variability which reaches statistical significance for end-systolic volume (4.4% to 9.2% versus 13.7% to 20.3%, $p < 0.001$).[4] This requires larger study population sample (55% to 93% larger than using MRI) to demonstrate statistically significant changes in LV volumes. In patients with poor ultrasound windows, contrast agents can be used intravenously to enhance border detection and, hence, accuracy and reproducibility of 2DE LV volumes.[5,6] Semi-automated detection of the LV

endocardial surface using full-volume 3DE data sets of the left ventricle (Fig. 18.1) is now available to obtain rapid and reproducible volume measurement.[7–9] In addition, test-retest variability of complete restudy by a separate operator has shown lower underestimation of LV volumes by 3DE than by 2DE in comparison with MRI.[7,10] Further minimization of the 3DE gap versus MRI can be obtained by tracing the endocardium such to include trabeculae in the LV cavity.[10,11]

18.2.2 Left Ventricular Mass and Geometry

The estimation of LV geometry and mass have been among the most studied issues by echocardiography in the epidemiologic studies and treatment trials dealing with uncomplicated hypertension in the last three decades. LV concentric remodeling and hypertrophy are independent predictors of morbidity and mortality in the general population. Changes of LV mass induced by anti-hypertensive treatments have been extensively studied. While LV mass measurements (indexed for body surface area or height) identify LV hypertrophy, relative wall thickness categorize LV geometry.[1]

All LV mass calculation algorithms (M-mode, 2DE, 3DE) are based upon the subtraction of LV cavity volume from the volume enclosed by the LV epicardium ("shell" volume) to obtain myocardial volume which is then multiplied by myocardium specific weight (1.055 g/mL) to obtain LV mass.

LV mass calculations can be made using linear primary measurements from 2DE guided M-mode or directly measured on 2DE views. The ASE formula for estimation of LV mass,[1] is appropriate for evaluating patients with normal LV geometry. Although it has been validated against post-mortem hearts, its accuracy is suboptimal, with standard error of estimate from 29 to 97 g (95% confidence interval [CI] 57 to 190 g) in comparison with LV mass at necropsy.[12] The operator dependence of this calculation is demonstrated by large inter-observer variability (SEE, from 28 to 41 g; 95% CI, 55 to 80 g).[12] The inter-study (test-retest) reproducibility is also poor, with standard deviations (SDs) of the difference between successive measurements from 22 to 40 g (95% CI, 45 to 78 g).[12] However, in the RES (Reliability of M-mode Echocardiographic Studies) trial (16 centers with good expertise for quantitative echo), the probability of a true change in LV mass over time for a single-reader difference was a change >18% of the initial value (90% interval of agreement of test retest between-observer variability = -26 to 30 g).[13] By using anatomically corrected 2DE linear measurements, the reproducibility of LV mass was similar

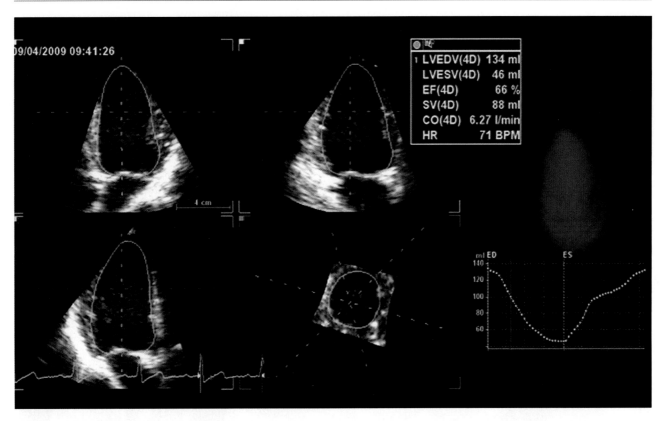

Fig. 18.1 3DE measurement of left ventricular volumes. Left ventricular endocardial surface is detected using a semi-automatic endocardial detection algorhythm both in longitudinal and in transversal planes of the left ventricle in order to develop a dynamic model of the left ventricle that it is independent on geometrical assumptions about its shape. Quantitative analysis panel and volume-time plot are provided on the right

in the echo core laboratory of the multicenter PRESERVE (Prospective Randomized Study Evaluating Regression of Ventricular Enlargement) trial: between-study LV mass change of ±35 g (18% of the baseline value) and 17 g, to have a likelihood of being true change >95% and >80%, respectively.[14]

The 2DE method of LV mass is based on the truncated ellipsoid model and area-length formula,[1] and relies on myocardial area measurements (= total area − cavity area) at the mid-papillary levels, excluding the papillary muscles from tracing. It has been validated with necropsy. Accuracy (SEE = 31–39 g) and reproducibility are moderately better than the calculation with linear measurements.

The 3DE calculation of LV mass removes geometric assumptions about LV shape (independence on geometric model) and reduces errors due to foreshortened views (Fig. 18.2).[15,16] 3DE derived LV mass has been validated with both post-mortem examination (concordance = 0.92) and with MRI (concordance = 0.91).[17] A much lower LV mass underestimation versus MRI has been found using 3DE than 2DE.[15,16] The very good reproducibility of LV mass calculation with 3DE (intra-observer variability = 7–12.5%)[16,17] can reduce sample size to assess LV mass changes.

18.2.3   Left Ventricular Global and Regional Systolic Function

LV ejection fraction is a well known prognosticator in epidemiologic studies on heart failure, valvular heart diseases and coronary artery disease, and is currently used for evaluating treatment effects on cardiac function.

The reproducibility of 2DE-derived LV ejection fraction has been rarely tested, but both ±7% of inter-observer variability[18] and ±5% of test-retest reliability[12] seem to be adequate for clinical purposes. Despite the better accuracy in the measurement of left end-systolic and end-diastolic volumes, 3DE does not show an additional value in estimating LV ejection fraction because of the constant underestimation of 2DE-derived volumes (either at end-systole and end-diastole) versus MRI.[7–9]

Longitudinal systolic function is an important component of LV global systolic function because it contributes to 60% of the stroke volume[19] and its alteration often precedes detectable ejection fraction reduction. It can be quantified by measuring systolic excursion of the mitral annulus with M-mode or, more simply, myocardial systolic velocity of the mitral annulus with pulsed Tissue Velocity Imaging.[20] Age-specific

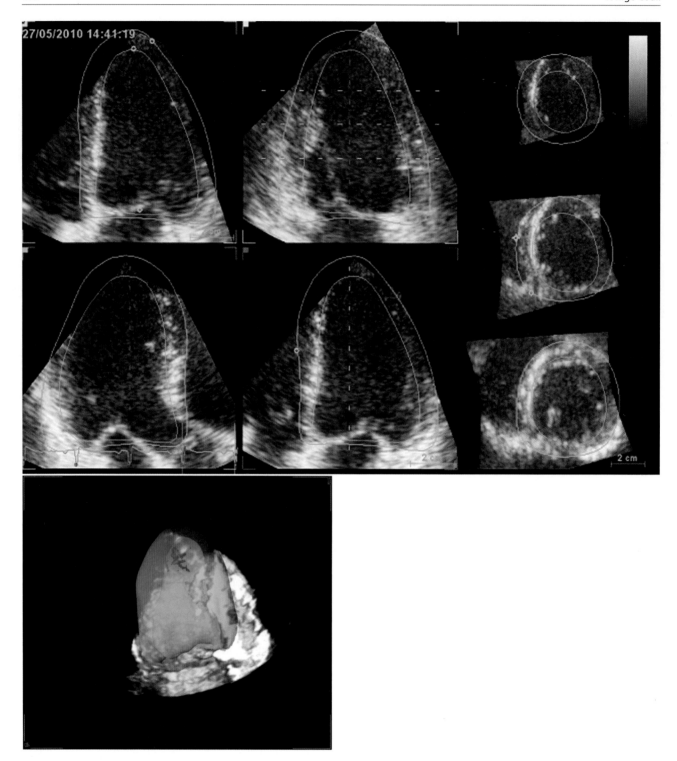

Fig. 18.2 Left ventricular mass is measured with 3D by subtracting the left ventricular endocardial volume from the left ventricular epicardial volume (*bottom panel*). The myocardial volume that is obtained (*top panel in green*) is then multiplied by 1.55 (myocardial specific weight) to obtain Left ventricular mass

reference values for tissue velocity imaging have been generated.[21] Longitudinal deformation imaging derived by 2D Speckle Tracking Echocardiography is a more robust and reproducible technique to assess LV longitudinal function, in particular in rounded shaped LV where the alignment of Doppler beam to obtain tissue velocity imaging is difficult, but reference values have not been yet obtained in large population size.

18.2.3.1 LV Regional Function

The assessment of regional wall motion is currently performed by visual, semiquantitative analysis (scoring) of both inward endocardial motion and myocardial thickening. In order to standardize wall motion and perfusion assessment among different imaging techniques, the American Heart Association recommends dividing LV wall into 17-segments also for echocardiography.[22] Accuracy of semiquantitative scoring and reproducibility of wall motion score index is heavily dependent on reader's experience. Attempts to quantify segmental LV function have resulted unsuccessful so far. 2D speckle-tracking-derived strain rate imaging is very promising[23] because of its technical advantages (absence of tethering effects of adjacent myocardial segments, no angle dependence when compared with tissue velocity imaging). However, the experience of this technique is still limited to restricted population sample sizes.

18.2.4 How to Increase Accuracy of Left Ventricular Measurements

18.2.4.1 Performance Recommendations

In order to increase accuracy and repeatability of 2DE LV volume measurements, the operator should avoid LV cavity foreshortening by reducing the difference of the LV long axes length in four- and two-chamber views to <10%. This is an important cause of LV volumes underestimation that does not affect, however, ejection fraction because underestimation involves at the same extent LV end-diastolic and end-systolic volumes. Images should be acquired either during held expiration or quiet respiration in order to minimize translational motion of the heart. LV cavity should be acquired at the lowest possible depth in order to display on the screen the LV as large as possible and the same field depth should be kept for both four- and two-chamber apical views. Larger sector width than needed should be avoided in order to preserve spatial and temporal resolution.[1] In the case of suboptimal visualization of endocardial borders of more than 2 LV segments, i.v. contrast agents can be used to improve accuracy and reproducibility.[6] Measurements of LV volumes from 3DE full volume datasets avoids most of the errors associated with 2DE echo calculation of LV volumes: i.e., long-axis foreshortening, image plane positioning by assuming orthogonality between the four- and the two-chamber views,

geometric assumptions about the shape of the LV; and tracing errors. When using 3DE full-volume, care should be taken to encompass the entire LV volume cavity in the digital data-set (consecutive four-beat ECG gated subvolumes) during end-expiratory apnoea. This can be verified using the multislice option that allows the operator to control that the entire cardiac structure has been comprehensively included in the data set (Fig. 18.3).

18.2.4.2 Reading Recommendations

2DE volumetric measurements should be the result of averaging measurements obtained over ≥3 heart beats in patients in sinus rhythm and ≥5 beats in atrial fibrillation. In order to calculate LV mass by using M-mode or 2DE, chamber dimensions and wall thicknesses can be measured by using direct 2DE measurements in parasternal long-axis view. This method prevents incorrect alignment of M-mode cursor (it should be perpendicular to both the septum and LV posterior wall). Novel 3DE LV analysis can be performed by rapid step-by-step softwares which provide automatic slicing of LV full-volume data-sets, manual alignment in order to identify LV central longitudinal axis, LV reference point identification, automated identification of endocardial borders at both end-diastole and end-systole and final data set display. 3DE analysis requires some technical caveats to avoid underestimation of LV volumes. Systematic border verification and manual correction is required to increase accuracy in LV volume measurements based on semi- or automated border detection.[11] Manual tracing of endocardial border should be performed outwards the black-white interface in order to include endocardial trabeculations.[24]

18.3 Right Ventricular Size and Function

Right ventricular (RV) function is an important predictor of exercise capacity and mortality in heart failure, pulmonary arterial hypertension and several systemic diseases involving the heart, independently of LV function.

18.3.1 Right Ventricular Size

The methods aiming to estimate RV size by 2DE are unreliable. Currently, RV volumes may be obtained from 3DE full-volume datasets (Fig. 18.4).[25]

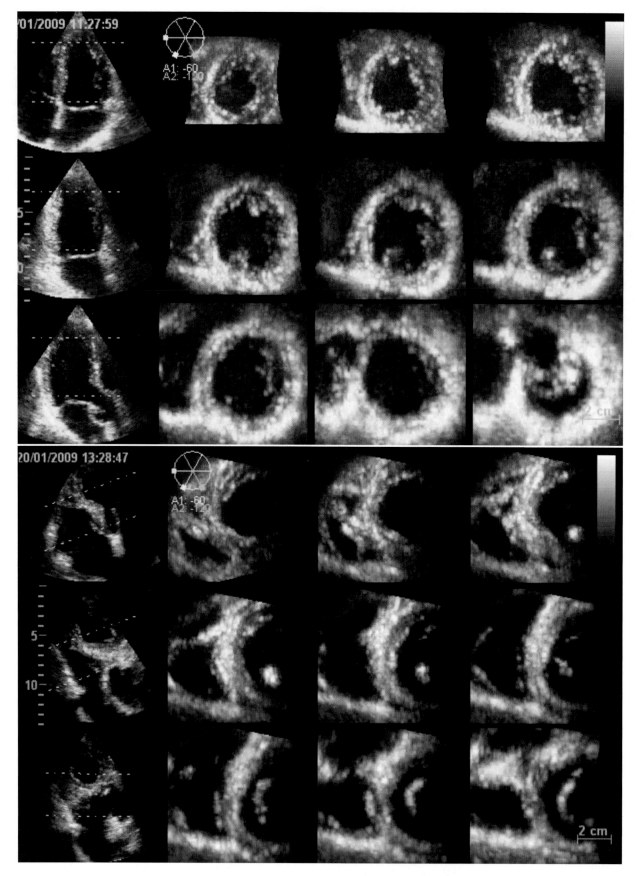

Fig. 18.3 Multislice display of the left (*top panel*) and right (*bottom panel*) ventricles showing three longitudinal and nine transversal planes from the base (lower cut plane on the bottom) to the apex (highest cut plane on the top). This display modality allows the operator to control that the cardiac chamber of interest is comprehensively contained in the data set

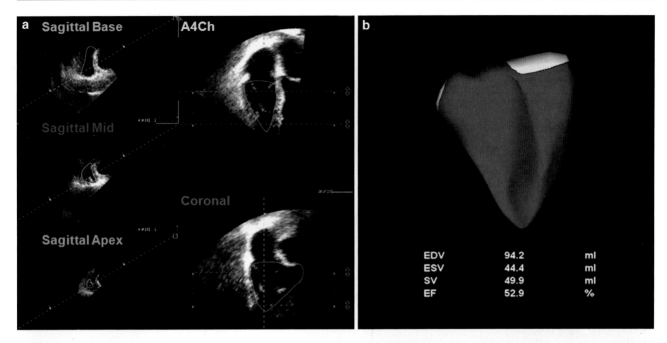

Fig. 18.4 3DE measurement of right ventricular volumes. In the left panel graphic demonstrating the five cut-plane images (sagittal base, mid and apex; apical four-chamber, coronal) used to trace right ventricular endocardial border. In the right panel, by software-enhanced analysis, a dynamic cast of the right ventricle is displayed. Right ventricular volumes (EDV and ESV), ejection fraction (EF) and stroke volume (SV) are shown

18.3.2 Right Ventricular Function

Tricuspid annular plane systolic excursion (TAPSE) has been proposed as an accurate index of RV global systolic function, taking into account that RV shortening occurs mainly along its longitudinal axis. TAPSE has been validated against RV ejection fraction obtained by radionuclide angiography and has an important prognostic role in population studies.[26] However, TAPSE does not assess accurately changes of RV systolic function after cardiac surgery: despite post-operative reduction of TAPSE, the absence of a decrease in 3DE-derived RV ejection fraction supports in fact the hypothesis of geometrical rather than functional RV changes under these circumstances.[27]

RV longitudinal function can be quantified using 2D speckle tracking-derived strain, or by simple pulsed tissue velocity imaging which allows to measure myocardial systolic velocity at the lateral tricuspid annulus.[28] Age-specific reference values have been generated for RV pulsed tissue velocity imaging[29] and its prognostic value has been demonstrated.[30] Very recently, semi-automated detection of the RV endocardial surface and volume measurements from 3DE has been validated against 3-Tesla MRI,[31] and has been found to be accurate and reproducible to assess RV ejection fraction.[32] This is mainly due to the enhanced ability of 3DE to include important volumes contributing to the RV inflow and outflow tracts, which may be missing by 2DE.[25] 3DE could fuel clinical research on RV function.

18.4 Left Atrial Size and Function

Left atrial cavity exerts three important physiologic roles: contractile pump (15–30% of LV filling), reservoir function (collection of pulmonary venous flow during ventricular systole) and conduit (passage from left atrium to ventricle during early diastole). Left atrial dilation occurs in response to impaired LV filling and as a consequence of mitral disease and/or atrial fibrillation, all conditions in which left atrial size could be a possible end-point in a clinical trial.

18.4.1 Left Atrial Volume

Changes in atrial size occur in three planes. Therefore, a single dimension (i.e., left atrial antero-posterior diameter), despite used for a long time and prognostically validated, cannot be taken as an accurate representation of actual left atrial size.[1] 2DE estimation of left atrial volume reflects better left atrial remodeling and has been validated against the cine-computerized tomography.[1] Left atrial maximal volume (at LV end-systole) can be measured by using either area-length or disc summation method, without significant difference between the two methods.[1] Reference values of left atrial volume and cut-off values to categorize left atrial enlargement (mild, moderate, severe) have been

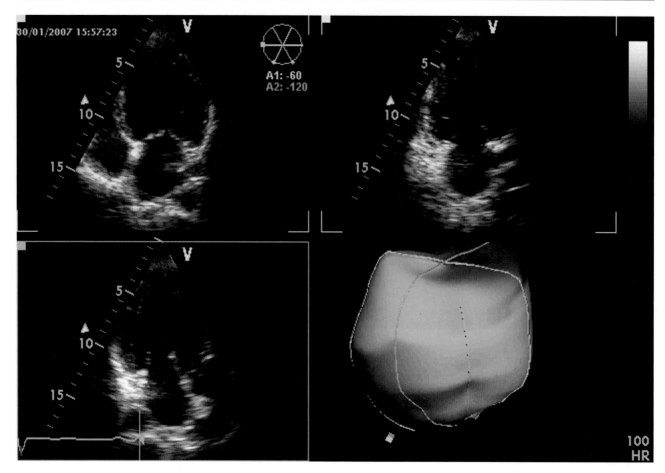

Fig. 18.5 3DE measurement of left atrial volume. Three apical cut planes are used to trace left atrial endocardial border. In the lower right panel a dynamic surface rendered model of the left atrium is displayed

established.[1] Despite systematic underestimation versus left atrial volumes obtained with 3DE[33,34] (Fig. 18.5) and MRI,[35] 2DE derived left atrial volume has satisfactory intra- and inter-observer variability (mean difference ± SD = 6 ± 6 mL and 8 ± 8 mL respectively).[36] The prognostic role of left atrial volume is also well demonstrated.[37] In patients in sinus rhythm, with no history of atrial arrhythmias or heart valve disease, left atrial size reflects LV diastolic function and left atrial pressure.[37] Based on this assumption, recommendations for the evaluation of LV diastolic function have introduced left atrial volume in the algorithm for the estimation of LV filling pressures.[38]

References

1. Lang RM, Bierig M, Devereux RB, Flachskampf FA, Foster E, Pellikka PA et al. American Society of Echocardiography's Nomenclature and Standards Committee; Task Force on Chamber Quantification; American College of Cardiology Echocardiography Committee; American Heart Association; European Association of Echocardiography, European Society of Cardiology. Recommendations for chamber quantification. *Eur J Echocardiogr.* 2006;7: 79–108.
2. Gottdiener JS, Bednarz J, Devereux R, Gardin J, Klein A, Manning WJ et al. American Society of Echocardiography. American Society of Echocardiography recommendations for use of echocardiography in clinical trials. *J Am Soc Echocardiogr.* 2004;17: 1086–1119.
3. Gardner BI, Bingham SE, Allen MR, Blatter DD, Anderson JL. Cardiac magnetic resonance versus transthoracic echocardiography for the assessment of cardiac volumes and regional function after myocardial infarction: an intrasubject comparison using simultaneous intrasubject recordings. *Cardiovasc Ultrasound.* 2009;7:38.
4. Grothues F, Smith GC, Moon JC, Bellenger NG, Collins P, Klein HU et al. Comparison of inter-study reproducibility of cardiovascular magnetic resonance with two-dimensional echocardiography in normal subjects and in patients with heart failure or left ventricular hypertrophy. *Am J Cardiol.* 2002;90:29–34.
5. Malm S, Frigstad S, Sagberg E, Larsson H, Skjaerpe T. Accurate and reproducible measurement of left ventricular volume and ejection fraction by contrast echocardiography: a comparison with magnetic resonance imaging. *J Am Coll Cardiol.* 2004;44: 1030–1035.
6. Senior R, Becher H, Monaghan M, Agati L, Zamorano J, Vanoverschelde JL, Nihoyannopoulos P. Contrast echocardiography: evidence-based recommendations by European Association of Echocardiography. *Eur Heart J.* 2009;10:194–212.

7. Jenkins C, Bricknell K, Hanekom L, Marwick TH. Reproducibility and accuracy of echocardiographic measurements of left ventricular parameters using real-time three-dimensional echocardiography. *J Am Coll Cardiol*. 2004;44:878–886.

8. Caiani EG, Corsi C, Zamorano J et al. Improved semiautomated quantification of left ventricular volumes and ejection fraction using 3-dimensional echocardiography with a full matrix-array transducer: comparison with magnetic resonance imaging. *J Am Soc Echocardiogr*. 2005;18:779–788.

9. Jacobs LD, Salgo IS, Goonewardena S et al. Rapid online quantification of left ventricular volume from real-time three-dimensional echocardiographic data. *Eur Heart J*. 2006;27:460–468.

10. Mor-Avi V, Jenkins C, Kühl HP, Nesser HJ, Marwick T, Franke A et al. Real-time 3-dimensional echocardiographic quantification of left ventricular volumes: multicenter study for validation with magnetic resonance imaging and investigation of sources of error. *JACC Cardiovasc Imaging*. 2008;1:413–423.

11. Muraru D, Badano L, Piccoli G, Gianfagna P, Del Mestre L, Ermacora D et al. Validation of a novel automated border-detection algorithm for rapid and accurate quantitation of left ventricular volumes based on three-dimensional echocardiography. *Eur J Echocardiogr*. 2010;11(4):359–368.

12. Gottdiener JS, Livengood SV, Meyer PS, Chase GA. Should echocardiography be performed to assess effects of antihypertensive therapy? Test-retest reliability of echocardiography for measurement of left ventricular mass and function. *J Am Coll Cardiol*. 1995;25:424–430.

13. de Simone G, Muiesan ML, Ganau A, Longhini C, Verdecchia P, Palmieri V et al. Reliability and limitations of echocardiographic measurement of left ventricular mass for risk stratification and follow-up in single patients: the RES trial. Working Group on Heart and Hypertension of the Italian Society of Hypertension. Reliability of M-mode Echocardiographic Studies. *J Hypertens*. 1999;17(12 Pt 2):1955–1963.

14. Palmieri V, Dahlöf B, De Quattro V, Sharpe N, Bella JN, de Simone G et al. Reliability of echocardiographic assessment of left ventricular structure and function: the PRESERVE study. Prospective Randomized Study Evaluating Regression of Ventricular Enlargement. *J Am Coll Cardiol*. 1999;34:1625–1632.

15. Mor-Avi V, Sugeng L, Weinert L, MacEneaney P, Caiani EG, Koch R et al. Fast measurement of left ventricular mass with real-time three-dimensional echocardiography: comparison with magnetic resonance imaging. *Circulation*. 2004;110:1814–1818.

16. Caiani EG, Corsi C, Sugeng L, MacEneaney P, Weinert L, Mor-Avi V et al. Improved quantification of left ventricular mass based on endocardial and epicardial surface detection with real time three dimensional echocardiography. *Heart*. 2006;92:213–219.

17. van den Bosch AE, Robbers-Visser D, Krenning BJ, McGhie JS, Helbing WA, Meijboom FJ et al. Comparison of real-time three-dimensional echocardiography to magnetic resonance imaging for assessment of left ventricular mass. *Am J Cardiol*. 2006;97: 113–117.

18. Himelman RB, Cassidy MM, Landzberg JS, Schiller NB. Reproducibility of quantitative two-dimensional echocardiography. *Am Heart J*. 1988;115:425–431.

19. Carlsson M, Ugander M, Mosén H, Buhre T, Arheden H. Atrioventricular plane displacement is the major contributor to left ventricular pumping in healthy adults, athletes, and patients with dilated cardiomyopathy. *Am J Physiol Heart Circ Physiol*. 2007;292:H1452–H1459.

20. Zacà V, Ballo P, Galderisi M, Mondillo S. Echocardiography in the assessment of left ventricular longitudinal systolic function: current methodology and clinical applications. *Heart Fail Rev*. 2010; 23:37.

21. Innelli P, Sanchez R, Marra F, Esposito R, Galderisi M. The impact of aging on left ventricular longitudinal function in healthy subjects: a pulsed tissue Doppler study. *Eur J Echocardiogr*. 2008;9:241–249.

22. Cerqueira MD, Weissman NJ, Dilsizian V, Jacobs AK, Kaul S, Laskey WK et al. American Heart Association writing group on myocardial segmentation and registration for cardiac imaging. Standardized myocardial segmentation and nomenclature for tomographic imaging of the heart: a statement for healthcare professionals from the Cardiac Imaging Committee of the Council on Clinical Cardiology of the American Heart Association. *J Nucl Cardiol*. 2002;9:240–245.

23. Choi JO, Cho SW, Song YB, Cho SJ, Song BG, Lee SC et al. Longitudinal 2D strain at rest predicts the presence of left main and three vessel coronary artery disease in patients without regional wall motion abnormality. *Eur J Echocardiogr*. 2009;10:695–701.

24. Mor-Avi V, Jenkins C, Kühl HP, Nesser HJ, Marwick T, Franke A et al. Real-time 3-dimensional echocardiographic quantification of left ventricular volumes: multicenter study for validation with magnetic resonance imaging and investigation of sources of error. *JACC Cardiovasc Imaging*. 2008;1:413–423.

25. Horton KD, Meece RW, Hill JC. Assessment of the right ventricle by echocardiography: a primer for cardiac sonographers. *J Am Soc Echocardiogr*. 2009;22:776–792.

26. Ghio S, Recusani F, Klersy C, Sebastiani R, Laudisa ML, Campana C et al. Prognostic usefulness of the tricuspid annular plane systolic excursion in patients with congestive heart failure secondary to idiopathic or ischemic dilated cardiomyopathy. *Am J Cardiol*. 2000;85: 837–842.

27. Tamborini G, Muratori M, Brusoni D, Celeste F, Maffessanti F, Caiani EG et al. Is right ventricular systolic function reduced after cardiac surgery? A two- and three-dimensional echocardiographic study. *Eur J Echocardiogr*. 2009;10:630–634.

28. Meluzín J, Spinarová L, Bakala J, Toman J, Krejcí J, Hude P et al. Pulsed Doppler tissue imaging of the velocity of tricuspid annular systolic motion; a new, rapid, and non-invasive method of evaluating right ventricular systolic function. *Eur Heart J*. 2001;22: 340–348.

29. Innelli P, Esposito R, Olibet M, Nistri S, Galderisi M. The impact of ageing on right ventricular longitudinal function in healthy subjects: a pulsed tissue Doppler study. *Eur J Echocardiogr*. 2009;10: 491–498.

30. Meluzín J, Spinarová L, Dusek L, Toman J, Hude P, Krejcí J. Prognostic importance of the right ventricular function assessed by Doppler tissue imaging. *Eur J Echocardiogr*. 2003;4:262–271.

31. Niemann PS, Pinho L, Balbach T, Galuschky C, Blankenhagen M, Silberbach M et al. Anatomically oriented right ventricular volume measurements with dynamic three-dimensional echocardiography validated by 3-Tesla magnetic resonance imaging. *J Am Coll Cardiol*. 2007;50:1668–1676.

32. Lu X, Nadvoretskiy V, Bu L, Stolpen A, Ayres N, Pignatelli RH et al. Accuracy and reproducibility of real-time three-dimensional echocardiography for assessment of right ventricular volumes and ejection fraction in children. *J Am Soc Echocardiogr*. 2008; 21:84–89.

33. Maddukuri PV, Vieira ML, De Castro S, Maron MS, Kuvin JT, Patel AR et al. What is the best approach for the assessment of left atrial size? Comparison of various uni-dimensional and two-dimensional parameters with three-dimensional echocardiographically determined left atrial volume. *J Am Soc Echocardiogr*. 2006;19: 1026–1032.

34. Jenkins C, Bricknell K, Marwick TH. Use of real-time three-dimensional echocardiography to measure left atrial volume: comparison with other echocardiographic techniques. *J Am Soc Echocardiogr*. 2005;18:991–997.

35. Keller AM, Gopal AS, King DL. Left and right atrial volume by freehand three-dimensional echocardiography: in vivo validation using magnetic resonance imaging. *Eur J Echocardiogr*. 2000;1: 55–65.

36. Lester SJ, Ryan EW, Schiller NB, Foster E. Best method in clinical practice and in research studies to determine left atrial size. *Am J Cardiol*. 1999;84:829–832.

37. Tsang TS, Abhayaratna WP, Barnes ME, Miyasaka Y, Gersh BJ, Bailey KR et al. Prediction of cardiovascular outcomes with left atrial size: is volume superior to area or diameter? *J Am Coll Cardiol*. 2006;47:1018–1023.

38. Nagueh SF, Appleton CP, Gillebert TC, Marino PN, Oh JK, Smiseth OA et al. Recommendations for the evaluation of left ventricular diastolic function by echocardiography. *Eur J Echocardiogr*. 2009;10:165–193.

Index

L.P. Badano et al. (eds.), *Textbook of Real-Time Three Dimensional Echocardiography*,
DOI: 10.1007/978-1-84996-495-1, © Springer-Verlag London Limited 2011